OXFORD MEDICAL PUBLICATIONS

Oxford Specialist Handbooks in Anaesthesia
Neuroanaesthesia

Oxford Specialist Handbooks published and forthcoming

General Oxford Specialist Handbooks

A Resuscitation Room Guide
Addiction Medicine
Hypertension
Perioperative Medicine, Second Edition
Post-Operative Complications, Second Edition
Pulmonary Hypertension
Renal Transplantation

Oxford Specialist Handbooks in Anaesthesia

Cardiac Anaesthesia
Day Case Surgery
General Thoracic Anaesthesia
Neuroanaesthesia
Obstetric Anaesthesia
Paediatric Anaesthesia
Regional Anaesthesia, Stimulation and Ultrasound Techniques

Oxford Specialist Handbooks in Cardiology

Adult Congenital Heart Disease
Cardiac Catheterization and Coronary Intervention
Cardiac Electrophysiology
Cardiovascular Magnetic Resonance
Echocardiography
Fetal Cardiology
Heart Failure
Nuclear Cardiology
Pacemakers and ICDs
Valvular Heart Disease

Oxford Specialist Handbooks in Critical Care

Advanced Respiratory Critical Care

Oxford Specialist Handbooks in End of Life Care

End of Life Care in Dementia
End of Life Care in Nephrology
End of Life in the Intensive Care Unit

Oxford Specialist Handbooks in Neurology

Epilepsy
Parkinson's Disease and Other Movement Disorders
Stroke Medicine

Oxford Specialist Handbooks in Paediatrics

Paediatric Dermatology
Paediatric Endocrinology and Diabetes
Paediatric Gastroenterology, Hepatology, and Nutrition
Paediatric Haematology and Oncology
Paediatric Intensive Care
Paediatric Nephrology
Paediatric Neurology
Paediatric Palliative Care
Paediatric Radiology
Paediatric Respiratory Medicine

Oxford Specialist Handbooks in Psychiatry

Child and Adolescent Psychiatry
Old Age Psychiatry

Oxford Specialist Handbooks in Radiology

Interventional Radiology
Musculoskeletal Imaging
Pulmonary Imaging

Oxford Specialist Handbooks in Surgery

Cardiothoracic Surgery
Colorectal Surgery
Hand Surgery
Liver and Pancreatobiliary Surgery
Operative Surgery, Second Edition
Oral Maxillofacial Surgery
Otolaryngology and Head and Neck Surgery
Paediatric Surgery
Plastic and Reconstructive Surgery
Surgical Oncology
Urological Surgery
Vascular Surgery

Oxford Specialist Handbooks in Anaesthesia

Neuroanaesthesia

Dr Michael Nathanson
Consultant Neuroanaesthetist, Nottingham University Hospitals NHS Trust, Queen's Medical Centre, Nottingham, UK

Dr Iain Moppett
Associate Professor and Honarary Consultant University of Nottingham and Nottingham University Hospitals NHS Trust, Queen's Medical Centre, Nottingham, UK

Dr Matt Wiles
Clinical Lecturer in Anaesthesia
University of Nottingham, Queen's Medical Centre, Nottingham, UK

OXFORD
UNIVERSITY PRESS

OXFORD
UNIVERSITY PRESS

Great Clarendon Street, Oxford OX2 6DP

Oxford University Press is a department of the University of Oxford.
It furthers the University's objective of excellence in research, scholarship,
and education by publishing worldwide in

Oxford New York

Auckland Cape Town Dar es Salaam Hong Kong Karachi
Kuala Lumpur Madrid Melbourne Mexico City Nairobi
New Delhi Shanghai Taipei Toronto

With offices in

Argentina Austria Brazil Chile Czech Republic France Greece
Guatemala Hungary Italy Japan Poland Portugal Singapore
South Korea Switzerland Thailand Turkey Ukraine Vietnam

Oxford is a registered trade mark of Oxford University Press
in the UK and in certain other countries

Published in the United States
by Oxford University Press Inc., New York

© Oxford University Press, 2011

The moral rights of the author have been asserted
Database right Oxford University Press (maker)

First edition published 2011

All rights reserved. No part of this publication may be reproduced,
stored in a retrieval system, or transmitted, in any form or by any means,
without the prior permission in writing of Oxford University Press,
or as expressly permitted by law, or under terms agreed with the appropriate
reprographics rights organization. Enquiries concerning reproduction
outside the scope of the above should be sent to the Rights Department,
Oxford University Press, at the address above

You must not circulate this book in any other binding or cover
and you must impose this same condition on any acquirer

British Library Cataloguing in Publication Data
Data available

Library of Congress Cataloging in Publication Data
Data available

Typeset by Glyph International, Bangalore, India
Printed in China
on acid-free paper by
Asia Pacific Offset

ISBN 978–0–19–922583–5

10 9 8 7 6 5 4 3 2 1

Oxford University Press makes no representation, express or implied, that the drug
dosages in this book are correct. Readers must therefore always check the product
information and clinical procedures with the most up-to-date published product
information and data sheets provided by the manufacturers and the most recent
codes of conduct and safety regulations. The authors and publishers do not accept
responsibility or legal liability for any errors in the text or for the misuse or misapplication of material in this work. Except where otherwise stated, drug dosages and
recommendations are for the non-pregnant adult who is not breastfeeding.

Preface

For some anaesthetists neuroanaesthesia carries with it an air of mystique – difficult, long operations, equally difficult anaesthetics complicated by the need to avoid swings in blood pressure and coughing, but requiring a fully awake patient as soon as the procedure is finished. For others it is just another branch of surgical anaesthesia performed with an eye to the underlying surgical pathology, the application of relevant pharmacology and physiology and careful attention to detail. Good neuroanaesthetic practice encompasses both these views.

The aim of this book is to provide trainees or those called upon to provide neuroanaesthesia on an occasional basis (such as colleagues working in non-neurosurgical centres who care for brain injured patients) with a contemporary guide to the underlying principles of neuroanaesthesia and their practical application.

We are indebted to our colleagues whose contributions to this book describe a common-sense, scientifically-based approach to neuroanaesthesia and neuro critical care. Their clarity of thought and careful writing demonstrate that neuroanaesthesia can be practiced to a very high standard by the application of relatively few rules and guidelines. We are also indebted to our many other colleagues, particularly in the neurosurgical department in Nottingham, who have read, discussed, or, indeed, co-written many sections of this book. In particular we thank the following who, while not listed as authors, have made substantial contributions – Richard Ashpole, Graham Dow, Andy Norris, Iain Robertson and Barrie White.

We have endeavoured to include all the commonly used techniques and to have been comprehensive enough to offer advice for most situations that might be encountered; we do not claim to have covered every eventuality but hope that the principles described in this book will stand the reader in good stead even so. Inevitably the techniques used most frequently in Nottingham will seem to take precedence, but we claim no superiority over others used elsewhere. As ever, it is the quality of the anaesthetic care provided and the attention to detail, rather than the choice of technique, that is most important for a good outcome.

Michael Nathanson
Iain Moppett
Matt Wiles

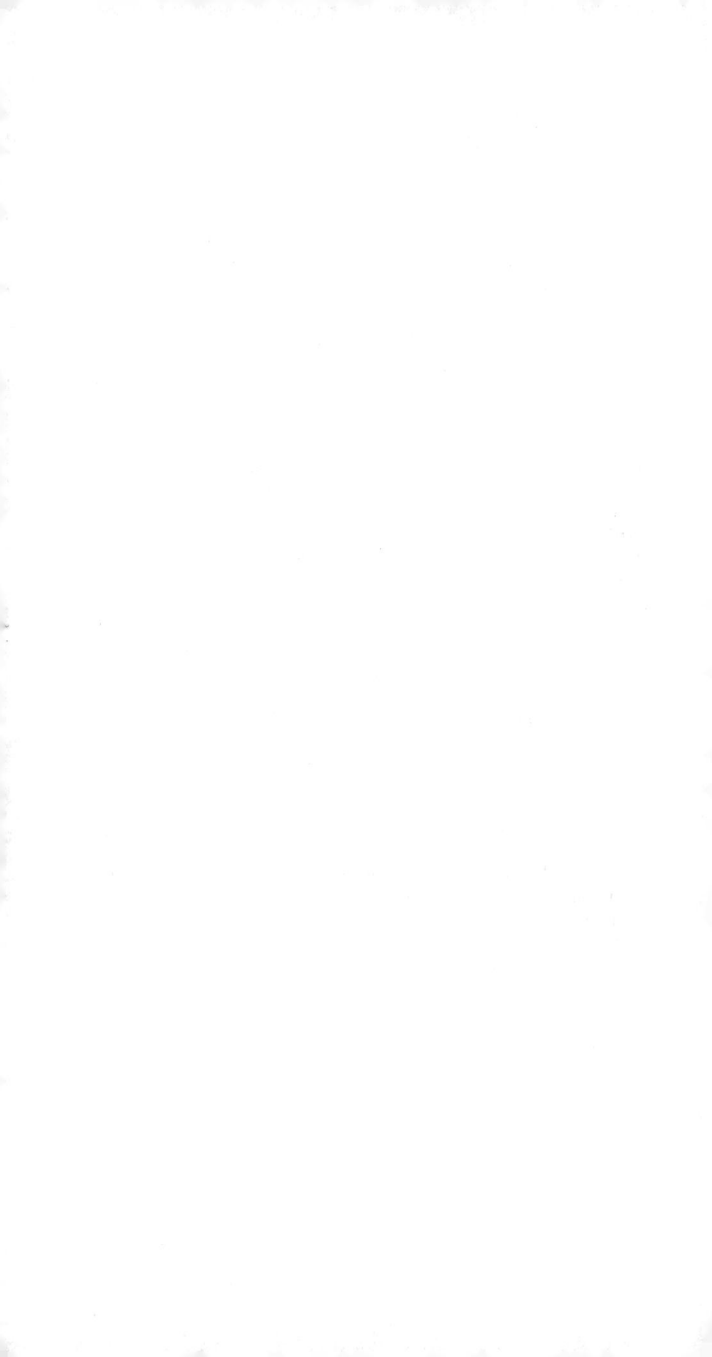

Contents

Detailed contents *ix*
Symbols and abbreviations *xv*
Contributors *xxi*

1. Anatomy and physiology 1
2. Pharmacology 29
3. Monitoring and imaging 67
4. General principles of neuroanaesthesia 103
5. Positioning and surgical approaches 161
6. Intracranial surgery (non-vascular) 179
7. Cerebrovascular surgery 257
8. Cranial surgery 285
9. Spinal surgery 291
10. Neurodiagnostics and interventional procedures 323
11. Acute brain injury 333
12. Postoperative management 383

Appendix *397*
Index *405*

Detailed contents

Symbols and abbreviations *xv*
Contributors *xxi*

1 Anatomy and physiology — 1

Anatomy *2*
Michael Nathanson

Control of the cerebral circulation *10*
Hannah Sycamore and Ravi Mahajan

Cerebral metabolism *18*
Iain Moppett

Intracranial pressure and CSF *22*
Iain Moppett

2 Pharmacology — 29

Inhalational agents *30*
Michael Nathanson

Intravenous agents *34*
Michael Nathanson

Mannitol and hypertonic saline *38*
Alison Chalmers

Glucocorticoids *42*
Alison Chalmers

Vasoactive drugs *44*
Asha Nandakumar

Opioids *52*
Michael Nathanson

Muscle relaxants *56*
Iain Moppett

Non-steroidal anti-inflammatory drugs and paracetamol *60*
Asha Nandakumar

Anti-emetics and PONV *62*
Asha Nandakumar

Vasopressin: argine vasopressin (AVP), antidiuretic hormone (ADH) *64*
Alison Chalmers

3 Monitoring and imaging — 67

Intracranial pressure *68*
Mark Ehlers

Electrophysiological monitoring *72*
Bernard Riley and Armagan Dagal

Transcranial Doppler ultrasonography *82*
Ravi Mehajan and Kumar Mekala

Multimodal monitoring *86*
Bernard Riley

Regional cerebral blood flow *92*
Mark Ehlers

Glasgow Coma Scale *98*
Michael Nathanson

4 General principles of neuroanaesthesia — 103

Pre-operative assessment *104*
Iain Moppett

General principles of neuroanaesthesia *110*
Philippa Veale

Paediatric neuroanaesthesia *120*
John Emery and Suzanne Wake

Cerebral protection *130*
Michael Nathanson

TIVA or volatile-based anaesthesia *134*
Michael Nathanson

Intra-operative temperature control *136*
Matthew Wiles

Management of intra-operative brain swelling *140*
Perm Bachra

Air embolism *142*
Sibylle Jürgens

Blood loss and cell salvage *146*
Sally Hancock

Glycaemic control *150*
Alison Chalmers

DETAILED CONTENTS **xi**

Thromboprophylaxis *152*
Asha Nandakumar
Pregnancy *156*
David Levy

5 Positioning and surgical approaches **161**
Positioning *162*
Sally Hancock
Surgical approaches *171*
Donald Macarthur

6 Intracranial surgery (non-vascular) **179**
Tumours in adults (meningioma, glioma, lymphoma, metastasis) *180*
Sibylle Jürgens and Surajit Basu
Tumours (children) *191*
John Emery and Suzanne Wake
Acoustic neuroma *196*
Michael Nathanson
Pituitary tumours *200*
Michael Nathanson
Posterior fossa surgery *206*
Iain Moppett
Shunts and ventricular drains *214*
Michael Nathanson
Neuroendoscopic surgery *220*
John Emery
Colloid cysts *222*
Iain Moppett
Midline surgery *224*
John Emery
Seizure surgery *228*
Surajit Basu and Sibylle Jürgens
Functional neurosurgery *234*
Sibylle Jürgens and Surajit Basu
Cranial neuralgias *238*
Iain Moppett
Awake craniotomy *242*
Sibylle Jürgens and Surajit Basu

Stereotactic surgery *246*
Iain Moppett

Cerebral abscesses *250*
Matthew Wiles

Decompressive craniectomy *254*
Iain Moppett

7 Cerebrovascular surgery 257

Extradural haematoma *258*
Iain Moppett

Subdural haematoma *262*
Iain Moppett

Intracranial haematoma *268*
Iain Moppett

Intracranial aneurysms and arterio-venous malformations (AVMs) *272*
David Levy

EC–IC bypass procedures *276*
John Emery

Carotid endarterectomy *278*
Iain Moppett

8 Cranial surgery 285

Cranioplasty *286*
Matthew Wiles

Craniofacial surgery in children *288*
John Emery and Suzanne Wake

9 Spinal surgery 291

Cervical spine surgery *292*
Sally Hancock

Lumbar surgery *298*
Michael Nathanson

Spinal cord masses and vascular malformations *302*
Sally Hancock

Spinal injury *308*
Sibylle Jürgens and Michael Grevitt

Baclofen pump implantation *314*
John Emery and Suzanne Wake

DETAILED CONTENTS xiii

Neural tube defects *316*
John Emery

Spinal haematoma and abscess *320*
Iain Moppett

10 Neurodiagnostics and interventional procedures — 323

Anaesthesia for neuroradiology *324*
Michael Bennett

Anaesthesia for MRI and CT scans *330*
Michael Bennett

11 Acute brain injury — 333

Pathophysiology *334*
Iain Moppett

Immediate care *340*
Iain Moppett

Transfers *346*
Katherine Ingram

General management *350*
Mark Ehlers

Cerebral protection *356*
Mark Ehlers

Subarachnoid haemorrhage *362*
Dale Gardiner

Systemic complications of brain injury *370*
Bernard Riley

Status epilepticus *374*
Bernard Riley

Death *378*
Dale Gardiner

12 Postoperative management — 383

Postoperative analgesia *384*
Iain Moppett

Postoperative fluid management *388*
Iain Moppett

Postoperative seizures *392*
Iain Moppett

Postoperative levels of care *394*
Dale Gardiner and Iain Moppett

Appendix 397

Guidance for transfers *398*
Iain Moppett

Drug infusions for ICU use *400*
Matt Wiles

Index *405*

Symbols and abbreviations

❶	warning
α	alpha
β	beta
δ	delta
θ	theta
AAGBI	Association of Anaesthetists of Great Britain and Ireland
ABG	arterial blood gases
ABL	allowable operative blood loss
ACCEPT	assessment, control, communication, evaluation, preparation and packing, transportation
ACT	activated clotting time
ADH	antidiuretic hormone
AJDO$_2$	arterio-jugular oxygen content difference
AMAN	acute motor axonal neuropathy
AMSAN	acute motor sensory axonal neuropathy
ANH	acute normovolaemic haemodilution
ARR	absolute risk reduction
ATP	adenosine triphosphate
AVF	arteriovenous fistula
AVM	arteriovenous malformation
AVP	argine vasopressin
BAEP	brainstem auditory evoked potential
BBB	blood–brain barrier
BIS	bispectral index
BOLD	blood oxygen level-dependent
BRW/CRW	Brown–Roberts–Wells/Cosman–Roberts–Wells
CABG	coronary artery bypass graft
CBF	cerebral blood flow
CBV	cerebral blood volume
CCF	congestive cardiac failure
CEA	carotid endarterectomy
CFAM	cerebral function analysing monitor
CFM	cerebral function monitor
cGMP	cyclic GMP

CIN	contrast-induced nephropathy
CM	cerebral microdialysis
CMAP	compound muscle action potential
$CMRO_2$	cerebral metabolic rate for oxygen
CMV	cytomegalovirus
CNS	central nervous system
COX	cyclo-oxygenase
CP	cerebello-pontine
CPAP	continuous positive airways pressure
CPP	cerebral perfusion pressure
CSDH	chronic subdural haematoma
CSF	cerebrospinal fluid
CSWS	cerebral salt-wasting syndrome
CT	computed tomography
CTG	cardiotocogram
CTZ	chemoreceptor trigger zone
CVA	cerebrovascular accident
CVC	central venous catheter
CVP	central venous pressure
CVR	cerebrovascular resistance
CVS	cardiovascular system
CXR	chest X-ray
DBP	diastolic blood pressure
DBS	deep brain stimulation
DCES	direct cortical electrical stimulation
DI	diabetes insipidus
DIC	disseminated intravascular coagulation
DNA	deoxyribonucleic acid
DVT	deep vein thrombosis
DWI	diffusion weighted imaging
EBV	estimated blood volume
ECF	extra-cellular fluid
ECG	electrocardiogram
EC–IC	extracranial–intracranial
ECoG	electrocorticography
EDAS	encephaloduroarteriosynangiosis
EDH	extradural haematoma
EEG	electroencephalogram
EMAS	encephalomyoarteriosynangiosis

EMG	electromyography
EP	evoked potential
ETCO$_2$	end-tidal carbon dioxide
EVD	external ventricular drain
FFP	fresh frozen plasma
fMRI	functional magnetic resonance imaging
FRC	functional residual capacity
FV	flow velocity
GA	general anaesthetic
GABA	γ-aminobutyric acid
GBS	Guillain–Barré syndrome
GCS	Glasgow Coma Scale
GCS	graduated compression stockings
GH	growth hormone
GI	gastrointestinal
GTN	glyceryl trinitrate
HA	hydroxyapatite
HDU	high dependency unit
HES	hydoxyethyl starch
HIV	human immunodeficiency virus
HR	heart rate
HTS	hypertonic saline
ICA	internal carotid artery
ICH	intracerebral haematoma
ICP	intracranial pressure
ICU	intensive care unit
IHAST	International Hypothermia for Aneurysm Surgery Trial
IJV	internal jugular vein
IM	intramuscular
INR	interventional neuroradiology
IPC	intermittent pneumatic compression
IPPV	intermittent positive pressure ventilation
ISAT	International Subarachnoid Haemorrhage Trial
LA	local anaesthetic
LMA	laryngeal mask airway
LMWH	low molecular weight heparin
LP	lumbar puncture
LP	lumboperitoneal
LPR	lactate:pyruvate ratio

LV	left ventricle
MAC	minimum alveolar concentration
MAP	mean arterial pressure
MCA	middle cerebral artery
MCAFV	middle cerebral artery flow velocity
MEP	motor evoked potentials
MG	myasthenia gravis
MI	myocardial infarction
MRI	magnetic resonance imaging
MS	multiple sclerosis
MUP	motor unit potential
NCA	nurse-controlled analgesia
NCS	nerve conduction studies
NG	nasogastric
NIPB	non-invasive blood pressure
NIRS	near infrared spectroscopy
NMB	neuromuscular block
NMDA	N-methyl-D-aspartate
NO	nitric oxide
NPPB	normal pressure perfusion breakthrough
NSAIDs	non-steroidal anti-inflammatory drugs
NTD	neural tube defects
NTS	nucleus tractus solitarius
NTV	neuroendoscopic third ventriculostomy
OEF	O_2 extraction fraction
OSA	obstructive sleep apnoea
PAE	paradoxical air embolism
PCA	patient-controlled analgesia
PCC	prothrombin complex concentrates
PE	pulmonary embolism
PEEP	positive end-expiratory pressure
PET	positron emission tomography
PFTs	pulmonary function tests
PFUCD	posterior fossa upper cervical decompression
PI	pulsatility index
PICC	peripherally inserted central line
PLED	periodic lateralized epileptiform discharges
PMMA	polymethylmethacrylate
PNET	primitive neuroectodermal tumours

PNS	parasympathetic nervous system
PONV	postoperative nausea and vomiting
PRBC	packed red blood cells
PRIS	propofol infusion syndrome
Prx	pressure reactivity
PTH	post-traumatic hyperthermia
PVA	polyvinyl alcohol
rCBF	regional cerebral blood flow
RNA	ribonucleic acid
ROI	regions of interest
RSI	rapid sequence induction
SAH	subarachnoid haemorrhage
SAP	sensory action potential
SBP	systolic blood pressure
SDH	subdural haematoma
SE	status epilepticus
SEP	somatosensory evoked potential
SHOT	Serious Hazards of Transfusion
SIADH	syndrome of inappropriate antidiuretic hormone hypersecretion
SOL	space-occupying lesion
SPECT	single photon emission computed tomography
SSEPs	somatosensory evoked potentials
STICH	Surgical Trial in Intracerebral Haemorrhage
SUDEP	sudden unexpected death in epilepsy
SVC	superior vena cava
SVR	systemic vascular resistance
TBI	traumatic brain injury
TCD	transcranial Doppler
TCI	target-controlled infusion
THAM	tromethamine
TIVA	total intravenous anaesthesia
TOE	transoesophageal echocardiography
TOR	tissue oxygen response
TRALI	transfusion-associated lung injury
U&E	urea and electrolytes
VA	ventriculo-atrial shunt
VAE	venous air embolism
vCJD	variant Creutzfeldt–Jakob disease

VEP	visual evoked potential
VNS	vagal nerve stimulator
VP	ventriculoperitoneal
VTE	venous thromboembolism
WFNS	World Federation of Neurological Surgeons

Contributors

Dr Armagan Dagal
Specialist Registrar in Anaesthesia
Nottingham University Hospitals
NHS Trust,
Queen's Medical Centre
Nottingham

Dr Perm Bachra
Consultant Neuroanaesthetist
Nottingham University Hospitals
NHS Trust,
Queen's Medical Centre
Nottingham

Mr Surajit Basu
Consultant Neurosurgeon
Nottingham University Hopitals
NHS Trust,
Queen's Medical Centre
Nottingham

Dr MIchael Bennett
Consultant Neuroanaesthetist
Nottingham University Hospitals
NHS Trust,
Queen's Medical Centre
Nottingham

Dr Alison Chalmers
Consultant Anaesthetist,
Queen Victoria Hospital NHS
Foundation Trust,
East Grinstead

Dr Rob Dineen
Consultant Neuroradiologist
Nottingham University Hospitals
NHS Trust,
Queen's Medical Centre
Nottingham

Dr Mark Ehlers
Consultant in Anaesthesia and
Intensive Care
Nottingham University Hospitals
NHS Trust,
Queen's Medical Centre
Nottingham

Dr John Emery
Consultant Paediatric Anaesthetist
Nottingham University Hospitals
NHS Trust,
Queen's Medical Centre
Nottingham

Dr Dale Gardiner
Consultant Intensivist
Nottingham University Hospitals
NHS Trust,
Queen's Medical Centre
Nottingham

Mr Mike Grevitt
Consultant Spinal Surgeon
Nottingham University Hospitals
NHS Trust,
Queen's Medical Centre
Nottingham

Dr Sally Hancock
Consultant Neuroanaesthetist
Nottingham University Hospitals
NHS Trust,
Queen's Medical Centre
Nottingham

Dr Katherine Ingram
Consultant Neuroanaesthetist
Nottingham University Hospitals
NHS Trust,
Queen's Medical Centre
Nottingham

Dr Sibylle Jürgens
Consultant Anaesthetist
Nottingham University Hospitals
NHS Trust,
Queen's Medical Centre
Nottingham

Dr David Levy
Consultant Neuroanaesthetist
Nottingham University Hospitals
NHS Trust,
Queen's Medical Centre
Nottingham

CONTRIBUTORS

Mr Donald Macarthur
Consultant Neurosurgeon
Nottingham University Hospitals NHS Trust,
Queen's Medical Centre
Nottingham

Professor Ravi Mahajan
Professor in Anaesthesia and Intensive Care,
University of Nottingham,
Nottingham

Dr Kumar Mekala
Specialist Registrar In Anaesthesia
Nottingham University Hospitals NHS Trust,
Queen's Medical Centre
Nottingham

Dr Iain Moppett
Associate Professor and Honorary Consultant
University of Nottingham and Nottingham University Hospitals NHS Trust
Queen's Medical Centre
Nottingham, UK

Dr Asha Nandakumar
Consultant Neuroanaesthetist
Sheffield Teaching Hospitals NHS Foundation Trust,
Royal Hallamshire Hospital
Sheffield

Dr Michael Nathanson
Consultant Neuroanaesthetist
Nottingham University Hospitals NHS Trust,
Queen's Medical Centre
Nottingham

Dr Bernard Riley
Consultant Intensivist
Nottingham University Hospitals NHS Trust,
Queen's Medical Centre
Nottingham

Dr Hannah Sycamore
Consultant Anaesthetist
Nottingham University Hospitals NHS Trust,
Queen's Medical Centre
Nottingham

Dr Philippa Veale
Consultant Neuroanaesthetist
Nottingham University Hospitals NHS Trust
Queen's Medical Centre
Nottingham

Dr Suzanne Wake
Consultant Paediatric Anaesthetist
Nottingham University Hospitals NHS Trust,
Queen's Medical Centre
Nottingham

Dr Matthew Wiles
Clinical Lecturer in Anaesthesia
University of Nottingham, Queen's Medical Centre
Nottingham

Chapter 1

Anatomy and physiology

Anatomy *2*
Control of the cerebral circulation *10*
Cerebral metabolism *18*
Intracranial pressure and CSF *22*

Anatomy

This chapter describes the basic structure of the central nervous system (CNS). This is important for the neuroanaesthetist to understand the effects of drugs and changes in physiology on the CNS, to understand the nature and risks associated with surgery and to understand the ways that patients may present for surgery and critical care.

The central nervous system is composed of the brain and spinal cord. These elements are surrounded for the most part by bony structures—the cranium and the spinal column.

Main structures

The brain

The brain comprises the brainstem (medulla and pons), the cerebellum, the midbrain, and the cerebrum (Figure 1.1).

Brainstem

The brainstem constitutes a highway of information between the brain and the spinal cord and contains many important structures including:
- respiratory and vasomotor (vital) centres
- ascending and descending nerve tracts
- lower cranial nerve nuclei
- reticular system, which is associated with consciousness.

A lesion or compression of the brainstem secondary to raised intracranial pressure produces abnormal functioning of the vital centres that is rapidly fatal (coning).

Cerebellum

The cerebellum occupies the posterior fossa of the cranium below the tentorium cerebelli (see p.4). It consists of two cerebellar hemispheres joined together with the vermis in between and is connected to the midbrain and the brainstem. The cerebellum co-ordinates balance and posture. Cerebellar lesions give rise to signs on the same side of the body.

Midbrain

The midbrain connects the brainstem and cerebellum to the hypothalamus, the thalamus, and the cerebral hemispheres. The thalamus contains the nuclei of the main sensory pathways.

Cerebrum

The cerebrum consists of the diencephalon and the two cerebral hemispheres.

The diencephalon is the central part of the forebrain and consists of the thalamus and the hypothalamus.
- The hypothalamus co-ordinates the autonomic nervous system and the endocrine systems of the body.
- The pituitary gland is below the hypothalamus. Pituitary tumours may produce the signs of a space-occupying lesion, or restrict the visual fields by compressing the optic chiasma or give rise to an endocrine disturbance.

The cerebral hemispheres comprise the cerebral cortex, the basal ganglia and the lateral ventricles. The surface of the cortex is thrown into folds or gyri which are separated from each other by clefts or sulci.

The central sulcus separates the main motor gyrus anteriorly from the main sensory gyrus posteriorly. Each hemisphere is divided into four areas or lobes: frontal; parietal: temporal; and occipital.
- The frontal lobe contains the motor cortex and areas concerned with intellect and behaviour.
- The parietal lobe contains the sensory cortex.
- The temporal lobe is concerned with auditory sensation and the integration of other stimuli.
- The occipital lobe contains the visual cortex.
- The medial part of the cortex also contains the limbic system, which is associated with emotion and behaviour.

Lesions of the cerebral hemispheres give rise to sensory and motor deficits on the opposite side of the body. Between the basal ganglia and the thalamus lies the internal capsule containing the descending motor tracts from the cerebral cortex.

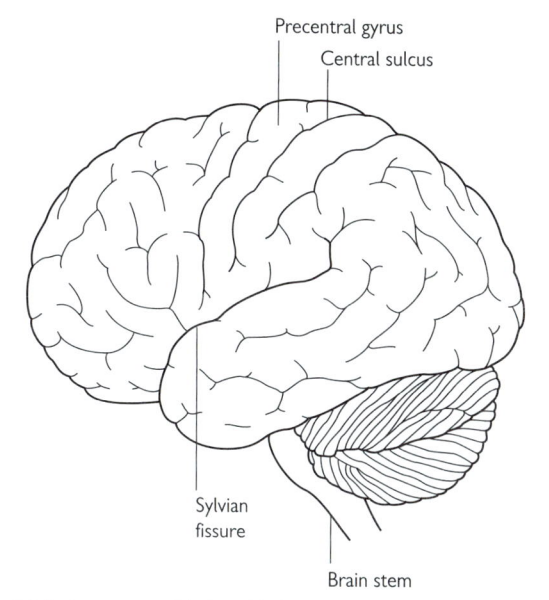

Fig. 1.1 Surface anatomy of the brain. The lateral sulcus (or Sylvian fissure) divides the temporal lobe from the parietal and frontal lobes. The central sulcus divides the frontal and parietal lobes. The motor cortex lies anterior to the central sulcus and the sensory cortex behind. The medial surfaces of the brain are joined by the corpus callosum and the inter-thalamic connection.

The spinal cord

The spinal cord is approximately 45 cm long and passes from the foramen magnum to a tapered end—the conus medullaris—at the level of the first or second lumbar vertebra. At each spinal level, paired anterior (motor) and posterior (sensory) spinal roots emerge on each side of the cord. The roots join at each intervertebral foramen to form a mixed spinal nerve. The collection of nerve roots below the end of the cord passing through cerebrospinal fluid (CSF) in the dural sac into the sacrum is called the cauda equina.

The cord constitutes:
- The central canal—normally a potential space—which may contain CSF in some disease states.
- Surrounding grey matter with anterior and posterior horns:
  - the anterior horns of grey matter contain the motor nerve cells
  - most peripheral sensory nerves synapse in the posterior horns
- White matter containing the ascending and descending tracts in anterior, posterior, and lateral columns (see p.5).

Meninges

CNS tissue is quite delicate and is protected by three layers—the meninges (or membranes) that surround the brain and the spinal cord. These are the dura mater, the arachnoid mater, and the pia mater. These layers also envelop, at their origin, the nerves as they leave the CNS.

The brain
- The dura mater is a thick, strong, double membrane which separates into its two layers in parts to form the cerebral venous sinuses.
  - The outer layer is strongly adherent to the skull bones and is the equivalent of the periosteum.
  - The inner layer is continuous with the dura which surrounds the spinal cord. This layer has projections which support the brain, including the falx cerebri which separates the two cerebral hemispheres and the tentorium cerebelli which separates the posterior fossa and its contents from the rest of the cranium.
  - The major artery supplying the dura mater is the middle meningeal artery which may be damaged in a head injury and skull fracture leading to the formation of an extradural haematoma.
- The arachnoid mater is a thin membrane normally adjacent to the dura mater. Cortical veins from the surface of the brain pass through the arachnoid mater to reach dural venous sinuses and may be damaged by relatively minor trauma leading to the formation of a subdural haematoma.
- The pia mater is a vascular membrane closely adherent to the surface of the brain and follows the contours of the gyri and sulci. The space between the pia and arachnoid mater is the subarachnoid space and contains CSF.

The spinal cord
The dura mater is a single layered structure around the spinal cord. It forms a sac which ends below the cord usually at the level of the second sacral vertebra. The space between the dura and the bony part of the spinal canal (the extradural or epidural space) is filled with fat, lymphatics, arteries, and an extensive venous plexus.

Blood supply

The arterial blood supply to the brain is derived from the two internal carotid arteries and the two vertebral arteries.

- The vertebral arteries are branches of the subclavian arteries and pass through foramina in the transverse processes of the upper six cervical vertebrae. They join together anterior to the brainstem to form the single basilar artery which then divides again to form the two posterior cerebral arteries. These vessels and the two internal carotid arteries form an anastamotic system known as the circle of Willis at the base of the brain (Figure 1.2).
- The main arteries supplying the cerebral hemispheres are the anterior, middle, and posterior cerebral artery for each hemisphere.
- Other important vessels supplying the brainstem and the cerebellum branch from the basilar artery.
- Venous blood drains into the cerebral venous sinuses whose walls are formed from the dura mater. These sinuses join and empty into the internal jugular veins.

The blood supply to the spinal cord comes from the single anterior spinal artery, formed at the foramen magnum from a branch from each of the vertebral arteries, and from the paired posterior spinal arteries.

- The anterior artery supplies the anterior two-thirds of the cord.
- There are additional supplies from segmental arteries and a direct supply from the aorta usually at the level of the eleventh thoracic intervertebral space. This artery is known as the artery of Adamkiewicz and is a major source of blood to the lower half of the spinal cord in most people.

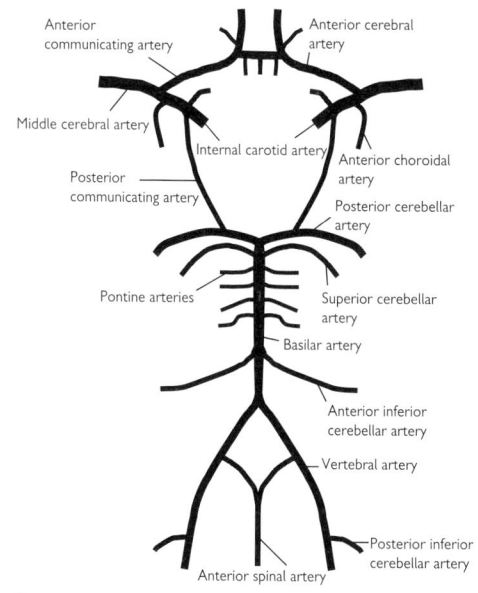

Fig. 1.2 The main arterial blood vessels supplying the brain.

Ascending and descending nerve tracts

The brain connects to the spinal cord via long tracts that arise deep within the cerebral hemispheres and pass down through the mid-brain and brainstem to enter the cord. These tracts have both descending (motor) and ascending (sensory) functions (Figure 1.3).

Motor pathways

Efferent motor impulses pass along the descending or pyramidal tracts which originate in the motor (pre-central) gyrus of the cerebral cortex.

- Fibres pass to the cranial nerve nuclei in the corticonuclear tracts and to the anterior horn cells in the spinal cord in the corticospinal tracts. The fibres pass between the basal ganglia and the thalamus in the internal capsule which is supplied by the medial and lateral striate branches of the middle cerebral artery.
- Most motor fibres decussate (cross) in the medulla and pass through the cord in the lateral corticospinal tract. Nerve fibres in the corticospinal tracts synapse with the lower motor neurons.
- The cell bodies of the lower motor neurons are in the anterior horn of the spinal cord and the fibres leave the cord in the anterior nerve root.
- Other descending tracts include the extrapyramidal tracts concerned with muscle tone, coordination and posture.

The effects of CNS lesions on motor function vary according to location.

- A lesion of the cord results in paralysis below the lesion on the same side of the body.
- A cerebral stroke will cause paralysis on the opposite side of the body.
- Some muscles groups (for example, muscles in the forehead supplied via the VIIth cranial nerves) are innervated from both cerebral hemispheres so may be spared after a stroke, but not in lesions affecting the motor nerves (a lower motor neurone lesion).

Sensory pathways

The two main ascending sensory tracts are the spinothalamic tracts and the posterior columns. Not all sensory nerves pass up through the cord; some supply afferent impulses to reflex arcs within the spinal cord itself.

Spinothalamic tracts

The anterior and the lateral spinothalamic tracts mainly serve light touch, pain and temperature sensation.

- Fibres serving pain and temperature synapse in the substantia gelatinosa in the posterior horn of the cord. They ascend in the cord for 1–3 segments before they decussate and ascend further in the lateral spinothalamic tract.
- Light touch fibres cross at the level of entry and ascend in the anterior spinothalamic tract. The ascending fibres synapse in the thalamus and third-order neurons pass to the sensory (postcentral) gyrus of the cortex. Pain sensation from the head is carried in fibres in the Vth, VIIth and IXth cranial nerves.
- Certain areas of the brain are closely associated with modification of the sensation of pain—these are the periventricular area of the diencephalon, the peri-aqueductal grey matter of the midbrain and some nuclei in the brainstem.

Posterior columns
The posterior columns contain fibres which carry vibration sensation, fine touch, and proprioception.
- The posterior column fibres are uncrossed and pass through the cord without synapsing to end in the gracile and cuneate nuclei in the medulla.
- Other ascending tracts include the spinocerebellar tracts which carry sensation from the muscle, tendon, and joint receptors to the cerebellum.

Damage to the spinal cord results in loss of sensation of vibration and proprioception on the same side as the lesion and loss of pain and temperature sensation on the opposite side of the body. Because the fibres supplying pain ascend for 1–3 segments before they cross the cord the 'level' may be different, as well as being on different sides.

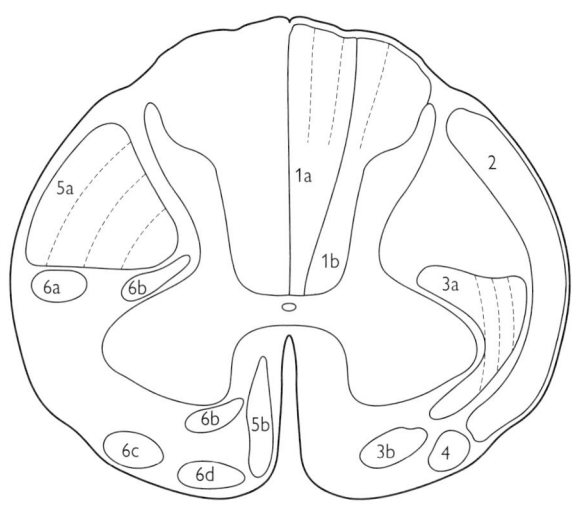

Fig. 1.3 Representative anatomy of spinal cord at cervical level. The motor tracts are shown on the left and the sensory tracts on the right.
Sensory tracts 1: Dorsal columns a, gracilis, b, cuneatus. These are crossed fibres, carrying discriminative touch and conscious proprioception. The medial side carries sacral and lumbar fibres, the lateral thoracic and cervical. 2: Spinocerebellar tracts (anterior and lateral or posterior). These crossed fibres carry 'unconscious proprioception'. 3: Spinothalamic tracts (a, lateral and b, anterior). These crossed fibres carry crude touch, pain, temperature and pressure. 4: Spino-olivary fibres: these convey proprioceptive information to the cerebellum.
Motor tracts 5: Pyramidal tracts: the majority of the motor pathways are crossed fibres which run in the lateral corticospinal tract, a. Cervical fibres are medial, sacral are lateral. b, The anterior corticospinal tract, and a small proportion of the lateral corticospinal tract consists of uncrossed fibres which cross at the level at which the spinal nerves exit. 6: Extrapyramidal tracts: these tracts are mainly concerned with maintenance of posture and co-ordination of movement: a, rubrospinal; b, reticulospinal; c, vestibulospinal; d, olivospinal.

CHAPTER 1 **Anatomy and physiology**

Autonomic nervous system

The autonomic nervous system is divided on anatomical and physiological grounds into the functionally opposing sympathetic and parasympathetic nervous systems. The central areas responsible for coordinating the autonomic nervous system are mostly in the hypothalamus and its surrounding structures, and in the frontal lobes.

Sympathetic nervous system

The sympathetic nerves emerge from the spinal cord between the first thoracic and second lumbar spinal segments.
- The neurons supplying the gut synapse in the coeliac ganglia and the superior and inferior mesenteric plexuses.
- The supply to the rest of the body synapses in the ganglia of the sympathetic chain lying alongside the vertebral column, and second-order neurons pass with spinal nerves or with the carotid vessels if they are supplying the head.
- There is also a sympathetic supply of first-order neurons to the adrenal medulla.

Parasympathetic nervous system

The neurones of the parasympathetic nervous system exit the central nervous system with the IIIrd, VIIth, IXth, and Xth cranial nerves and from the 2nd–4th sacral segments of the spinal cord. The neurons usually synapse in ganglia or plexuses near, or in, the organ concerned.

The autonomic nervous system also has an afferent component for both the sympathetic and parasympathetic systems which generally follows the same pathways as the efferent system.

The cranial nerves

There are twelve paired cranial nerves, arising mostly from the base of the brain. Cranial nerves I, II, and VIII are entirely sensory, nerves III, IV, VI, XI and XII are entirely motor and the rest are mixed. The nuclei of the cranial nerves are within the midbrain and the brainstem.

I: the olfactory nerve

A specialized tract carrying afferent fibres for smell sensation from the nasal mucosa.

II: the optic nerve

This nerve and the retina are derived from the developing forebrain and the nerve is not therefore a true nerve. The two optic nerves join in the optic chiasm anterior to the pituitary gland. Fibres from the medial (nasal) half of the retina cross in the optic chiasm to enter the opposite optic tract and join fibres from the ipsilateral lateral retina.

III, IV, VI: the oculomotor, trochlear and abducent nerves

These nerves control the extraocular eye muscles. Raised intracranial pressure causes compression of the oculomotor (IIIrd) nerve leading to pupillary dilatation on the affected side.

V: the trigeminal nerve

Carries sensation from the face, orbit, nose, and mouth via three divisions: ophthalmic; maxillary; and mandibular. It also supplies motor fibres (via the mandibular branch) to the muscles of mastication and the anterior belly of the digastric muscle.

VII: the facial nerve
A mixed sensory and motor nerve. The motor supply is to the muscles of facial expression and the stapedius muscle in the ear. The facial nerve has secretomotor fibres for the lacrimal, submandibular and sublingual glands, and transmits taste sensation from the anterior two-thirds of the tongue. That part of the facial nerve nucleus which controls the upper facial muscles receives innervation from both cerebral cortices.

VIII: the vestibulocochlear or auditory nerve
Supplies the ear. As well as cochlear fibres for hearing there are vestibular fibres concerned with balance.

IX: the glossopharyngeal nerve
Contains sensory fibres for the pharynx and the posterior one-third of the tongue, secretomotor fibres for the parotid gland, innervation for the carotid body and carotid sinus, and motor fibres to the stylopharyngeus muscle.

X: the vagus nerve
Carries motor, sensory and secretomotor fibres. Its motor supply is to the pharynx and larynx, heart and lungs, and the gut as far as the splenic flexure of the colon. The sensory supply is to the epiglottis, airway, heart, and gut, and the secretomotor supply is to the bronchi and the gut.

XI: the accessory nerve
Has two components—a cranial component which innervates the muscles of the pharynx and larynx via the vagus nerve and a spinal component derived from the upper part of the cervical spinal cord which provides motor innervation to the sternomastoid and trapezius muscles.

XII: the hypoglossal nerve
Entirely motor and supplies the muscles of the tongue.

Control of the cerebral circulation

Adequate blood flow to the brain is essential to maintain substrate delivery and waste product removal. Cerebral blood flow (CBF) accounts for 20% of the cardiac output (approximately 700 ml min^{-1} in an adult) and 20% of the body's basal oxygen consumption is consumed by the brain.
- Mean CBF is approximately 50 ml 100 g brain tissue^{-1}
  - grey matter: 70 ml 100 g^{-1} min^{-1}
  - white matter: 20 ml 100 g^{-1} min^{-1}

Constant delivery of glucose as substrate for aerobic metabolism to generate ATP is necessary to support neuronal electrical activity. This relatively high oxygen consumption, coupled with the absence of significant oxygen reserves in the brain, means that any interruption to cerebral perfusion rapidly results in unconsciousness as the oxygen tension and substrate levels fall. Without oxygen, energy-dependent processes cease, leading to irreversible cellular injury if blood flow is not re-established promptly (see Cerebral metabolism, p.18).

Under normal circumstances CBF is tightly controlled, with regulatory responses to changes in the local or systemic environment. At times this control may be disordered, or the regulatory mechanisms themselves may be detrimental to other areas of the brain.

The cerebral circulation exists within a non-compliant space and the verebral veins are relatively collapsible. For this reason, the pressure gradient driving CBF is dependent not only on the outflow pressure (central venous pressure, CVP) but also on the intracranial pressure (ICP). The relationship is complex but a pragmatic approach is to define cerebral perfusion pressure (CPP) as the difference between mean arterial pressure (MAP) and ICP or CVP (whichever is greater).
- CPP = MAP—ICP or
- CPP = MAP—CVP if CVP>ICP.

Autoregulation

This is the ability of the cerebral circulation to maintain a relatively constant blood flow over a range of perfusion pressures by altering cerebrovascular resistance (CVR) (Figure 1.4).

Various factors interact to generate the autoregulatory response:
- myogenic responses of the smooth muscle cells of the arteriolar wall to stretch induced by variations in transmural pressure.
- shear stress (blood velocity) induced changes in vascular tone—increased blood velocity may result in vasoconstriction.
- metabolic factors such as oxygen delivery to tissues, neuronal and glial metabolism and the autonomic nervous system also modulate the response.

The response is not immediate; estimates of the latency period for compensatory changes in CVR range from 10–60 s.

CBF (ml 100 g⁻¹ min⁻¹)

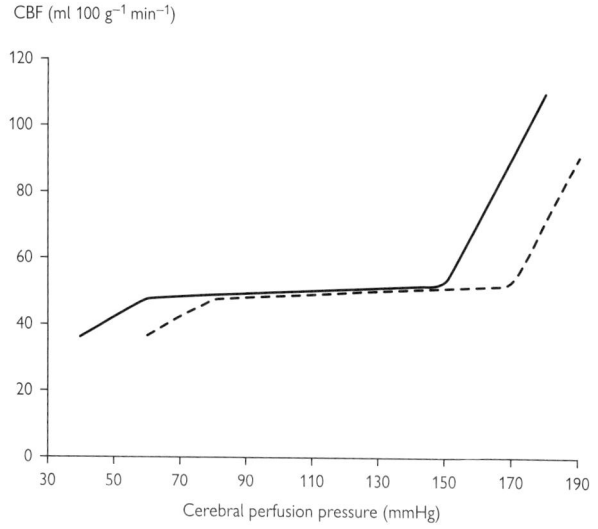

Fig. 1.4 The effect of cerebral perfusion pressure on cerebral blood flow. The solid line is the relationship in a normotensive patient, the dashed line is the relationship in a patient with chronic hypertension.

Cerebral blood flow remains approximately constant over a CPP of between 60–150 mmHg in normotensive individuals. A reduction in arterial blood pressure induces cerebral pre-capillary vessel dilation and results in a decreased CVR. Near the lower limit of autoregulation, cerebral vasodilatatory responses are insufficient to maintain CBF if CPP falls. CBF becomes pressure dependent, with a decrease in MAP producing a similar decrease in CBF. Conversely, increased arterial blood pressure induces net cerebral pre-capillary vessel constriction and an increased CVR. Around the upper limit, the vasoconstrictive response is insufficient to prevent significant rises in CBF when CPP rises. Elevated intraluminal pressure may cause passive vessel dilatation, leading to an increase in CBF and damage to the blood–brain barrier.

Disease processes, such as TBI, CVA or hypertension, impair autoregulation. Drugs that cause cerebral vasodilatation (see Chapter 2) such as volatile anaesthetic agents and glyceryl trinitrate also diminish the autoregulatory response. The curve is shifted to the right in chronic uncontrolled hypertension (see Figure 1.4) and to the left with induced hypotension.

Biochemical

Carbon dioxide

Cerebral blood vessels vasodilate and vasoconstrict in response to increases and decreases in $PaCO_2$. The effect of $PaCO_2$ is mediated through CSF pH. Changes in pH influence cerebral vascular tone via second messenger systems and by direct alteration of the concentration of calcium ions in vascular smooth muscle. The system of mediators that link extracellular pH to cerebral vascular tone is complex and interrelated; prostaglandins, nitric oxide (NO), cyclic nucleotides, potassium channels and intracellular Ca^{2+} have all been implicated as chemical mediators.

- In the physiological range, there is an approximately linear relationship between $PaCO_2$ and CBF (Figure 1.5).
  - With hypercapnia, 1 kPa change in $PaCO_2$ increases cerebral blood flow approximately 25–35%.
  - With hypocapnia, 1 kPa change in $PaCO_2$ decreases cerebral blood flow approximately 15%.
  - Above ~10–11 kPa there is no further increase in CBF due to maximal vasodilatation.
  - Below around 2.5 kPa there is no further vasoconstriction. This is believed to be due to counteracting effects of tissue hypoxia promoting vasodilatation.
- The response to changes in $PaCO_2$ is relatively prompt, with a half-time of around 20 s.
  - The effect of changes in $PaCO_2$ wanes over time, effectively resetting the 'normal' $PaCO_2$ for the individual.
  - Under normal conditions brain $PaCO_2$ is slightly higher, and pH and bicarbonate levels slightly lower, than arterial values. During acute hyperventilation, alkalosis results in cerebral vasoconstriction, resulting in a reduction in CBF, cerebral blood volume (CBV) and ICP.
  - After 6–12 h of sustained hypocapnia, extracellular brain pH recovers to near baseline. This influences cerebrovascular tone and thus restores CBF and CBV to baseline.
  - Normalization of CBF is mediated by a reduction in CSF and extracellular bicarbonate concentration, and correction of extracellular pH. Glial cells, which contain large amounts of the enzyme carbonic anhydrase, appear to be important in the regulation of extracellular bicarbonate concentration.
- The neonatal and adult cerebral circulations respond to CO_2 in a similar fashion, although the magnitude of the response may be less in neonates.
  - Vasodilator prostaglandins derived from vascular endothelium are important in the response to hypercapnia in the neonate.
  - Cyclo-oxygenase products appear to play a less important role in regulation of the adult cerebral circulation.
  - NO, on the other hand, produced by a family of NO-synthase enzymes found in brain vascular endothelial cells, parenchymal neurons and glia, exerts a profound influence on adult cerebral vascular tone.

CBF (ml 100 g^{-1} min^{-1})

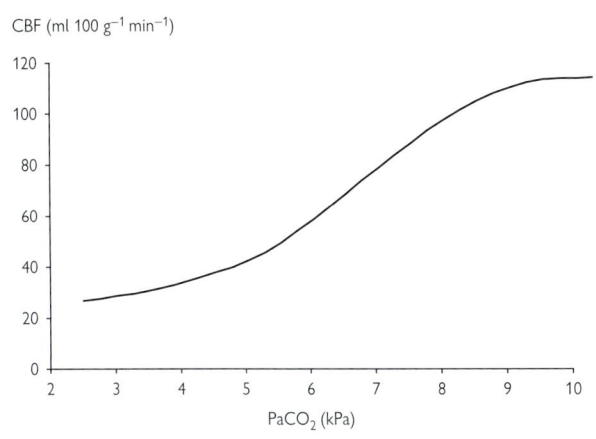

Fig. 1.5 The effect of PaCO$_2$ on cerebral blood flow.

Oxygen

Cerebral blood flow is responsive to blood oxygen content with vasodilatation in response to reduced oxygen delivery.

- As a consequence of the shape of the oxyhaemoglobin dissociation curve, there is little change in CBF seen with physiological changes in PaO$_2$ (Figure 1.6).
- The relationship between blood oxygen content (CaO$_2$) and cerebral blood flow is relatively independent of the cause of the change in CaO$_2$ (e.g. acute or chronic anaemia, hypoxia, hyperoxia).
- There are small (~10%) but significant decreases in CBF with hyperoxia. The clinical implications of this are unclear.

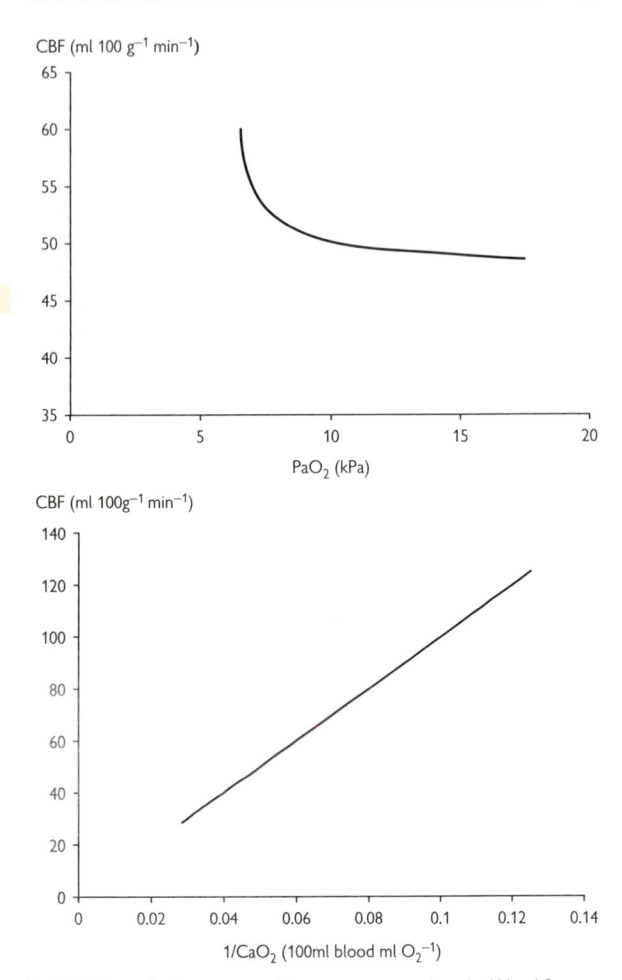

Fig. 1.6 Relationship between arterial oxygen content and cerebral blood flow.

Flow-metabolism coupling

Changes in cerebral blood flow and metabolism tend to follow each other. Local increases in metabolic demand are met rapidly by an increase in CBF and substrate delivery, and vice versa. Under normal circumstances, local CBF may change but global flow remains constant. When activity in a particular region of the brain increases, activity within another region tends to decrease and blood flow is diverted from one area to another. Conditions that cause a global increase in cerebral metabolic rate (CMR), such as pyrexia and convulsions, cause a corresponding increase in CBF. Conversely, factors such as anaesthetic drugs, hypothermia and coma will reduce CMR and CBF.

- Increases in cerebral blood flow in areas of increased neuronal activity match CMR_{glu} but are far in excess of the increase in oxygen consumption.
- Astrocytes may play an important role in the regulation of cerebral metabolism, by utilizing glucose *anaerobically*, reducing the local oxygen extraction ratio and producing lactate that can be used by neurons as substrate in the citric acid cycle.
- Flow-metabolism coupling occurs very promptly (~1 s). Numerous factors are involved:
  - local concentrations of K^+ and adenosine, which increase secondary to neuronal depolarization
  - neurogenic pathways. Cerebral blood vessels are innervated by a network of nerve fibres that utilize a number of different neurotransmitters to regulate flow-metabolism coupling. Dopaminergic pathways may be of particular importance.

Autonomic nervous system

Cerebral blood vessels are richly innervated and there are a number of different neurotransmitters involved in neural pathways within the cerebral circulation. Neurogenic factors play an important role in modulation of the response of the CBF to metabolic demands and in certain pathological states. There is some controversy concerning the relative importance of autonomic control of CBF.

Sympathetic nervous system

- Stimulation (or denervation) of the carotid baroreceptors or arterial chemoreceptors, does not cause significant alterations in resting CBF or dynamic responses to $PaCO_2$, MAP and PaO_2.
- Sympathetic innervation of cerebral vessels via the release of norepinephrine, serotonin and neuropeptide Y causes vasoconstriction. This may confer an important role in limiting the increase in intravascular pressure in the capillaries and in the smaller cerebral arterioles during arterial hypertension, thus preventing damage to the blood–brain barrier.
- The sympathetic nerves may also serve a protective function during periods of hypoxia as well as having trophic effects on cerebral vessels.

Parasympathetic nervous system
The role of the parasympathetic nervous system (PNS) is less well defined.
- Acetylcholine, vasoactive intestinal polypeptide and NO are the transmitters involved in the parasympathetic innervation of cerebral blood vessels.
- The PNS may control vasodilatation during certain pathological conditions such as ischaemia/reperfusion.

Trigeminovascular nerves
An additional vasodilatory influence on cerebral circulation arises from the trigeminovascular fibres. These originate from the first division of the trigeminal ganglion and from the somatosensory pathways relaying in the thalamus.
- Neurotransmitters include substance P, calcitonin gene-related peptide, cholecystokinin and neurokinin A.
- They influence cerebral vasodilatation in post-ischaemia reperfusion conditions, such as post-seizure hyperaemia or arterial hypotension.
- They may also protect against vasospasm in subarachnoid haemorrhage.

Flow dynamics

Changes in blood rheology may have complex effects on CBF, cerebral blood volume (CBV), and cerebral oxygen delivery.
- Resistance arterioles are responsive to shear stress, which is a function of blood flow velocity. Pharmacological interventions and pathological conditions can increase flow velocity, which results in vasoconstriction.
- Conversely, reduced blood viscosity reduces resistance to flow.
- In some circumstances these two effects may be clinically useful. Mannitol (which decreases blood viscosity) may increase blood flow through reduced viscosity and also result in reduced CBV through vasoconstrictive effects.
- The effects of acute anaemia are complex. Cerebral blood flow increases, maintaining cerebral oxygen delivery. This is in part due to changes in blood viscosity, but NO mediated vasodilatation is also important.

Cerebral metabolism

A significant focus of the neuroanaesthetist is on maintaining an appropriate balance between cerebral metabolic demand and supply in an attempt to minimize the risk of neurological injury. A basic understanding of cerebral metabolism will support the anaesthetist and intensivist in making appropriate decisions about use of drugs, sedation and anaesthetic techniques in the operating room and in intensive care. Spinal cord physiology is broadly similar, so the same principles apply to the management of the 'at risk' cord.

The brain is highly metabolically active taking:
- 20% of cardiac output
- 25% of total body glucose consumption
- 20% of total body oxygen consumption.

The energy expenditure of the brain is classically divided into:
- basal (45%): cellular integrity, ionic gradients, protein synthesis
- activation (55%): generation of electrical signals.

When the EEG is isoelectric (flat), energy expenditure reflects purely basal activity. Increasing sedation beyond this will not result in any further decrease in energy expenditure.

Substrates
- Glucose is the preferred substrate, but ketone bodies, lactate, glycerol, fatty acids, and amino acids can also be used.
- Aerobic metabolism is through oxidative phosphorylation.
- 99% of resting ATP production is from oxidative phosphorylation.
- Anaerobic metabolism is through glycolysis.
- Neural activation is associated with an increase in glycolysis.
- Ketone bodies supply <1% of energy normally, but during prolonged fasting may provide up to 60%.

Blood flow dependence
- Normally there is tight coupling between blood flow and metabolism.
- If coupling is lost or blood flow is too low then oxygen extraction may increase, resulting in low capillary oxygen levels.
- If blood flow is too low, relative to metabolic demand, then there is an increase in anaerobic metabolism.
- Prolonged ischaemia results in cellular ATP depletion and failure of membrane ion gradients.
- Critical thresholds of blood flow leading to irreversible tissue damage have been described:
  - traumatic brain injury: 15 ml 100 g^{-1} min^{-1}
  - ischaemic stroke: 5–8.5 ml 100 g^{-1} min^{-1}.

Neural–glial energy coupling
- Glial cells are non-neuronal cells found in the brain and spinal cord which provide supportive and metabolic functions.
- Astrocytes (a type of glial cell) are an active partner to the neural tissue with regard to metabolism, with cycling of substrates and metabolites

between the two cell types. The result is close coupling of neural and glial metabolism.
- Glucose is taken up and metabolized anaerobically by astrocyte glycolysis.
- Lactate from astrocytes then diffuses to coupled neural cells and is metabolized aerobically.
- Neural activation leads to release of potassium and glutamate, which are taken up by astrocytes.
- The energy for potassium and glutamate uptake is provided by increased glycolysis.

Factors affecting cerebral metabolism

Cerebral metabolism can be influenced by physiological changes, drugs and disease. Some of these effects can be modified deliberately in an attempt to match supply and demand.
- Neural activation—this tends not to affect overall cerebral metabolic rate for oxygen ($CMRO_2$) but produces regional changes in $CMRO_2$ and CBF.
  - wakefulness
  - movement
  - sensory input
  - pain
  - seizures.
- Temperature
  - ~5–10 % change in $CMRO_2$ per °C change in temperature
  - there may be greater change with lower temperatures
  - isoelectric EEG occurs at ~20° C.
- Pathology
  - $CMRO_2$ is reduced in dementia
  - variable changes in $CMRO_2$ following head injury
  - $CMRO_2$ is reduced after subarachnoid haemorrhage, though seizures may cause increases
  - $CMRO_2$ is not affected directly by endotoxin.

Measurement of cerebral metabolism

Cerebral metabolism can be measured in various ways. Global measures assess the change in concentration of oxygen, glucose or lactate between the arterial inflow and venous outflow. Regional techniques can measure metabolism in defined regions of interest (ROI) or the local concentrations of metabolites and substrates. Local oxygen delivery can also be assessed using oxygen sensing catheters.

Global techniques

If a substance is consumed or produced by a tissue of interest (brain) at a rate proportional to metabolic rate, then the difference between arterial and venous concentrations can be used to estimate metabolic rate. The difference is also affected by blood flow: high blood flow will lead to a smaller difference for the same metabolic rate, low blood flow to a higher difference. Arteriovenous differences, therefore, more strictly reflect the balance between supply and demand.

Common techniques include:
- arteriovenous oxygen or glucose difference
- arteriovenous lactate difference
- jugular venous oxygen saturation (SjO_2)
  - assuming that cerebral blood flow and arterial oxygen content are constant, then SjO_2 is an estimate of the amount of oxygen consumed by the brain overall. This represents a global average so is relatively insensitive to focal abnormalities. (📖 This is covered in more detail in Chapter 3.)

Regional techniques

Imaging techniques which can identify different regions of interest can be used to estimate regional metabolism. These are generally intermittent positron emission tomography (PET) techniques performed using radioactive substrates. Microdialysis catheters can be placed in neuronal tissue to measure metabolites, which can give some indication of the relative amount of aerobic and anaerobic metabolism. 📖 Microdialysis is covered in more detail in Chapter 3.

- $CMRO_2$—lactate metabolism by neural tissue (PET)
- CMRglc—glucose metabolism by astrocytes (PET)
- Lactate/pyruvate ratio (microdialysis).

Table 1.1 Values for cerebral metabolism

Measured factor	Normal values	In head injury
CBF (ml 100 g^{-1} min^{-1})	54 (Kety–Schmidt) 40 (PET) 48 (Grey matter, PET) 22 (White matter, PET)	Variable
SjO_2 (%)	62 (50–75)	70 (Variable)
$CjVO_2$ (ml O_2 dl^{-1})	14.0	Variable
$AVDO_2$ (ml O_2 dl^{-1})	7.3	Variable
$CMRO_2$ (ml 100 g^{-1} min^{-1})	3.8 – 5 (PET) 4 (Grey matter, PET) 2 (White matter, PET)	Variable
Oxygen extraction ratio (OER (%))	40 (independent of $CMRO_2$)	Variable
Arterio-venous difference—glucose (AVDG) (μmol dl^{-1})	53	40
Arterio-venous difference—lactate (AVDL) (μmol dl^{-1})	19	5
Microdialysis:		
Lactate (mmol l^{-1})	2.9	Variable
Pyruvate (μmol l^{-1})	166	Variable
Lactate/Pyruvate ratio	23	Variable
Glycerol (μmol l^{-1})	82	Variable

Intracranial pressure and CSF

The brain and spinal cord exist within a relatively non-compliant box (the bony-ligamentous cranio-spinal space). The pressure within the space is termed intracranial pressure (ICP) and is generally higher than atmospheric pressure.

Monroe–Kellie doctrine
This simple model of the pressure-volume relationships of the brain, cerebral blood volume and cerebrospinal fluid assumes that (Figure 1.7):
- the cerebrospinal structures are contained with in a non-compliant box.
- four volumes are present:
  - brain
  - intravascular blood
  - cerebrospinal fluid
  - additional space occupying lesions (extra-vascular blood, tumour, oedematous tissue).
- brain, blood and cerebrospinal fluid are incompressible, but they can move according to pressure gradients:
  - CSF can move from the intracranial compartment into the more compliant spinal compartment.
  - the brain can be compressed against or between rigid structures if there are pressure gradients.

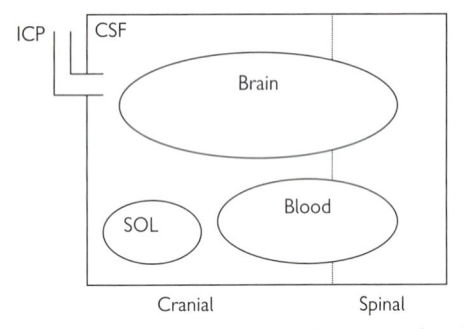

Fig. 1.7 Model to demonstrate the compartments in the cranium and spinal cord.

- Cerebral blood volume (CBV) can change in response to vasodilatatory or vasoconstrictive mechanisms.
- If the volume of one component increases then the pressure inside the 'box' will increase. This may result in a compensatory shift of another component (e.g. CSF) which may limit the increase in pressure (Figure 1.8 A).
- If the ability to compensate for an increase in intracranial content volume is exhausted, then there will be a large increase in intracranial pressure. (Figure 1.8 B).
- If ICP is raised then a reduction in cerebral perfusion pressure may occur (📖 Control of the cerebral circulation, p. 10). If ICP is sufficiently high then cerebral blood flow will cease.

There are a number of important features to note about the model.

- The axes are generally drawn without scale. Different individuals have differently positioned elastance curves (elastance is the reciprocal of compliance), so an individual ICP value does not provide much information about the relative intracranial volume or the effect of changes in that volume.
- Long term increases in intracranial volume, such as caused by tumours, allow more time for adaptive effects so the elastance curve is shifted to the right.
- Head trauma may reduce intracranial compliance, thereby shifting the curve upwards and to the left.

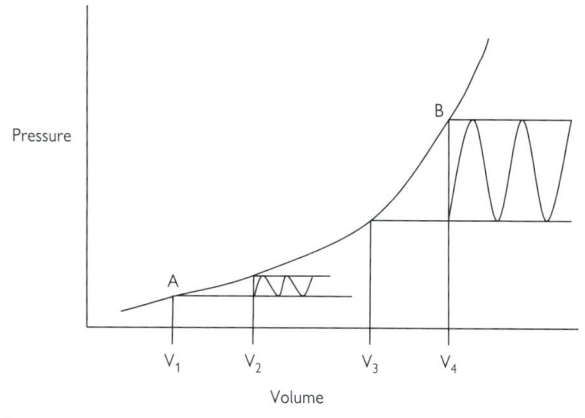

Fig. 1.8 Intracranial elastance curve.

Manipulation of intracranial pressure

On the basis of the Monroe–Kellie doctrine, it is fairly straightforward to reduce ICP.
- Reduce cerebral blood volume (CBV)
- Reduce brain volume
- Reduce CSF volume
- Reduce space-occupying lesion volume.

Reduction of cerebral blood volume

As detailed in the earlier (📖 p. 10), control of CBF is mediated through changes in arteriolar diameter. Factors which increase CBF will increase CBV. Venous blood volume may also affect ICP. Methods to reduce CBV and ICP include:
- Avoidance of cerebral activation
  - analgesia
  - adequate anaesthesia/sedation.
- Temporary reduction of $PaCO_2$
  - although a reduction in $PaCO_2$ may reduce ICP, there is evidence from PET studies in traumatic brain injury (TBI) that there may be an increase in ischaemic brain volume, due to reduction of flow in at-risk areas.
  - long term hypocapnia is associated with a gradual return of CBF/CBV to normal. When $PaCO_2$ is then allowed to return to normal, this is sensed as a hypercapnic episode and so will tend to increase ICP.
- Avoidance of hyper- and hypotension
  - when autoregulation is intact, systemic hypotension will cause cerebral vasodilation and may increase ICP
  - if autoregulation is impaired, hypertension may result in pressure dependent expansion of blood vessels or increasing cerebral oedema which may increase ICP.
- Avoidance of hypoxia
- Avoidance of severe anaemia (causes vasodilation)
- Avoidance of pharmacological cerebral vasodilation
  - various drugs increase CBV, notably high dose volatile anaesthetics, nitrous oxide and nitrates. (📖 More details are provided in Chapter 2).
- Increasing CBF, leading to reflex cerebral vasoconstriction
  - this may be one of the mechanisms by which mannitol exerts its effects.
- Ensuring adequate venous drainage
  - moderate held-up tilt
  - avoidance of constricting ties around the neck and removal of hard cervical spine collars.

Reduction of brain/space occupying lesion volume

Acute brain injury (trauma, stroke) and chronic space-occupying lesions (meningioma, intrinsic tumour, lymphoma) may all result in increased ICP due to so called 'mass effect'. A decision to operate to reduce mass volume is influenced by many factors. In some instances this may be essentially curative (e.g. meningioma), in other cases, 'making space' purely buys time. This may allow time for an acute condition such as TBI or stroke to improve, or it may allow increased duration of survival from intrinsic tumours.

Reduction of CSF volume
CSF is produced constantly (~0.4 ml min^{-1}). If it is not reabsorbed at the same rate, then CSF volume will increase.
- Various pathological conditions may result in acute or chronic decreases in CSF absorption including:
  - subarachnoid haemorrhage
  - trauma
  - infection
  - normal pressure hydroecephalus.
- Intracranial CSF can either be removed (usually using an external ventricular drain) or diverted (shunts from the cerebral ventricles to a site of absorption—peritoneum, pleura or atrium, see Shunts and ventricular drains, Chapter 6, p. 214).
- CSF production can also be reduced using acetazolamide.

Temporal variation in ICP
Intracranial pressure is not a static value. There are cyclical changes in ICP. The amplitude and temporal relationships of these pressure waves may vary in pathological conditions.

Pulse waves

ICP pulse pressure.
Intracranial pressure follows the pulsatile changes in cerebral blood volume caused by the arterial pulse.

The amplitude of the ICP pulse (ICP pulse-pressure) may give an indication of the relative compliance of the intracranial space. In Figure 1.8, when compliance is high {A}, for a given change in volume (V_1–V_2) the ICP pulse pressure is relatively small. When compliance is low {B} for the same change in volume (V_3–V_4) the pulse pressure is greater.

B- and C-waves.
These are slower oscillations in ICP related to rhythmic changes in $PaCO_2$, MAP and lower brainstem related rhythms.
- B-waves and C-waves occur with a frequency of 1–2 and 4–8 per minute, respectively, and cause relatively small changes in ICP.
- The clinical importance of B- and C-waves is debated.

A-waves (plateau waves)
These are pathological. They are abrupt rises in ICP from near normal values of ICP to 50 mmHg or greater.
- They last around 5–20 min and then usually terminate spontaneously.
- They are probably the consequence of a low compliance intracranial space which is perturbed by some event causing an increase in intracranial content volume.
- Various feedback mechanisms may serve to maintain the high ICP even though the original stimulus has gone.
- They are often accompanied by neurological deterioration as a consequence of the prolonged high ICP.

ICP phase analysis

If autoregulation is intact then when MAP increases, cerebral vasoconstriction should ensue, causing a reduction in cerebral blood volume (CBV) and ICP. There should be a strong negative correlation between slow changes in MAP and ICP. If autoregulation is sufficiently disturbed then global CBV will follow MAP, and ICP will correlate directly with MAP. Pressure reactivity (Prx) is a mathematical description of the strength of this correlation. The minimum value is −1, the maximum is +1. Various groups have associated high values (>0.2–0.3) with poor outcome after traumatic brain injury.

Cerebrospinal fluid

Cerebrospinal fluid (CSF) fills the cerebral ventricles and the subarachnoid space around the brain and the spinal cord and acts as a buffer separating the brain and spinal cord from the hard bony projections inside the skull and the vertebral canal.

- CSF is produced by the choroid plexus mainly in the lateral and third ventricles by a combination of filtration and secretion.
  - There is probably a significant amount of extra-choroidal production as well.
- CSF is produced at a rate of around 0.4 ml min^{-1} in adults. Production is proportional to cerebral metabolism and falls with age.

CSF volume

Estimates of total CSF volume have changed over the years as measurement techniques have become more precise. More recent estimates using magnetic resonance imaging (MRI) studies suggest that adult intracranial CSF volume is around 170 ml. The ventricles contain around 25 ml. Spinal CSF volume is estimated to be around 100 ml.

CSF flow

Under normal circumstances, CSF flows from the lateral ventricles into the third ventricle and then into the fourth ventricle through the narrow aqueduct of Sylvius. It leaves the fourth ventricle through the lateral and midline foramina (of Luschka and Magendie, respectively). Most of the CSF flows around the basal cisterns and then upwards to the superior sagittal sinus. Some flows over the cord down to the lumbar sac. Free flow between the various CSF spaces is important for allowing compensation for increases in intracranial volume and the avoidance of pressure gradients. Where this free flow is disturbed (TBI, Arnold–Chiari malformations, non-communicating hydrocephalus) pathological pressure gradients occur.

CSF absorption

CSF passes back in to the venous blood through arachnoid villi which are diverticuli of the arachnoid mater through the dura mater into the dural venous sinuses.

- The absorption of CSF is a one-way, essentially passive process; raised venous pressure or reduced ICP reduces the rate of CSF absorption.
- The resistance to CSF absorption can be estimated using CSF infusion tests with normal values of around 6–10 mmHg ml^{-1} min^{-1}.

- In some pathological conditions (e.g. normal pressure hydrocephalus) CSF may leak directly into the brain parenchyma from where it is subsequently absorbed.

CSF pressure

CSF pressure is dependent on the relative site of measurement (intracranial vs. lumbar) and patient factors such as position and movement.

- Intracranial pressure in normal subjects is 7–15 mmHg when supine, falling to −10 mmHg when erect.
- Lumbar CSF pressure is the same as ICP when supine (7–15 mmHg) and is greater when subjects are seated.
- CSF pressure fluctuates as a result of respiration and arterial pressure.
- Changes are also seen as a result of changes in venous pressure, for example an increase in pressure in the intrathoracic veins after coughing.

CSF composition

CSF is produced actively. It therefore has a different cellular and ionic composition to blood.

CO_2 and bicarbonate

The CSF bicarbonate concentration is slightly lower than that of plasma, whereas PCO_2 and hydrogen ion concentration are slightly greater. *In vitro* CSF has very poor buffering capacity, but *in vivo* the inter-relationship between CSF and plasma bicarbonate, means that CSF pH is buffered.

Cations

CSF sodium concentration is approximately the same as blood. Potassium is about 60% and calcium about 50% that of plasma, whereas magnesium is somewhat greater.

Anions

Chloride concentration is higher in CSF than plasma.

Glucose

Glucose is usually about half to two-thirds of plasma concentration. Lower relative values are suggestive of bacterial meningitis.

Proteins

Total protein concentration is much lower in CSF than plasma. Very high concentrations (1–3 g l^{-1}) may be seen in Guillain–Barré syndrome. Abnormal oligoclonal bands may be seen in patients with multiple sclerosis.

Cells

In an atraumatic (non-bloody) sample there should be <5 white cells mm^{-3}, with very few polymorphs. Acute haemorrhage will lead to all components of blood being present. CSF samples taken >12 h after subarachnoid haemorrhage may be xanthochromic due to the presence of haem breakdown products.

Chapter 1 Anatomy and physiology

Box 1.1 Comparison of plasma and CSF constituents

	Plasma (mmol⁻¹)	CSF (mmol⁻¹)	Comments
Sodium	140	140	Not usually measured, of research relevance only.
Potassium	4.5	2.8	
Calcium	2.1	1.1	
Magnesium	0.8	1.1	
Chloride	102	112	
pH	7.4	7.3	
Bicarbonate	25	22	
Glucose	5	2.5–3	50–66% of blood taken at the same time. Lower in bacterial meningitis
Protein	60–80 g/L⁻¹	0.2–0.4 g/L⁻¹	Raised in Guillain–Barré (1–3 g/L⁻¹). May also be raised in the presence of infection and inflammation. Abnormal bands on electrophoresis in multiple sclerosis.
Pressure		7–15 mm Hg lying (adults) >–10 mm Hg vertical (ICP) 3–7 mm Hg (children) 1.5–6 mm Hg (term infants)	

Chapter 2

Pharmacology

Inhalational agents *30*
Intravenous agents *34*
Mannitol and hypertonic saline *38*
Glucocorticoids *42*
Vasoactive drugs *44*
Opioids *52*
Muscle relaxants *56*
Non-steroidal anti-inflammatory drugs and paracetamol *60*
Anti-emetics and PONV *62*
Vasopressin: argine vasopressin (AVP), antidiuretic hormone (ADH) *64*

Inhalational agents

Volatile agents are used for maintenance of anaesthesia in the majority of general anaesthetics in the UK. In neuroanaesthesia volatile-based inhalational anaesthesia or propofol-based TIVA techniques are used in approximately equal proportions. Nitrous oxide has mostly been replaced by remifentanil infusion if an analgesic agent is required, or by a greater dose of maintenance agent when analgesia is less important—for example, interventional neuroradiology procedures.

Nitrous oxide

The observed effect of nitrous oxide on the brain depends on the baseline state of the brain while it is being studied—in other words the effect will depend on whether cerebral metabolism is already maximally depressed from the use of volatile or intravenous anaesthetic agents.

- Added to 'low-dose' anaesthesia, nitrous oxide may further depress cerebral metabolism.
- Given to an awake individual nitrous oxide increases cerebral metabolism and cerebral blood flow.
- Administered alone, or with volatile agents, nitrous oxide impairs cerebral autoregulation.
- Administered with propofol, autoregulation is preserved.

Further potential disadvantages of nitrous oxide include:

- Increased risk of postoperative nausea and vomiting
- Expansion of air emboli
- Expansion of air in the head to create a pneumo-encephalocoele
- Disruption of vitamin B_{12} metabolism (long duration cases).

Effects of volatile agents on the cerebral vasculature and metabolism

Cerebral blood flow

All the volatile agents have a direct action on cerebral blood vessels leading to vasodilatation. However, these agents also depress cerebral metabolism (see p.31) and it is the balance between these two effects that determines the effect on blood vessel diameter and CBF.

- At low concentrations the vasodilatory effect may be outweighed by the reduction in cerebral metabolic activity secondary to the state of anaesthesia, and cerebral blood flow and blood volume will decrease.
- At higher doses the vasodilatory actions override the reduction in metabolism, blood flow, and brain metabolism become uncoupled (metabolism is decreased while flow increases) and flow and blood volume increase.
  - acute hypocapnia may reverse these vasodilatory effects.

Following the introduction of isoflurane, it became apparent that different volatile agents affect the brain differently and that cerebral vasodilatation and impairment of autoregulation are less with isoflurane than halothane.

- Sevoflurane has the least effect of all the currently available agents.
- Desflurane affects the cerebral vasculature to a similar degree as isoflurane.

Autoregulation

Volatile anaesthetic agents depress normal cerebral autoregulation in a dose-dependent manner. However, the agents differ in the potency of this effect.

- At normocapnia, 1 MAC (minimum alveolar concentration) of halothane significantly depresses autoregulation.
- There is little effect from sevoflurane up to 1.5 MAC.
- The order of potency for disturbance of autoregulation is:
    halothane > isoflurane = desflurane > sevoflurane.
- At high concentrations of any inhalational agent autoregulation is lost and blood flow becomes pressure-dependent.
- Acute hypocapnia may restore autoregulation.

Carbon dioxide reactivity

At clinical concentrations carbon dioxide reactivity is only minimally affected by volatile anaesthetic agents. This is important as hypocapnia induced by hyperventilation can be used (if necessary) to control ICP or to counteract the effect of those agents with more vasodilatory actions such as halothane. Hypocapnia is also used in exceptional circumstances to manage raised ICP intra-operatively.

ICP

As volatile agents lead to some degree of cerebral vasodilatation they produce an increase in blood flow and, therefore, blood volume. In a healthy brain the result is usually a small increase in ICP. In situations where the ICP is already raised, or the patient is on the inflexion point of the ICP elastance curve, the increase may be more significant.

Cerebral metabolism

Inhalational agents, by their nature as anaesthetics, decrease cerebral metabolism. At MAC multiples of around 2, the brain is maximally anaesthetized and the EEG will be isoelectric. At this point metabolism will be approximately half that of awake values.

Cerebral protection

There are no outcome studies to support the use of volatile agents as neuroprotective agents. There is, however, a body of laboratory evidence which suggest that they may be beneficial, through various mechanisms, for example:

- Reduction in $CMRO_2$
- Suppression of excitatory and enhancement of inhibitory pathways
- Regulation of intracellular calcium during ischaemia.

Specific agents

Halothane

Although the vasodilatory effects of halothane can be overcome by hypocapnia, this agent has now all but been replaced by newer agents. It may have a role for inhalational induction in children—although sevoflurane seems a better alternative. The use of hypocapnia has, itself, fallen into disrepute (see Chapter 4) except in exceptional circumstances.

Isoflurane

After its release isoflurane was seen as the ideal neuroanaesthetic as its use was associated with less vasodilatation than halothane, and recovery from anaesthesia was quicker. It has been replaced by sevoflurane but remains a widely used and acceptable alternative.

Sevoflurane

Sevoflurane has replaced isoflurane as the 'gold standard' volatile anaesthetic agent for neuroanaesthesia.

- It has minimal vasodilatory effects and no action on autoregulation up to 1.5 MAC.
- It has a low blood-gas solubility making for easy dose titration, rapid inhalational induction (if required) and rapid recovery.
- It is well tolerated at high concentrations contributing to its acceptability for inhalational induction.
- Seizure-like EEG activity has been seen in children during inhalational induction but the significance of this is unclear.
- Although prolonged use at low fresh gas flows is limited in some countries due to the build up of a breakdown product in circle systems containing carbon dioxide absorbers, these concerns appear to be theoretical only.

Desflurane

- The actions of desflurane on the cerebral vasculature (vasodilation and changes to autoregulation) are very similar to that seen with isoflurane. The low blood-gas solubility of desflurane leads to very rapid recovery even after long-duration cases.
- It is poorly tolerated by spontaneously breathing patients and is, therefore, unsuitable for inhalational induction.
- Rapid changes in inspired concentration are associated with sympathetic stimulation unless the patient is also receiving an opioid.

Tips and pitfalls

- There are no outcome studies to suggest that one agent is truly beneficial.
- Nitrous oxide is generally avoided for intracranial procedures but is used by some for spinal column surgery.
- All volatile agents affect cerebral blood flow, cerebral blood volume and autoregulation at high doses.
- Volatile agents are usually combined with high-dose opioids (for example, remifentanil) and the MAC value is then reduced.

Intravenous agents

Intravenous anaesthetic agents are used for induction of anaesthesia, maintenance of anaesthesia, sedation for painful or unpleasant procedures and sedation on the intensive care unit (ICU). The available agents include thiopental, propofol, etomidate, and ketamine. However, etomidate is less commonly used. Ketamine was thought to have been contraindicated for neuroanaesthesia, although recent work on its possible neuroprotective properties has led to a re-evaluation.

The advantages and disadvantages of TIVA compared with inhalational anaesthesia are discussed elsewhere (p. 134).

Uses

Induction of anaesthesia
Induction is most commonly performed with an intravenous agent—the advantages of rapid, smooth induction and early onset of airway control apply to neuroanaesthesia as much as to other types of surgery. Although inhalational induction may seem counter-intuitive (due to vasodilation and possible changes in ICP), if intravenous induction is contraindicated (e.g. in children without intravenous access) it is a reasonable alternative.

Maintenance of anaesthesia
Propofol may be used for maintenance of anaesthesia because its pharmacokinetic profile makes it suitable for total intravenous anaesthesia (TIVA). Changes in the infusion rate are soon followed by changes in plasma concentration and, a little later, by changes in effect site concentration. On stopping the infusion the elimination is rapid, with predictable awakening of the patient.

Sedation
Propofol infusions are used for sedation in the ICU in many patients including those with head injuries. Even after prolonged infusion, recovery can still be measured in minutes or hours. Propofol infusions can also be use for sedation during 'awake craniotomy' or for minor procedures.

Infusions of thiopental are used to suppress cerebral metabolic activity in patients with uncontrolled, raised ICP or with status epilepticus (see p. 374). The pharmacokinetics of thiopental mean that recovery, once the infusion has been stopped, will be slow (several days).

Cerebral effects

Metabolism
As a rule the intravenous agents reduce cerebral metabolism—the expected anaesthetic effect. This effect is dose-dependent until metabolism is fully suppressed and the EEG is isoelectric (a flat line). At this point the only cerebral metabolism continuing is that to preserve cellular integrity, not function.

- The maximal suppression of $CMRO_2$ that can be achieved with anaesthetic agents is about 60%.
- There are regional differences in the degree of metabolic suppression but these are not important clinically.

Autoregulation

Autoregulation is preserved with the intravenous agents at clinically relevant doses. However, these agents do have an effect on systemic blood pressure and may secondarily affect cerebral blood flow if the autoregulatory limits are exceeded.

Vasodilation/coupling

The intravenous agents act as direct vasodilators but their *in vivo* effect is determined by their action on cerebral metabolism
- Metabolism and blood flow remain coupled at clinical doses, so the net effect is for CBF to reduce in a dose-dependent manner.
- If blood flow (and hence, blood volume) reduces, so will ICP.
- There is experimental evidence that etomidate, and possibly propofol, may be associated with a reduction in blood flow greater than expected for the reduction in metabolism, with the possibility that these may become mismatched and relative ischaemia induced.

Carbon dioxide reactivity

At clinical concentrations there is little or no change in carbon dioxide reactivity following administration of any of these agents.

EEG

The overall effect is to reduce electroencephalogram (EEG) activity as cerebral metabolism is suppressed. The exact changes in the EEG are agent-specific.

ICP

Except for ketamine, these agents usually lead to a reduction of elevated ICP. However, the reduction in systemic blood pressure may be greater than the reduction in ICP, leading to a reduction in cerebral perfusion pressure.

Neuroprotection

Although there is much animal evidence of neuroprotection against ischaemic episodes from the use of intravenous agents, there is scant evidence that this is significant in clinical practice. There is some evidence that thiopental may protect against focal ischaemia.

Thiopental

Thiopental has been used in neuroanaesthesia for many years. It remains popular due to its action on cerebral metabolism and cerebral vasculature.
- It reduces $CMRO_2$ and concomitantly reduces cerebral blood flow.
- It is an anti-epileptic.
- It can be used to induce anaesthesia and to provide some small degree of cerebral protection during periods of ischaemia (see p. 130 and p. 356)
- Hypotension may complicate its use in head injured patients and the standard dose used (3–5 mg kg^{-1}) should be reduced in these patients—particularly those shocked due to concomitant injuries.
- Thiopental is uncommonly used as a first line sedative in ICU due to accumulation (its terminal half-life is ~11 h), but it is used by bolus therapy to reduced peaks of raised ICP.

Propofol

Propofol is the most commonly used induction agent in neuroanaesthesia.
- The usual dose is 1.5–2.5 mg kg^{-1}, but, in common with other anaesthetic practice, the dose should be reduced in shocked patients or those with cardiovascular comorbidities.
- $CMRO_2$ is reduced, as is cerebral blood flow, in a dose-dependent manner until an isoelectric EEG is obtained.
- Its use has been associated with epileptiform movements. There is no evidence that this represents cortical seizure or epilepsy.
- Although the terminal half-life is 3–4 h, the effective half-life is much shorter.
- Prolonged infusions of propofol maybe associated with propofol infusion syndrome (PRIS), a syndrome of metabolic acidosis, cardiovascular collapse and rhabdomyolysis:
  - critically ill neurological patients (including those with acute head injury) are at greater risk of PRIS
  - other risk factors include propofol sedation for >48 h and doses >5 mg kg^{-1} hr^{-1}.

Etomidate

Etomidate was popular as an induction agent, as a mode of pharmacological neuroprotection and as a bolus therapy to reduce ICP in severe head injury. Its popularity was due to its minimal effects on systemic haemodynamics.
- There is now experimental evidence that etomidate is associated with a reduction in cerebral blood flow in excess of the reduction in cerebral metabolism possibly leading to cerebral tissue hypoxia.
- Etomidate is now no longer used as a sedative as prolonged intravenous infusions have been shown to have suppressive effects on adrenal corticosteroid production in critically unwell patients.
- Seizures may be unmasked in susceptible patients with low doses of etomidate.

Ketamine

Ketamine has different neurophysiological effects to the other intravenous agents.
- Due to a degree of cerebral stimulation, $CMRO_2$, CBF, and ICP may increase.
- Its NMDA antagonist activity may provide some protection from ischaemia.
- The potentially harmful effects on metabolism and blood flow usually outweigh any protective effects.

Benzodiazepines
- Although cerebral metabolism and blood flow are reduced when a benzodiazepine is given, the effect is less than that seen with propofol or thiopental.
- These agents may be useful for sedation (in ICU or for surgical procedures), for co-induction, or as anticonvulsants.
- Benzodiazepines should be used with caution in patients receiving intrathecal baclofen due to the risk of excess sedation.

Tips and pitfalls
- Reduce the dose of intravenous agents in the elderly, shocked patients or those with co-morbidities.

Mannitol and hypertonic saline

Hyperosmolar agents are used during intracranial surgery and in the management of traumatic brain injury to reduce brain volume and hence ICP, and to improve cerebral perfusion. Although they are effective in reducing cerebral blood volume, convincing data supporting improved outcome in either elective surgery or emergency situations are lacking.

Mannitol

Indications
- Treatment of raised intracranial pressure in patients with severe head injury (GCS ≤ 8).
- Urgent treatment of patients with clinical signs of raised intracranial pressure (dilated pupil(s), Cushing's response) when ICP is not being monitored or during transfer.

Doses and routes of administration
- 0.25–1 g kg^{-1} given intravenously over 15–30 min.
- 10% and 20% solutions are available; there is no evidence that one is better than the other, though many units use 20% to reduce the volume load.
- The effect of mannitol lasts 1–4 h.
- Repeat doses should be given according to response and guided by serum osmolality, which should be kept <320 mosmol kg^{-1}.

Mechanism of action
Mannitol is a low molecular weight (182 Daltons) six-carbon sugar that acts as an osmotic diuretic and free radical scavenger. It is freely filtered by the glomerulus and not re-absorbed by the renal tubules. It increases the osmolality of the renal tubular fluid, increasing urine volume by an osmotic effect. It increases serum osmolality causing fluid to shift from the intracellular space to the extracellular space resulting in acute intravascular volume expansion.

Mannitol decreases intracranial pressure by several complementary actions.
- It reduces blood viscosity by dilution and increasing the deformability of red cells. The increased flow results in vasoconstriction secondary to increased oxygen delivery.
- In the presence of an intact blood–brain barrier it acts to withdraw brain extracellular fluid into the plasma.
- It decreases the rate of cerebrospinal fluid formation.

Neurological effects
- Mannitol reduces intracranial pressure when the blood–brain barrier is intact.
- It maintains cerebral blood flow in patients with preserved autoregulation.
- When the blood–brain barrier is damaged, mannitol can pass directly into the brain extracellular fluid and may lead to increased cerebral volume and paradoxical increase in ICP. This may be counteracted in part by increased local blood flow leading to increased clearance of water from surrounding tissue.

- When autoregulation is disturbed the increased flow due to reduced viscosity is not matched by vasoconstriction and CBF may increase.

Systemic effects
- Mannitol increases plasma volume. This may result in increased cardiac output and mean arterial blood pressure (MAP) is generally stable. The subsequent diuresis may lead to hypovolaemia.
- A significant minority of patients experience a transient drop in MAP following bolus administration of mannitol due a drop in systemic vascular resistance.
- Mannitol increases renal blood flow and leads to a diuresis generally maximal 1–3 h following administration.
- In addition to a diuresis, administration of mannitol results in increased excretion of sodium, chloride and bicarbonate ions, resulting in electrolyte disturbance after prolonged administration.
- Serum osmolality >320 mosmol kg^{-1} is associated with an increased risk of renal failure.

Special monitoring
- Various expert guidelines recommend that mannitol is used in patients with severe head injury as part of a written protocol for the management of raised intracranial pressure. Therefore, patients should have an ICP monitor *in situ* unless treatment is deemed necessary before this can be inserted.
- Serum osmolality should be monitored at least daily, and mannitol administration should cease when serum osmolality reaches 320 mosmol kg^{-1}.

Hypertonic saline

The role of hypertonic saline (HTS) in neuroanaesthesia and in the management of traumatic brain injury is still under debate and yet to be fully defined.

- Although not an osmotic diuretic by definition, HTS is as effective as mannitol in reducing cerebral oedema and ICP and improving cerebral regional blood flow in traumatic brain injury.
- The benefits of HTS, however, are not seen in patients with other conditions, for example, subarachnoid haemorrhage. Its main role may lie in the resuscitation of the hypotensive poly-trauma patient with severe head injury.
- Small volume (<250 ml; 2 ml kg^{-1}) resuscitation with HTS (7.5% solution) of these patients is associated with increased survival.

Dose and route of administration
Adults: Intravenous boluses of 2 ml kg^{-1} 7.5% HTS.
Children: 0.1–1.0 ml.kg^{-1}.hr^{-1} of 3% HTS to a maximum osmolality of 360 mosm kg^{-1}.

Mechanism of action
Hypertonic solutions of saline are not strictly defined and the term has been used for concentrations ranging from 3% to 20%. All work in the same way.
- In the presence of an intact blood–brain barrier, an osmotic gradient for sodium and water is created, thus water leaves the brain parenchyma resulting in reduced brain volume.
- Dehydration of endothelial cells may result in small increases in internal vascular diameter leading to increased perfusion.
- Complementary effects may also include restoration of neuronal membrane potential, and reduction of endothelial leucocyte adhesion, which may affect the inflammatory response.

Neurological effects
- Hypertonic saline effectively reduces intracranial pressure in patients with intracranial hypertension.
- Rebound cerebral oedema in patients with disrupted blood–brain barrier has been reported after prolonged infusion.
- Brain volume as assessed by surgical conditions at craniotomy is reduced.

Systemic effects
- There is a transient (20 min) expansion of intravascular volume following administration. Cardiac output increases, possibly due to a direct inotropic effect. Systemic vascular resistance is not altered. MAP is increased due to increases in blood volume and cardiac output.
- The cardiovascular effects can be prolonged by the administration of hyperoncotic colloids.
- A natriuresis and diuresis occurs as a consequence of increased renal perfusion pressure, increased glomerular filtration rate and increased atrial natriuretic peptide release.
- Hypernatraemia is inevitable with repeated dosing.
- Hyperchloraemic acidosis may occur with large saline loads.
- Hypokalaemia may occur due to increased renal loss of potassium.

Tips and pitfalls
- Some units administer mannitol or hypertonic saline routinely to every craniotomy (elective and emergency) arguing that it is likely to be beneficial without evidence of harm. Many units take the opposing view that there is no need to administer potentially harmful drugs unless there is a clear indication.
- There is no evidence that the routine use of mannitol in elective surgery or traumatic brain injury is beneficial.
- Good direct evidence for 'rescue' use of hypertonic fluids in patients with intracranial hypertension is lacking, but clinical experience suggests some short-term benefit.
- Mannitol is available as a 10% or 20% solution, both of which are hypertonic solutions. Care should be taken to administer the correct one.
- 0.5 g kg^{-1} mannitol is 40 g for an 80 kg subject:
  - this equates to 200 ml of 20% mannitol or 400 ml of 10%.

- The degree of reduction in brain volume is not related to the amount of diuresis induced.
- Extensive tissue necrosis can occur if extravasation of hypertonic fluids occurs.
- Care should be exercised when using hypertonic fluids in elderly patients or those with poor cardiac function as cardiac failure can be precipitated.
- Currently there is no conclusive evidence to suggest whether use of HTS is safe or dangerous in the presence of hyponatraemia.
- The validity of trials suggesting that high-dose mannitol is beneficial have been questioned.

Glucocorticoids

Dexamethasone is used widely in neurosurgical practice to reduce the swelling associated with tumours and abscesses. High-dose methylprednisolone has been advocated previously in the management of acute spinal cord injury. Currently high-dose steroids are not a standard of care for spinal cord injury, but may be considered as one of the therapeutic options.

Indications

Dexamethasone
- Reduction of perilesional swelling in patients with cerebral and spinal tumours or infective intracranial lesions.
- Prophylaxis of postoperative nausea and vomiting.
- The use of steroids including dexamethasone is not recommended for improving outcome or reducing ICP in patients with severe head injury.

Methylprednisolone
- Spinal cord injury: intravenous 30 mg kg^{-1} bolus followed by 5.4 mg kg^{-1} hr^{-1} for 23 hours. **(Currently not recommended).**

Doses and routes of administration
Dexamethasone can be given orally or intravenously. The usual dose for adults is 4 mg four times daily orally, or 8–32 mg given IV at induction. For children the dose range is 200–500 µg kg^{-1} day^{-1}.

There is debate regarding the optimal dose (both oral and intravenous) of dexamethasone. Lower-dose regimens may be as efficacious as high doses with a lower incidence of adverse side effects.

Mechanism of action
Dexamethasone and methylprednisolone are synthetic corticosteroid compounds with predominant glucocorticoid activity. Dexamethasone in particular has minimal mineralocorticoid activity making it ideal for the treatment of cerebral oedema.

The activity of the steroid compound is mediated via specific intracellular receptors in the cytoplasm or nucleus. The steroid-receptor complex binds to deoxyribonucleic acid (DNA) and regulates the formation of specific messenger ribonucleic acid (RNA) molecules which modulate the synthesis of proteins. Steroid receptors are found in virtually all tissues. A reduction in oedema is largely brought about by the anti-inflammatory action of dexamethasone. Production of inflammatory cells and mediators such as histamine, interleukin-1 and interleukin-2 are reduced and anti-inflammatory mediators such as lipocortin increased. Lipocortin inhibits phospolipase A$_2$ decreasing arachidonate synthesis from which virtually all inflammatory mediators are produced.

Neurological effects
- The improvement in symptoms in patients given dexamethasone pre-operatively can be marked.
- Steroids can also alter mood and can induce psychosis.
- Adverse events following stereotactic brain biopsy are reduced when steroids are given.
- The CRASH study was a prospective randomized controlled trial of 10,008 patients. Methylprednisolone treatment given routinely

following traumatic brain injury (2 g followed by 0.4 g hr^{-1} for 48 hours) was associated with **increased mortality** compared with placebo. The relative risk of death at 2 weeks and 6 months following injury was higher in the corticosteroid group (relative risk ~1.15).

Systemic effects
- Metabolic effects:
  - carbohydrate metabolism is altered. Gluconeogenesis and liver glycogen deposition are increased resulting in increased glucose output from the liver. In addition, there is decreased peripheral glucose utilization resulting in the tendency to develop hyperglycaemia
  - protein catabolism is increased leading to muscle wasting
  - fat redistribution occurs resulting in the classic Cushingoid appearance in patients on longer-term steroid therapy.
- Renal effects:
  - the mineralocorticoid activity of steroids causes an increase in sodium re-absorption. Potassium and hydrogen ion excretion by the kidney increases resulting in hypokalaemia.
- Cardiovascular effects:
  - sodium and water retention secondary to any mineralocorticoid activity results in hypertension and peripheral oedema.
- Immune system effects:
  - there is increased susceptibility to infection and patients taking steroids will not mount the normal immune response to infection, potentially delaying diagnosis.
- Adrenal suppression:
  - steroid treatment suppresses intrinsic adrenal activity resulting in an inability to mount the appropriate response to stress. Patients taking more than the equivalent of 10 mg of prednisolone a day will require additional steroid cover peri-operatively.
- Gastric ulceration:
  - minor symptoms of gastrointestinal (GI) irritation are common and the risk of GI bleeding and perforation is increased
  - concurrent proton pump inhibitors are usually prescribed.

Tips and pitfalls
- Dexamethasone is an ideal anti-emetic for patients undergoing neurosurgery. A dose of 4 mg is suitable for adult patients.
- 5 mg prednisolone is equivalent to 750 µg dexamethasone.
- Hyperglycaemia is common after administration of dexamethasone, and tends to occur a few hours after IV administration (i.e. postoperatively). Blood glucose should be checked regularly and may require the use of a temporary insulin sliding scale.
- Acute administration causes redistribution of the neutrophil pool leading to an increase in blood neutrophil count in the absence of infection.
- Prolonged dexamethasone administration may cause sufficient regression of lymphoma to result in non-diagnostic biopsy. In patients with suspected cerebral lymphoma the use of dexamethasone should be discussed with the surgeon prior to administration.
- There is continuing controversy over the use of low-dose steroid 'replacement' therapy in critically ill patients.

Vasoactive drugs

Maintenance of an adequate cerebral perfusion pressure (CPP) is dependant on several factors as described in Chapter 1. A stable mean arterial pressure assists maintenance of an appropriate CPP. Vasoactive substances may be required in both neuro-intensive care and in the operating theatre. Their use should follow the institution of other interventions such as altering the position of the patient, correction of hypovolaemia, optimizing ventilator settings and adjusting the dose of other agents: sedation; anaesthesia; analgesia; neuromuscular blockade; and anticonvulsants.

Drugs used to treat hypertension

Some aspects of surgery may cause transient but marked hypertension, such as traction on the trigeminal nerve or pressure on the spinal cord. These episodes are usually indications of potential neural damage, which should be communicated to the surgeon immediately. Other parts of the operation are predictably stimulating, such as Mayfield pin placement. Sufficient depth of anaesthesia and analgesia may blunt these responses. Following craniotomy raised blood pressure is seen in around 50% of patients and there is an association between systolic blood pressure >160 mmHg and intracranial bleeding. Patients undergoing arteriovenous malformation (AVM) resection are particularly prone to cerebral hyperaemia. Patients with subarachnoid haemorrhage have a high incidence of myocardial ischaemia. Numerous drugs have been used for treatment and prevention of hypertension and there is little evidence to suggest which is better in terms of patient outcome.

β antagonists

There are a number of drugs in this category and they have varying degrees of receptor selectivity. Some have intrinsic sympathomimetic activity, while others have membrane stabilizing activity. The agents used most commonly are labetalol and esmolol.

Mechanism of action
- Esmolol is relatively selective for β_1-receptors and has almost no intrinsic sympathomimetic activity.
- Labetolol acts by selective antagonism of α_1, β_1 and β_2 receptors. It also has some intrinsic sympathomimetic activity at β_2.

Dose and duration

Esmolol
- Usually administered as an infusion 50–150 µg kg^{-1} min^{-1} titrated to response; 300 µg kg^{-1} min^{-1} has been used to attenuate post-craniotomy hyperaemia.
  - peak effect seen within about 6–10 min of administration
  - lasts around 20 min after stopping infusion.

Labetolol
- 5–20 mg IV bolus injected over 2 min with subsequent increments to a maximum adult dose of 200 mg
  - onset in 5–30 min
  - lasts around 2–4 h
  - infusion at a rate of 20–160 mg h^{-1}.

Neurological effects
- No direct effects on cerebral blood flow or cerebral autoregulation.
- Esmolol blunts the cerebral hyperaemia sometimes seen on emergence after craniotomy, which may be distinct from its antihypertensive effect.

Systemic effects
- Reduction in heart rate and cardiac output leading to reduction in systolic blood pressure (SBP), diastolic blood pressure (DBP) and MAP
  - MAP reduced by around 0.1 mmHg mg^{-1} labetolol.
- Labetolol and esmolol do not affect airway smooth muscle tone.

Calcium channel antagonists

The dihydropyridine group of drugs include nifedipine, nicardipine, and amlodipine. Nimodipine is used for prevention of vasospasm in patients following subarachnoid haemorrhage (SAH) rather than for its antihypertensive properties.

Mechanism of action
- Blockade of vascular smooth muscle calcium channels.
- Little effect on cardiac output, due to baroreceptor-mediated tachycardia.
- No effect on cardiac conduction with dihydropyridines.

Dose and duration

Nifedipine
- 10–20 mg orally or sublingual (remove contents of capsule and place under tongue; use with care)
  - limited buccal absorption, effect is due to gastric absorption
  - peak effect seen within about 15–30 min of administration
  - lasts around 6 h.

Neurological effects
- Small increase in cerebral blood flow due to vasodilation.

Systemic effects
- Reduction in vascular tone leading to reduction in SBP, DBP and MAP
- Cardiac output not usually affected.
- May cause reflex tachycardia.
- There are concerns that sublingual nifedipine is poorly absorbed and is associated with serious adverse events (including cerebral ischaemia and myocardial infarction) when used for acute hypertension. Careful consideration of the risk:benefit ratio of this agent and route should precede its use.

Nitrates
- Glyceryl trinitrate (GTN) is the nitrate most commonly used, though sodium nitroprusside has been used in the past. Nitrates are generally avoided due to risks of cerebral vasodilation and increased ICP.

Mechanism of action
- Activation of guanyl cyclase (via nitric oxide) leading to increased cyclic GMP and smooth muscle relaxation.

Dose and duration

GTN
- 300 µg sublingual
- Infusion 10–400 µg min^{-1}
  - peak effect seen 3 mins after sublingual administration
  - onset 90–120 s after iv administration
  - lasts around 15–30 min.

Neurological effects
- Vasodilation
- Maintenance of cerebral perfusion pressure
- Increase in ICP, particularly where compensatory mechanisms are exhausted.

Systemic effects
- Reduction in venous tone leading to reduction in preload
- Reduction in arterial tone leading to reductions in SBP and MAP
- Cardiac output not usually affected
- May cause reflex tachycardia.

Hydralazine
- Thought to act directly on vascular smooth muscle by interfering with calcium entry into the cell or the release of intracellular calcium.
- As with other vasodilators may have detrimental effects on ICP.

Mechanism of action
- Inhibition of calcium entry/release in vascular smooth muscle.

Dose and duration
- Slow intravenous bolus 20–40 mg
  - onset around 15–20 min
  - lasts around 2–6 h.

Neurological effects
- Cerebral vasodilator
- Inhibits cerebral autoregulation.

Systemic effects
- Reduction in arterial tone leading to reductions in SBP and MAP
- Cardiac output may increase as a consequence of reduced afterload
- May cause reflex tachycardia
- Additive hypotensive effect with volatile anaesthetic agents.

α_2 agonists
Clonidine has been used but dexmedetomidine may a better alternative, though it is not yet licensed in the UK.

Mechanism of action
- Peripheral stimulation of α_{2B} receptors leading to an early increase in MAP.
- Central inhibition of sympathetic activity (α_2 and imadazoline receptors).

Dose and duration

Clonidine
- 5 µg kg^{-1} orally the night before surgery and repeated 90 min before surgery
- 150–300 µg by slow iv injection. Effects may last for up to 8 h.

Dexmedetomidine
- Bolus 10 µg iv
- Loading dose of 1 µg kg^{-1} followed by infusion 0.1–0.5 µg kg^{-1} hr^{-1}. Effects persists beyond duration of infusion.

Neurological effects
- Sedation
- Analgesia
- No effect on cerebral autoregulation
- May cause cerebral vasoconstriction
- Reduction in cerebral blood flow and CMRO$_2$.

Systemic effects
- Reduction in MAP (15%)
- Reduction in heart rate (15%)
- Cardiac output maintained
- Little effect on respiratory drive.

ACE inhibitors

Enalaprilat has been used with good effect to prevent hypertension following craniotomy.

Mechanism of action
- Inhibition of conversion of angiotensin-1 to angiotensin-2, blocking the renin–angiotensin system.

Dose and duration

Enalaprilat
- 1.25 mg or 15 µg kg^{-1} bolus
- Onset within 15 min
- Lasts >4 h.

Neurological effects
- Cerebral blood flow generally maintained despite fall in MAP
- Reduction in cerebral blood flow and CMRO$_2$.

Systemic effects
- Reduction in MAP
- Increase in cardiac output.

Tips and pitfalls
- As with all anaesthetic pharmacology, the safest drug is often the one with which the user is most familiar.
- Antihypertensives do not treat pain, nausea, or anxiety.
- Labetolol is commonly used and in clinical practice does not tend to cause catastrophic hypotension.

- Hypertension following craniotomy is common, particularly in the elderly, and the anaesthetist should endeavour to prevent it occurring.
- Peri-extubation hypertension may be obtunded by the use of opioids, such as continuing a remifentanil infusion during this period.
- Nitrates and hydralazine should be avoided in patients with an increased ICP.

Drugs used to treat hypotension

Neuroanaesthetists aspire to stable haemodynamics throughout the intra- and postoperative period in order to reduce the risk of neurological or systemic injury. Neurosurgical operations can quickly proceed from very stimulating (e.g. pin insertion) to unstimulating, and hypotension may be troublesome. Sudden large blood loss may complicate matters further, as may the effects of positioning or the release of high ICP. The ideal vasoactive agent would be easily titrated to maintain cardiac output, systemic blood pressure, and regional perfusion and have no detrimental effects on the cerebral circulation. Such agents do not exist but the sympathomimetic agents, when used appropriately, are generally adequate.

Sympathomimetics

These drugs vary in their mode of action (direct or indirect) and their receptor selectivity. Most are licensed for administration through peripheral cannulae, though epinephrine, norepinephrine, and dopamine should ideally be administered into central veins.

Mechanism of action
- Phenylephrine is an almost pure α agonist.
- Metaraminol and norepinephrine are predominantly α with some β activity.
- Ephedrine is predominantly β with some α effects.

Dose and duration

Phenylephrine
- Bolus doses of 50–100 µg
- Can be administered as an infusion of 0.5–10 mg hr^{-1}
- Peak effect seen within 1–2 min
- Lasts around 5–10 min.

Metaraminol
- Bolus doses of 0.5–1 mg
- Peak effect seen within 1–2 min
- Lasts around 5–10 min.

Ephedrine
- Bolus doses of 3–15 mg. Can be given by infusion 60 mg in a 500–1000 ml bag of saline, titrated to effect
- Onset after 1–2 min
- Duration 5–10 min.

Norepinephrine
- Intravenous infusion into central vein, 0.05–0.5 µg kg^{-1} min^{-1}
- Onset within one circulation time
- Cardiovascular effects gone within 5–10 min of stopping infusion.

VASOACTIVE DRUGS

Neurological effects
- Small decrease in cerebral blood flow in healthy brains with systemic administration of catecholamines.
- No effects on dynamic autoregulation in healthy volunteers.
- Cerebral blood flow increases with increase in MAP if autoregulation is lost (e.g. MAP below lower limit of autoregulation, high dose volatile anaesthetics, trauma).
- In the traumatized brain increases in CPP may not always be associated with increases in oxygen delivery.
- Little evidence for increased oedema formation when used to keep CPP ~ 70 mmHg.

Systemic effects
- α stimulation results in increased SVR and MAP.
- Without β stimulation this may lead to reflex bradycardia.
- β stimulation results in inotropy and increase in HR.
- High dose of vasoconstrictor may lead to regional systemic hypoperfusion due to excessive vasoconstriction.

Vasopressin analogues (see also p. 64)

Vasopressin and terlipressin have been used in patients with catecholamine resistant shock and as part of cardiopulmonary resuscitation. Their use in patients with 'at risk' brains remains controversial due to uncertainty over the overall effects on cerebral blood flow and metabolism.

Mechanism of action
- Agonist at ADH receptors causing systemic vasoconstriction.
- Terlipressin is a prodrug, converted to lysine vasopressin.

Dose and duration

Vasopressin
- Intravenous infusion 0.01-0.04 U min^{-1}
  - plasma half-life is 24 min.

Terlipressin
- Bolus dose of 1–2 mg IV
  - effective half-life is 6 h.

Neurological effects
- Preferentially vasodilates large intracranial arteries (circle of Willis) whilst constricting smaller vessels.

Systemic effects
- Increase in SVR leading to increased MAP
- Pulmonary vasodilator
- Augments sensitivity of vasculature to catecholamines
- May lead to coronary vasoconstriction, though less than catecholamines
- Antidiuresis
- Releases endothelial von Willebrand factor.

Tips and pitfalls
- As with all anaesthetic pharmacology, the safest drug is often the one with which the user is most familiar.
- In theatre phenylephrine, metaraminol, and ephedrine are the most commonly used drugs.
- Ephedrine is the most commonly used first line drug, particularly in the period following induction of anaesthesia.
- Vasopressin is still considered an experimental drug for the treatment of sepsis induced vasodilatation.
- Patient positioning, bleeding, and excessive sedation or anaesthesia should be corrected rather than relying on vasoactive drugs, though they may be needed in the short term to maintain perfusion pressure.

Opioids

Opioids are an essential part of neuroanaesthetic and neurocritical care practice. They are used to obtund cardiovascular and cerebral responses to stimulation, to reduce the requirements for other anaesthetic or sedative agents, to suppress respiration deliberately (in theatre or ICU) and to provide analgesia.

Although short-acting agents are commonly used, longer-acting agents were used successfully for many years and there is little evidence of superiority of one agent over another.

Remifentanil is the most popular agent for intra-operative use and has in general replaced nitrous oxide. Morphine is used for postoperative analgesia and sedation in critical care.

Cerebral effects

Apart from their analgesic effects, the actions of opioids on the central nervous system are minor and there are few direct effects.

Cerebral metabolism

All opioids depress cerebral metabolic rate (and cerebral blood flow) at high doses. However, at clinical doses there is no effect on carbon dioxide reactivity or cerebral autoregulation.

ICP

If an opioid results in respiratory depression and hypercapnia, ICP will increase. Any direct effects on ICP are insignificant.

Neuroprotection

There is some evidence that opioids have some neuroprotective effects although the clinical significance is unclear.

EEG

All opioids change the EEG. Usually, these effects will be combined with those from the other anaesthetic agents being used. Very high-dose opioids may cause epileptiform activity. This is of no concern at 'normal' doses. This effect may be used, however, to induce seizure activity as part of cortical mapping for seizure surgery.

Available opioids

Fentanyl

- Experience with fentanyl is the longest of any of the short-acting opioids.
- Fentanyl is unsuitable for use by infusion and boluses are used at induction and prior to stimulating parts of the operative procedure such as skin incision, dural incision, and dural repair.
- Some analgesic action may be present at emergence, but postoperative analgesia is short-lived.

Alfentanil

- Because of its pharmacokinetics, alfentanil can be infused, although prolonged infusions are associated with longer recovery.

- Its very short onset time (1–2 min) make it ideal for use before very stimulating procedures such as laryngoscopy or Mayfield frame pin insertion.

Remifentanil

Remifentanil is the most commonly used short-acting opioid for intra-operative use.

- Its very short context-sensitive half-life makes it ideal to titrate by intravenous infusion.
- Its potency allows its use as a replacement for nitrous oxide and it may be used in combination either with intravenous anaesthesia (propofol) or with inhalational anaesthesia.
- The offset of remifentanil is rapid so it must be accompanied by administration of a long-acting opioid prior to emergence and tracheal extubation
  - the only exception may be a patient with a depressed conscious level pre-operatively who needs to be awoken to determine their neurological status. However, many of these patients may go on to be sedated and ventilated in ICU.
- Boluses of remifentanil ($\geq 0.5 \, \mu g \, kg^{-1}$) should be administered with care; they may result in a fall in blood pressure (and heart rate) that may compromise CPP.
- Target-controlled infusion algorithms are now available for suitably-equipped syringe driver pumps. Either a plasma or effect site target is chosen and a bolus followed by an infusion is given according to a weight, height, and gender-based formula.
- Prolonged intraoperative administration of remifentanil may result in acute opioid tolerance and patients may require increased doses of postoperative analgesia to compensate for this.
- Some anaesthetists use the respiratory depressant effects of remifentanil to reduce or avoid the use of intra-operative muscle relaxation.
- Some anaesthetists continue a low dose infusion of remifentanil until after tracheal extubation in order to reduce the pressor response at that time.

Codeine

Codeine given intramuscularly was, until recently, the mainstay of postoperative analgesia following craniotomy, largely because of a belief that it did not affect consciousness or impair neurological assessment. Most units have now switched to morphine-based regimes because of the well-recognized disadvantages of codeine.

- It can not be given intravenously so rapid titration of analgesia is difficult.
- A significant proportion of patients can not metabolize codeine and so obtain little analgesia.
- The dose of codeine administered is usually insufficient to provide adequate analgesia.
- There is no evidence, at equi-analgesic levels, that codeine behaves any differently to other opioids with regards to respiratory depression of neurological assessment.

Morphine
- Morphine remains the most commonly-used opioid analgesia for postoperative use though pethidine has been successfully used.
- If remifentanil has been used, a dose of morphine—slightly less than that used in non-neurosurgical anaesthetic practice (e.g. 0.05–0.1 mg kg^{-1}) is given approximately 30 min prior to emergence
  - an anti-emetic should also be administered.
- Postoperatively, morphine can be given by bolus subcutaneous injection, intravenous infusion, patient-controlled analgesia (PCA) or orally.
- For the majority of patients concerns about excess sedation or respiratory depression are unwarranted and good practice mandates adequate pain relief
  - care should be taken with patients who have depressed conscious levels or significant co-morbidities.
- Morphine infusions are used on ICU to provide sedation, and cough and respiratory depression in ventilated patients.

Tips and pitfalls
- Remifentanil is a useful drug when used properly. When used badly significant swings in blood pressure and heart rate will occur.
- If remifentanil is a significant component of the anaesthetic technique then the same risks of awareness apply as with propofol infusion. Continuous intravenous infusion into the patient must be assured.
- There is no good evidence that any one intra-operative opioid results in a better patient outcome than any other.
- Codeine has largely been abandoned in adult neuroanaesthesia practice though it is still used sometimes in children.

Muscle relaxants

Most patients having a neurosurgical procedure will receive a muscle relaxant at some point either to facilitate intubation, ensure safe transfer and surgery or help control intracranial pressure. There is little to choose between the agents on offer, though specific circumstances may dictate the use of particular agents.

Indications
- To facilitate emergency tracheal intubation in the obtunded patient following trauma, intracranial bleeding, surgery, fitting etc.
- To facilitate safe inter- and intrahospital transfer of neurosurgical patients.
- To facilitate tracheal intubation for elective neurosurgery and interventional procedures requiring a secured airway.
- To facilitate surgical access (e.g. to the abdomen for peritoneal shunt procedures).
- To prevent movement and coughing during neurosurgical procedures.
- As part of a multimodal strategy to reduce intracranial pressure in acute brain injury.

Side effects
Neurological effects
- No effect of vecuronium, rocuronium or atracurium on ICP or CPP.
- Laudanosine (atracurium metabolite) is epileptogenic but there is no clinical evidence that this is a concern; levels in clinical use are very low.

Systemic effects
- Small increase in heart rate after bolus administration of rocuronium.
- Small decrease in MAP after bolus administration of atracurium due to histamine release.
- Atracurium metabolism, via Hofmann elimination, is independent of renal function, so atracurium may be the preferred drug in patients at risk of renal dysfunction.

Monitoring required
- Neuromuscular monitoring is suggested by Association of Anaesthesists of Great Britain and Ireland (AAGBI) guidelines.
- Around 50% of UK neuroanaesthetists aim for deep paralysis throughout surgery (train of four, (TOF) 0), others opt for less profound
(TOF 2), or no relaxation, particularly when remifentanil is used.

Reversal
- No evidence that either neostigmine or sugammadex (used to 'reverse' rocuronium or vecuronium only) affect ICP or CPP.
- Glycopyrrolate does not dilate pupils but atropine does, which may hinder neurological assessment.
- Sugammadex is more effective at reversing deep block than neostigmine.

Suxamethonium has a limited role in neuroanaesthetic practice, mainly because of concerns about its effect on ICP, as well as its other well documented side effects. It is still used where the risks associated with the use of slower onset and offset muscle relaxants outweigh the effects of suxamethonium on ICP.

Indications
- To facilitate emergency tracheal intubation in the obtunded patient following trauma, intracranial bleeding, surgery, fitting etc.
- To facilitate elective tracheal intubation in the neurosurgical patient with a high risk of gastric aspiration.

Side effects
Neurological effects
- Possibly a small increase in ICP (4–6 mmHg) if the patient is not already paralysed, though some studies have demonstrated no change in ICP.
- Increase in ICP may be related to increased afferent activity from muscle spindles.

Systemic effects
- Repeated doses may lead to significant bradycardia.
- Risk of hyperkalaemia especially with conditions causing increase in extra-junctional acetylcholine receptors:
  - Spinal cord injury—suxamethonium is generally viewed as safe within 72 h of injury or after 9 months from injury.
  - Guillain–Barré—isolated case reports.
  - Critical hyperkalaemia has not been observed soon after SAH
  - Normal neurological examination does not exclude risk of hyperkalaemia.
  - Patients with status epilepticus may be hyperkalaemic so suxamethonium is probably best avoided.

Monitoring required
- In practice most anaesthetists do not monitor onset or offset of suxamethonium unless concerned about delayed recovery.

Tips and pitfalls
- Clinical experience suggests that rocuronium has a rather abrupt offset so regular monitoring or infusion may avoid problems.
- Some basal skull surgery requires the use of VIIth nerve stimulation and pharmacological paralysis should be avoided.
- Bispectral index (BIS) monitoring may be affected by changes in degree of muscle relaxation.
- Following (cranial) neurosurgery patients are at high risk of postoperative pulmonary complications, which may be exacerbated by inadequate reversal.
- Sugammadex may be particularly useful in situations where prompt and complete reversal is needed. It only works after rocuronium or vecuronium.

CHAPTER 2 Pharmacology

- Hypoxia is a more serious hazard than a small rise in ICP so if suxamethonium is the best drug to aid intubation it should be used.
- Some neuroanaesthetists advocate using high dose rocuronium (0.9–1.0 mg kg^{-1}) instead of suxamethonium, but this is a matter of clinical judgement.

Non-steroidal anti-inflammatory drugs and paracetamol

This group of drugs is used mainly for their analgesic properties. Some units also use non-steroidal anti-inflammatory drugs (NSAIDs) for their inhibitory effect on new bone formation. Different units have different views on their peri-operative use due to their effects on platelet function.

NSAIDs
Mechanism of action
- Inhibition of cyclo-oxygenase (COX) enzyme system leading to prevention of production of prostaglandins and thromboxanes from membrane phospholipids.
- COX exists as two isoenzymes. COX-1 is constitutive and responsible for the production of prostaglandins that control renal blood flow, haemostatic function and form the protective gastric mucosal barrier. COX-2 is the inducible form and is produced in response to tissue damage and facilitates the inflammatory response.

Dose and duration

Diclofenac
- Oral or iv 150 mg day^{-1} in divided doses
  - Peak effect seen within about 10 min of iv administration
  - Onset time around 1 h after oral administration
  - Lasts ~8 h.

Ibuprofen
- Oral 20 mg kg^{-1} day^{-1} or 1.2–2.4 g day^{-1} in divided doses
  - Onset time around 1 h after oral administration
  - Lasts ~ 6 h.

Indomethacin
- Oral 50–200 mg day^{-1} in divided doses, 0.2 mg kg^{-1} iv
  - Onset time of around 1 h after oral administration
  - Lasts around 12 h.

Neurological effects
- Indomethacin reduces cerebral blood flow by up to 40% and reduces carbon dioxide reactivity.
- Indomethacin reduces ICP in patients with tumours and traumatic brain injury; this effect is attenuated by concomitant use of propofol.
- Indomethacin has no effect on CMRO$_2$.
- Other NSAIDS have no effect on CBF or CMRO$_2$.

Systemic effects
- Anti-inflammatory
- Analgesia
- Antipyretic
- Inhibition of platelet function which may lead to increased bleeding time
- Reduction in renal blood flow, especially in the hypovolaemic patient
- Inhibition of new bone formation
- Gastric/duodenal irritation, ulceration, perforation and bleeding.

Paracetamol

Paracetamol is an excellent analgesic and antipyretic, which is well tolerated by most patients and under-used by many clinicians.

Mechanism of action
- Poorly understood, but it is thought to be a potent inhibitor of prostaglandin synthesis within the CNS, accounting for its antipyretic effect.
- Peripherally it acts by blocking impulse generation within the bradykinin-sensitive chemoreceptors responsible for the generation of nociceptive impulses.

Dose and duration
- Oral or iv 4 g day^{-1} (adult) or 90 mg kg^{-1} (children) in divided doses
  - Peak effect seen within about 15 min of iv administration
  - Peak effect seen at around 60–90 min after oral administration
  - Longer duration of analgesia with oral than iv.

Neurological effects
- None

Systemic effects
- Analgesic
- Antipyretic

Tips and pitfalls
- NSAIDs provide good analgesia for bony surgery and are safe after straightforward discectomy or laminectomy.
- Risk of bleeding is such that most units do not prescribe NSAIDs until 2 days after craniotomy.
- Bleeding risks may be less with COX-2-specific NSAIDs, but there are concerns about increased cardiovascular events associated with their use.
- The risk of GI disturbance or renal dysfunction is higher in the elderly.
- Some units routinely prescribe NSAIDs after cervical arthroplasty in an attempt to reduce the risk of bony fusion.
- The cerebrovascular effects of indomethacin are unique to indomethacin and not a NSAID effect. Some units use this effect to reduce CBF/CBV.
- Paracetamol can be given safely orally pre-operatively.
- Rapid iv infusion of paracetamol (<5 min) is associated with nausea and hypotension in awake patients.

Anti-emetics and PONV

Postoperative nausea and vomiting (PONV) are common with all types of surgery. Factors in the neurosurgical population influencing PONV include hypotension, raised ICP, CSF leak at surgery, use of lumbar CSF drains, drugs, vestibular disease, surgery near the cerebellopontine angle and infratentorial surgery, fear, pain, and migraine. It is vital in all patients to look for a cause of the nausea and vomiting while treating it. Avoidance is important in the neurosurgical population in particular, as excessive elevation of ICP may occur secondary to vomiting. Overall rates of PONV after craniotomy have been quoted to be as high as 50%, whereas they are lower for trans-sphenoidal hypophysectomy (7.5%) and higher for microvascular decompression procedures (> 60%).

Mechanism of action

Inhibition of various pathways involved in nausea and vomiting:
- D_2 receptors in the chemoreceptor trigger zone (CTZ) and nucleus tractus solitarius (NTS): prochlorperazine, droperidol.
- 5 HT_3 receptors in the stomach, small intestine, CTZ : ondansetron, granisetron.
- Histamine receptors in the NTS and vestibular pathway: cyclizine.
- Muscarinic receptors in the NTS, vestibular pathway and CTZ: cyclizine.

Dose and duration

Cyclizine
- 50 mg iv
- Onset time ~ 30–60 min
- Lasts ~8 h.

Ondansetron
- 4 mg iv
- Onset time ~30–60 min
- Lasts ~8–12 h.

Droperidol
- 1.25–2.5 mg iv
- Onset time unclear, but recommended to be given at end of surgery
- Lasts ~8 h.

Dexamethasone
- 4–8 mg iv
- Onset time unclear, but recommended to be given at induction
- Single dose used.

Neurological effects

- Cyclizine may cause sedation or confusion, particularly in the elderly.
- Ondansetron may cause headache.
- Droperidol at the low doses used for PONV is not associated with sedation or extra-pyramidal symptoms.
- Dexamethasone may exacerabate pre-existing hyperglycaemia, though this effect is not usually seen intra-operatively.

Systemic effects
- Cyclizine causes some vasodilation and tachycardia particularly if given as a fast bolus.
- Ondansetron has been associated with bradycardia.
- Droperidol at high doses has been associated with prolonged QTc. This is not a concern with licensed doses for PONV.

Tips and pitfalls
- There is conflicting evidence regarding the benefit of single agent prophylaxis in neurosurgery.
- The efficacy of antiemetic therapy for either prevention or treatment of PONV may be enhanced by combination therapy.
- Sedation associated with cyclizine and droperidol is not normally sufficient to interfere with neurological assessment.
- TIVA is associated with lower rates of PONV than volatile-based anaesthesia.

Vasopressin: argine vasopressin (AVP), antidiuretic hormone (ADH)

Vasopressin and its analogues are used for three reasons in neuroanaesthetic practice:
- replacement in cases of temporary or permanent posterior pituitary dysfunction (pituitary diabetes insipidus)
- an experimental vasoconstrictive agent, particularly in patients with catecholamine resistant sepsis
- to increase circulating von Willebrand Factor and factor VIII levels in von Willebrand's disease and haemophilia.

Mechanism of action

Vasopressin is a neuropeptide synthesized *in vivo* in the cell bodies of the supraoptic and paraventricular nuclei. It is transported via their axons to the posterior pituitary gland from where it is secreted. Vasopressin acts via vasopressin receptors, which are G-protein linked. Its main action is as an antidiuretic, acting at the renal collecting duct to increase water permeability. At high doses, vasopressin is a potent vasoconstrictor due to a direct effect on vascular smooth muscle. It increases plasma levels of factor VIII and von Willebrand factor.

Desmopressin is a synthetic analogue of ADH. It has minimal vasoconstrictor activity, but an antidiuretic potency twelve times that of ADH.

Doses and duration

Vasopressin
- Intravenous infusion 0.01–0.04 U min^{-1}
  - plasma half-life is 24 min.

Desmopressin (DDAVP)
- For the treatment of pituitary diabetes insipidus, desmopressin should be used in a dose of 1–4 µg daily by subcutaneous, intramuscular or intravenous route
  - plasma half-life 2–4 h.

Terlipressin
- Bolus dose of 1–2 mg iv
  - effective half-life is 6 h.

Neurological effects
- Preferentially vasodilates large intracranial arteries (circle of Willis) whilst constricting smaller vessels.

Systemic effects
- Increase in systemic vascular disease (SVR) leading to increased MAP.
- Augments sensitivity of vasculature to catecholamines.
- May lead to coronary vasoconstriction, though less than catecholamines.
- Antidiuresis.
- Releases endothelial von Willebrand factor.

Tips and pitfalls
- Start with a low dose first and titrate to effect, as the antidiuretic activity can be dramatic.
- Monitor urine output and electrolytes closely.
- Diabetes insipidus after trauma and surgery is often short-lived. The need for desmopressin should be reviewed regularly.

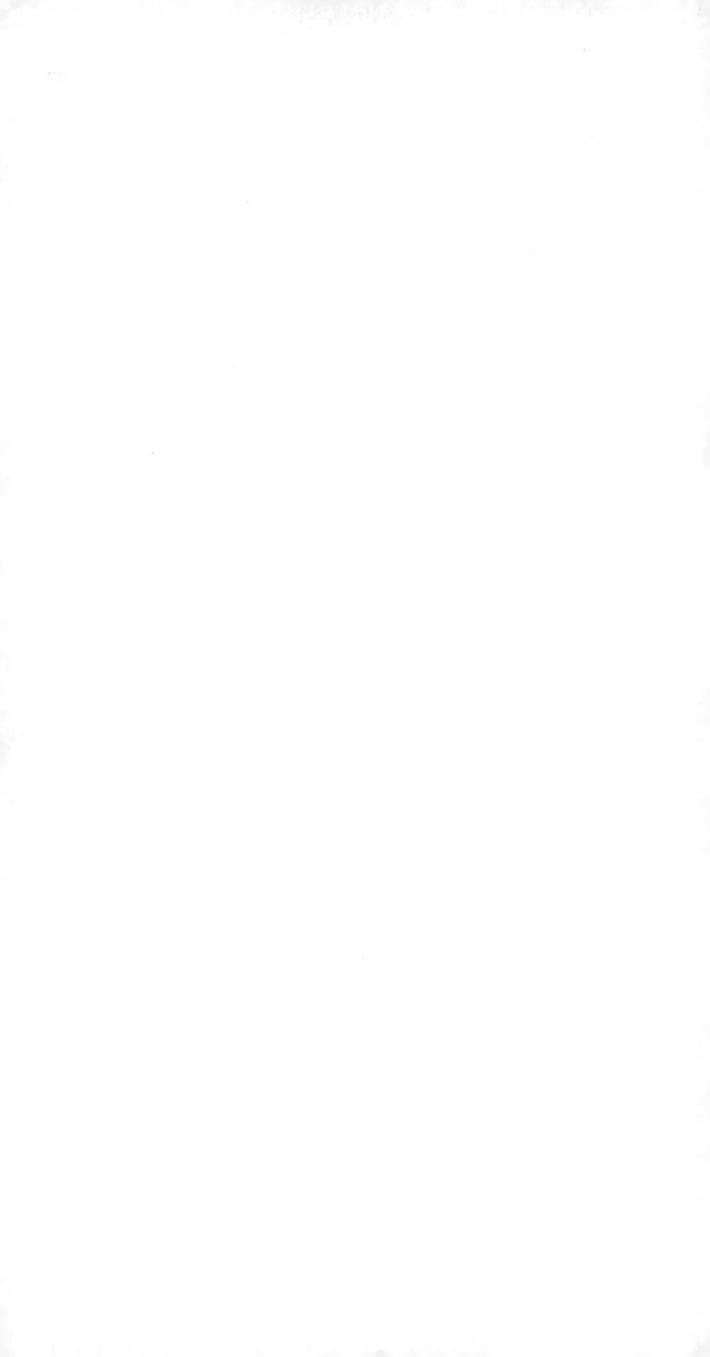

Chapter 3

Monitoring and imaging

Intracranial pressure *68*
Electrophysiological monitoring *72*
Transcranial Doppler ultrasonography *82*
Multimodal monitoring *86*
Regional cerebral blood flow *92*
Glasgow Coma Scale *98*

Intracranial pressure

Intracranial pressure (ICP) and mean arterial pressure (MAP) can be used to derive cerebral perfusion pressure CPP = MAP–ICP.

Although the measurement of ICP and its derivative CPP are widely used in patients with acute brain injury, there is no Level I evidence to support their use. However, systemic hypotension, intracranial hypertension and a CPP <50 mmHg are all individually associated with a poor outcome following traumatic brain injury (TBI).

Devices for ICP measurement

There are several types of device available for measurement of ICP (Table 3.1). The two most accurate and most commonly used are the ventricular catheter connected to an external strain gauge and the solid state parenchymal microcatheter with a strain gauge tip (ICP 'bolt'). The former is cheaper, more reliable and accurate, and remains the reference standard. ICP bolts are commonly inserted on ICU under local anaesthesia, thus avoiding the risks of a transfer to theatre. These two devices are compared in Table 3.2.

Indications for ICP monitoring

There are two main indications for ICP monitoring: acute brain injury and the investigation of various types of hydrocephalus.

Acute brain injury

TBI is the commonest indication for acute ICP monitoring. Other less common indications include:
- elective postoperative monitoring following craniotomy
- subarachnoid haemorrhage or intracranial haematoma
- encephalopathies, e.g. hepatic, Reye's syndrome.

In general terms TBI in a ventilated patient with an abnormal computed tomography (CT) scan requires an ICP monitor. The Brain Trauma Foundation (BTF) recommends ICP monitoring for:
- severe TBI (GCS 3–8/15) with an abnormal CT scan
- severe TBI with an apparently normal CT scan and at least two of the following:
  - age >40 yr
  - unilateral or bilateral motor posturing
  - SBP <90 mmHg.

ICP monitoring in acute brain injury is used for various reasons:
- in sedated patients where clinical assessment (e.g. GCS) is impaired
- to calculate CPP
- to guide therapies (and prevent their overuse) for manipulation of CPP
- early detection of expanding mass lesions
- to prompt early neurosurgical intervention
- determining prognosis.

Normal pressure hydrocephalus (NPH)

There is no consensus on the best method to diagnose or exclude NPH in patients with suggestive symptoms. Some centres advocate continuous ICP monitoring in all, or selected, possible cases. A waves and frequent B-waves are associated with good outcome from shunting, as are high amplitude CSF waves. Other centres feel that similar information can be obtained from less invasive approaches.

Interpretation

The ICP should not be viewed as an isolated number, though treatment thresholds are described, e.g. the BTF recommends treating ICP > 20–25 mmHg. ICP should be interpreted in relation to other physiological factors (notably blood pressure, $PaCO_2$, pain and arousal). The cyclical changes in ICP should also be observed as these may provide more information than a single mean value (see p.22).

Tips and pitfalls

- The use of ICP monitoring in non-neurosurgical centres is controversial. It can prevent unnecessary transfer of patients, but subsequent transfer of patients with high ICP may be too late for treatment.
- Malfunction, obstruction or malposition are complications that can result in inaccurate measurements. These should be suspected when the trace is unusual in appearance or when the ICP is not in keeping with the clinical picture.
  - The measured ICP should rise when the jugular vein is temporarily compressed.
  - Tube ties and hard cervical collars are common iatrogenic causes of an elevated ICP.
- When the ICP measurement does not correlate with the clinical picture, a repeat CT scan is useful.
- The ICP monitor is usually positioned in the non-dominant frontal lobe, regardless of the site of injury.
- The ICP measurement from a ventricular catheter should be taken at the level of the external auditory meatus.
- Clinically significant infection (colonization rate 8–14%) and haemorrhage (0.5% requiring surgery) are rare complications and should not deter the use of ICP monitoring.
- Infection rates plateau after 4 days of monitoring and are not reduced by routine monitor change. Prophylactic antibiotics are not recommended.
- Coagulopathy is a relative contraindication to ICP monitoring.

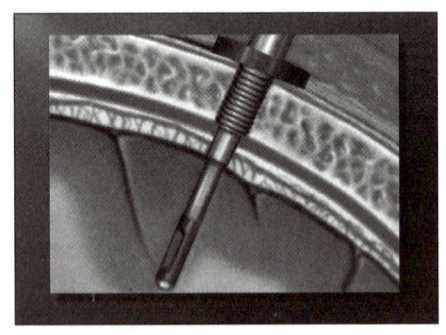

Fig. 3.1 An ICP bolt. (Image supplied courtesy of Codman, Johnson & Johnson Medical Ltd.)

Table 3.1 Devices for ICP measurement

Fluid coupled	
Type	Site
External strain gauge	Ventricular, subarachnoid, subdural, epidural
Micro strain gauge in catheter tip	Ventricular
Fibre-optic	Ventricular

Solid state	
Type	Site
Micro strain gauge in catheter tip	Parenchymal, subdural
Fibre-optic	Parenchymal, subdural

Other	
Type	Site
Pneumatic	Ventricular, parenchymal, epidural

Table 3.2 Comparison of two common ICP measurement devices

Fluid coupled ventricular	Solid-state parenchymal
Technically more difficult to place, especially when ventricles are compressed	Technically easier to place
Does not require calibration prior to insertion	Must calibrate prior to insertion
Can recalibrate *in situ*	Cannot re-calibrate *in situ*, thus affected by baseline drift (may change by 1 mmHg /day)
Must recalibrate with change in patient position	Not affected by patient position
Accurate measure of global pressure	Regional pressure differences reduce accuracy; less accurate when placed in areas of damaged brain
Loss of integrity of fluid column (e.g. due to blockage, air, kinking) results in damped trace	Trace not prone to damping
Allows withdrawal of CSF for therapeutic or diagnostic purposes	
Risk of infection from repeated access	
Cheaper	

CHAPTER 3 **Monitoring and imaging**

Electrophysiological monitoring

The electrical activity of the nervous system can be assessed in awake patients using clinical methods such as sensory testing, visual fields, and motor power. During anaesthesia or when patients are sedated, these approaches are impractical or insufficiently sensitive. In these cases, direct recording of electrical activity can be used, analogous to the use of electrocardiography as a diagnostic tool in cardiology.

In neuroanaesthetic practice, two main modalities are used: electroencephalography (EEG) and evoked potentials (EP). In the ICU additional modalities such as the cerebral function analysing monitor (CFAM), nerve conduction studies (NCS) and electromyography (EMG) are used. In the ICU setting neurophysiological monitoring may be used for either prognosis (e.g. to determine if the brain is functioning, the integrity of the spinal cord, the presence of seizures or in assessing depth of drug-induced coma) or diagnosis (e.g. brain death, 'locked-in' syndrome, Guillain–Barré syndrome or critical illness polyneuropathy).

Electroencephalography (EEG)

EEG

EEG is the non-invasive, continuous recording of the weak electrical activity generated by the brain, detected by surface electrodes placed on the scalp. Electrical activity originates from excitatory and inhibitory post-synaptic potentials of the pyramidal cells found in layers II, III, and V of the cerebral cortex.

EEG characteristics

The EEG is described with relation to frequency, amplitude (normally 20–200 µV), paroxysmal activity and position of the electrodes.
- Delta (δ): 0–4 Hz
  - Very low frequency. Occurs during stage 4 slow-wave sleep. Also occurs with depressed functions (coma, deep anaesthesia, hypoxia, ischaemia, infarction).
- Theta (θ): 4–8 Hz
  - Low frequency. Seen under general anaesthesia.
- Alpha (α): 9–12 Hz
  - Medium frequency, higher amplitude.
- Beta (β): 13–30 Hz
  - High frequency, low amplitude.

The healthy adult EEG in an awake state has the following characteristics:
- frequency of 9 Hz (α)
- amplitude of 50–100 µV
- disappears with eye opening or mental arithmetic (sometimes)
- with eyes closed, the alpha waves are symmetrical and located in the posterior two quadrants.

Pathological EEG patterns

Seizures may be convulsive and non-convulsive in nature. The majority (90%) of seizures in ICU patients are non-convulsive and more common than previously recognized. Detection and early effective management of

seizure activity may avoid potentially irreversible insults to already vulnerable brain.
- Seizure activity:
  - focal or generalized spikes, sharp waves, or spike and wave
  - absence seizures 3 Hz spike and wave
  - juvenile myoclonic epilepsy 4 Hz spike and wave.
- Herpes encephalitis:
  - periodic lateralized epileptiform discharges (PLED).
- Burst suppression:
  - periods of 'suppressed' EEG between 'bursts' of high-voltage slow, sharp spiking activity
  - may be drug-induced (hypnotics, benzodiazepines) or deep coma
  - may represent deterioration of generalized status epilepticus
  - associated with poor prognosis.

Effects of anaesthetic drugs on the EEG

Inhalational anaesthetics
- Nitrous oxide results in activation of the EEG even when added to burst suppressing doses of isoflurane. Somatosensory evoked potentials (SSEPs) (see below) are reduced.
- At 1.0 MAC, isoflurane, desflurane, sevoflurane, and halothane produce limited β activity.
- At 1.5 MAC isoflurane generates burst suppression while desflurane, sevoflurane, halothane generate limited α activity.
- At 2.0 MAC isoflurane creates electrical silence, desflurane burst suppression or electrical silence, sevoflurane δ activity and burst suppression, halothane θ and δ activity.

Intravenous anaesthetics
- Barbiturates: increase β activity at low doses; as the dose increases initially the EEG slows followed by burst suppression and then electrical silence.
- Propofol: initially produces an increase in the amplitude of the alpha rhythm, followed by an increase in δ and θ activity and burst suppression in some patients. SSEPs better preserved with propofol than with volatile agents.
- Etomidate: there is no association between myoclonic movements and epileptogenic activity on the EEG. At high doses etomidate increases θ wave amplitude and slows the α rhythm.
- Opioids: in lower doses there is an increase in the amplitude of both α and β frequency bands. In higher doses, θ and δ frequencies develop. May be proconvulsant at high doses in some subjects with epilepsy. Small reduction and increase in latency of SSEPs.
- Benzodiazepines: in low doses benzodiazepines decrease the percentage of α activity while increasing the prevalence of β waves. At high doses, θ and δ activity occurs.

Indications for EEG
- Investigation of epilepsy, location of seizure origin, and assessment of drug effects.
- Localizing damaged areas following head injury, stroke, tumour, etc.

- Monitoring pharmacologic depression of brain for 'cerebral protection'.
- Monitoring sedation, coma, and assessment of prognosis.
- Brain death: not a requirement in the UK but may be used as supportive test.

Limitations
- Expert knowledge required to interpret.
- Different anaesthetic agents cause different effects on the EEG
- Difficulty in differentiating EEG changes between drug-only effects and the patient's clinical condition (e.g. hypotension, hypoxaemia, hypercapnia).
- 30% of the cortex is inaccessible for measurement, e.g. the indentations (the sulci), the basal surface, or the large folds of the brain.
- Cumbersome equipment.
- Interference from other electrical equipment.

Electrocorticography (ECoG)
To improve the spatial resolution of the EEG it is possible to place electrodes on the cortical surface during craniotomy, either extra- or subdurally. These can either be attached by joints to a fixed frame or halo, or incorporated into a flexible grid as an array of 4 to 64 electrodes.

- Temporal resolution is around 5 ms and spatial resolution is around 1 cm.
- Depth electrodes can also be used to access deeper structures such as the hippocampus and can have a spatial resolution of <1 mm.
- The grids are flexible enough to allow brain pulsation without injury, and can be left in place postoperatively to lengthen the recording time.
- Direct cortical electrical stimulation (DCES) techniques are often used in conjunction with ECoG to aid identification of epileptogenic foci and 'eloquent areas' of cortex. This can be performed before, during and after resection surgery.

Indications
- Functional mapping of cortex
- Identification of epileptogenic foci
- Assessing success of surgical resection.

Limitations
- Limited sampling time if used intra-operatively
- Invasive, requiring craniotomy
- Limited 'field of view'
- Requires expert for interpretation
- Affected by anaesthetics and anti-epileptic drugs.

Cerebral function analysing monitor (CFAM)
The cerebral function analysing monitor (CFAM) is a development of the earlier cerebral function monitor (CFM). It produces a continuous display of an analysed (processed) EEG signal from two symmetrical pairs of scalp electrodes. Fast Fourier transformation is used to calculate the relative proportions of different EEG frequency bands. These are displayed continuously; the unprocessed EEG can also be displayed. The advantage is that it is easier for non-experts to interpret than the raw EEG.

Clinical applications
- Monitoring burst suppression in ICU during drug-induced coma
- Detection of subclinical fitting
- Adequacy of cerebral perfusion during carotid endarterectomy or aneurysm clipping
- Monitoring and quantifying intravenous anaesthesia.

CFAM is particularly useful when monitoring the depth of drug-induced coma in patients with intractably raised intracranial pressure secondary to head injury. The dose of sedation is titrated to produce burst suppression. Increasing the dose beyond this has no proven benefit and runs the risk of brainstem anaesthesia and causes prolonged duration of coma. Other monitors of the 'depth' of sedation such as the Advanced Depth of Anaesthesia Monitor and the Bispectral Index monitor are not widely used in ICU practice.

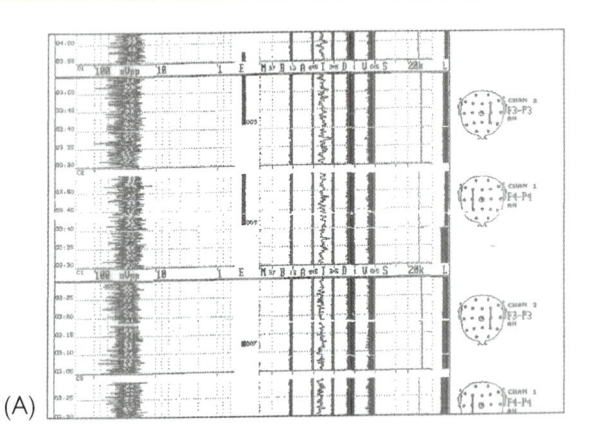

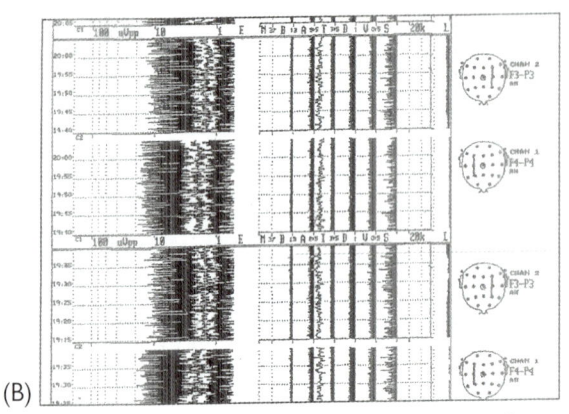

Fig. 3.2 CFAM trace in anaesthesia (A) and burst suppression (B). From left to right the recording displays: Time (minutes); Raw EEG in microvolts on a logarithmic scale; E, Event marker; M, Muscle activity; B, Beta activity; A, Alpha activity; T, Theta activity; D, Delta activity; V, Very low frequency activity; S, Burst suppression. Note that with anaesthesia there is a shift of the EEG towards lower amplitudes but greater relative variability.

Evoked potentials (EP)
Evoked potential monitors measure electrical activity of the nervous system in response to stimulation of specific nerve pathways. They can be somatosensory (SEP), visual (VEP), brainstem auditory (BAEP) or motor-evoked potentials (MEP). Evoked potential recordings constitute a minimally- to non-invasive, objective and repeatable measurement to supplement the clinical examination. In barbiturate coma and drug overdoses, EPs can help to separate drug effects from true CNS damage. This is possible because barbiturates and benzodiazepines have little effect on short latency EPs, even for drug doses sufficient to produce an isoelectric EEG.

Indications
- Nervous system integrity during surgery, e.g. complex spinal deformity surgery
- Monitoring head injury and coma
- Depth of anaesthesia
- Investigation of demyelinating disease
- Neuropathies and brain tumours.

Classification of evoked potentials
EPs are defined according to type of stimulation, site of stimulation and recording, amplitude, latency between stimulus and signal and polarity of the potential (positive or negative).

Stimulation
- Electrical—electrodes applied to the scalp, over the spinal column or over peripheral nerves, or epidurally during surgery.
- Magnetic—used for MEPs, avoids problems with electrode contact but is cumbersome.
- Visual (reversing chequerboard pattern) or auditory (clicks).

Site
- Cortical
- Spinal cord above and below area of concern
- Mixed peripheral nerves
- Muscle (for MEPs).

Latency
- Long (hundreds of milliseconds): these are suppressed under surgical anaesthesia, and are not useful for monitoring of sedation.
- Medium (tens of milliseconds): these are recordable under anaesthesia, and can be affected by anaesthetic state.
- Short (milliseconds): these are most commonly studied during surgery as they are influenced least by anaesthesia and sedation.
- Increase in latency >10% or a decrease in amplitude >50% indicates increased risk of complications.

Polarity
- Each type of EP has its own characteristic waveform. Specific peaks are used to define the responses to injury or drugs.

Visual evoked potentials
Visual evoked potentials (VEP) are the cortical response to visual stimulation with either a flashing light or reversing chequerboard pattern, recorded from the occipital area (Figure 3.3).
- Visual evoked potentials (VEP) are recorded during operations involving the optic nerve, optic chiasm and cranial base surgery and in the diagnosis of multiple sclerosis.
- VEP are generally thought to be less reliable than other modes.

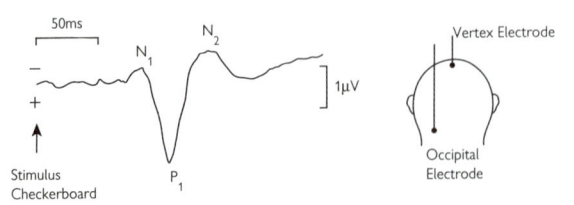

Fig. 3.3 Normal visual evoked potential (VEP).

Brainstem auditory evoked potentials
Brainstem auditory evoked potentials (BAEP) test acoustic conduction through the ear, the VIIIth cranial nerve, into the lower pons, and rostrally in the lateral lemniscus up the brain-stem (Figure 3.4).
- Used in procedures in the posterior cranial fossa
- BAEPs can be recorded easily in patients who are comatose or sedated and may be useful in assessing brain stem injury in the absence of other causes of depressed consciousness.

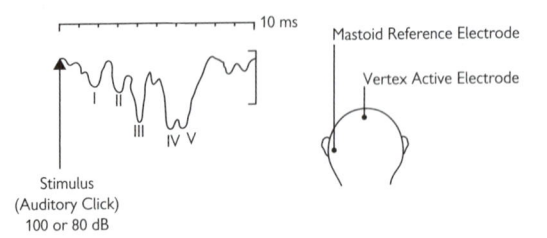

Fig. 3.4 Normal BAEP.

Somatosensory evoked potentials
Somatosensory evoked potentials (SEP) are the recordings from the brain or spinal cord in response to electrical stimulation of a peripheral sensory nerve (Figure 3.5). Commonly median, ulnar, and posterior tibial nerves are used during operations on the spine, spinal cord, and brachial plexus.

Fig. 3.5 Normal SEP.

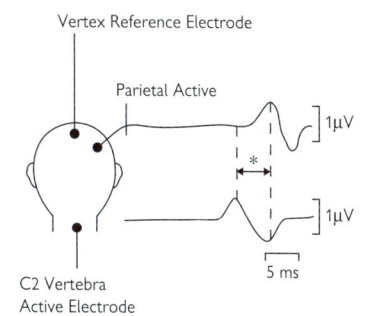

* Subtraction of latencies can assess conduction speed from dorsal columns to parietal cortex

All of these tests need to be performed by experienced personnel and their interpretation in an ICU is complex as underlying disease (e.g. deafness or blindness), hypothermia, hypoxaemia, hypotension, hypercapnia, and neural ischaemia may cause abnormal results.

Motor evoked potentials (electromyography, EMG)

- This measures the electrical potential produced by muscle cells when they are at rest or active. The motor unit potential (MUP) is measured on insertion of needle electrodes into the muscle area under investigation to determine if the muscle is normal, myopathic or neuropathic.
- In conscious patients, measurements are taken on insertion, at rest, during weak muscle movement and maximal muscle movement. Twenty different MUPs must be recorded from at least ten separate sites.
- Following insertion of the electrode there is a brief period of electrical activity of less than 500 µV in amplitude followed by no activity in normal muscle which remains at rest.
- Occasionally there is background motor endplate activity.
- Biphasic fibrillation generally suggests that the muscle is denervated although fibrillation from a single site may be seen even in normal muscle.
- Fasiculations (unless secondary to suxamethonium) are always pathological and are commonly seen in anterior horn cell disease but may occur secondary to nerve root or peripheral muscle disease.

Nerve conduction studies (NCS)

In nerve conduction studies the nerves are electrically stimulated using a narrow pulse (100–200 µs) with a repetitive stimulation that may range from 0.5 to 50 Hz. NCS are often carried out in conjunction with EMG and measure the amplitude and velocity of action potentials along the nerve innervating a muscle—the compound muscle action potential (CMAP). The tests may be subdivided into sensory or motor NCS, F wave or H reflex studies and Small Pain Fibre studies. In each case the latency, amplitude and velocity of the CMAP is recorded along with the sensory action potential (SAP).

Indications
- Diagnosis of acute-onset neuropathy
- Diagnosis of neuromuscular transmission disorders.

Critical illness polyneuropathy
This is a peripheral neurological disorder that arises *de novo* while a patient is in the ICU for other, primarily non-neurological conditions. Its features include severe diffuse muscular wasting and weakness, areflexia or hyperreflexia and variable sensory loss but with predominant preservation of sensation in those patients able to communicate. Extra-ocular and facial muscle weakness is rare. There is evidence to suggest that its incidence is increased in multiple organ failure, sepsis and prolonged ventilation, particularly in combination with the use of steroids and infusions of non-depolarizing muscle relaxants.

The NCS findings are of low-amplitude SAPs and CMAPs, although 24% of patients may have normal median and sural nerve SAPs, normal conduction velocity CMAPs from the abductor pollicis brevis and normal muscle EMG studies. The clinical picture can be very mixed with predominantly pure or mixed motor loss with widespread denervation, axonal peripheral neuropathy, neuromuscular junction dysfunction and simple atrophy.

Acute onset neuropathies

Guillain–Barré syndrome (GBS)
The most common form is an acute motor axonal neuropathy with a multi-focal inflammatory demyelination which results in EMG findings of motor abnormality exceeding sensory changes, prolonged distal motor latencies, particularly of the median nerve at the wrist and the common peroneal nerve at the ankle. Motor conduction velocities are characteristically reduced to around 30–40 m s^{-1}.

An acute motor axonal neuropathy (AMAN) variant of GBS exists which has characteristic NCS findings of normal SAPs and no evidence of demyelinating change with normal motor conduction velocities and distal motor latencies. There is an additional sensory variant (AMSAN) where severe sensory axonal damage and Wallerian degeneration occurs. The Miller–Fisher variant of GBS (characterized by ophthalmoplegia, areflexia and ataxia) has normal distal CMAPs but abnormal BAEPs where brain stem features are present.

Acute intermittent porphyria
Peripheral neuropathy occurs in several forms of porphyria and may be precipitated by numerous drugs including barbiturates, carbamazepine, phenytoin, and benzodiazepines. NCS in such patients with acute onset neuropathy do not show slow conduction velocity or temporal dispersion of CMAPs.

Botulism
This bacterial toxin-mediated disorder of neuromuscular transmission may occur following food poisoning or, more recently, in drug addicts who have run out of veins and resort to 'popping'—the subcutaneous injection of drugs—contaminated with *Clostridium botulinum*. Botulinum toxin reduces the presynaptic availability of acetylcholine thereby blocking

neuromuscular transmission at synaptic level. This results in preserved nerve conduction with normal sensory conduction studies, low-amplitude CMAPs with normal or near-normal conduction velocities paradoxically in severely weak limbs. Post-tetanic facilitation of baseline CMAP amplitude by greater than 50% to a supramaximal stimulus after 15 to 20 s of sustained voluntary effort is almost diagnostic.

Myasthenia gravis (MG)
The synaptic aetiology of both GBS and MG results in the diagnostic specificity of NCS and EMG studies being very low.

Channelopathies
This group of neuromuscular disorders includes the familial periodic paralyses, paramyotonia congenita, etc. The sensory conduction studies are normal but during the acute phase muscle cannot contract either voluntarily or by electrical stimulation. CMAP is either of very low or absent amplitude.

Tips and pitfalls
- The range of neurophysiological monitoring available to neurocritical care practice is extensive and in specific cases may provide assistance for both diagnosis and prognosis in neurological disease. This is particularly useful where the patient's clinical condition is such that conventional neurological assessment is not feasible.
- The ICU environment produces electromagnetic interference, difficulties in patient access, and a vast diversity of pathology. The data derived from neurophysiological monitoring is complex and subject to both data analysis and modification by the effects of multiple organ failure and the drug treatment that this requires.
- While it is tempting to consider the result of neurophysiological monitoring as analogous to simple ECG analysis in cardiovascular disease, the reality is often different. Specialist input is required for the choice of investigation, its specificity, sensitivity, and the interpretation of the results obtained.

Transcranial Doppler ultrasonography

Transcranial Doppler ultrasonography (TCD) was first introduced in 1982 and has since become a widely used technique for monitoring cerebral blood flow. Although it is not a perfect technique, it has the advantage of being non-invasive, repeatable and real-time, without requiring the patient to be moved.

Principles
TCD uses pulsed ultrasound to measure the velocity of moving objects in its path.
- Typically 1–2 MHz probes are used which provides adequate bone penetration.
- The ultrasonic beam crosses the skull at points known as 'windows' (temporal, orbital, and foramen magnum) and is reflected back from the moving erythrocytes in blood vessels in its path.
- By varying the time interval between transmitting and receiving, the depth of assessment can be varied.
- The change in frequency of the reflected signal is the Doppler shift:

    Doppler frequency shift = 2 × V × Ft × cosθ/C
    - V is the velocity of the reflector (red cells)
    - Ft is the transmitted frequency (fixed; 1–2 MHz depending upon the probe)
    - C is the speed of sound in soft tissue (fixed; 1540 m s^{-1})
    - θ is the angle of insonation.
- Frequency shift is dependent upon red cell velocity and the angle of insonation.
- The relationship between angle of insonation and frequency shift is non-linear so maintaining a constant angle of insonation is important.
    - cos 0° = 1; cos 15° = 0.96; cos 30° = 0.87; cos 45° = 0.71
- Measured velocity is dependent upon both blood flow and blood vessel area
    - FV (cm s^{-1}) = blood flow (cm^3 s^{-1})/vessel area (cm^2)
    - Changes in FV may occur due to changes in one or both of these factors.

Technique
The middle cerebral artery (MCA) carries 50–60% of ipsilateral carotid artery flow and so is the most commonly studied vessel. Numerous techniques are described.
- The temporal window is usually found within 2cm of a line drawn between the lateral canthus and the tragus.
- The artery is identified by systematically varying the site, angle, and depth of insonation to find the strongest signal.
- The MCA is identified when:
    - there is blood flow towards the probe at a depth of 35–60 mm
    - the signal can be followed for at least 10 mm
    - there is reduction in flow velocity (FV) with compression of the ipsilateral carotid artery.

Other vessels can also be identified using various characteristics.

Table 3.3 Typical patterns of identification of cerebral arteries. These are 'normal' patterns expected in individuals with 'normal' Circle of Willis anatomy and without vascular or intracranial pathology. Individual examinations may differ

Vessel	Probe direction	Depth (mm)	Direction of flow	Ipsilateral carotid compression	Contralateral carotid compression
Anterior cerebral artery	Anterior	60–75	Away	Flow reversal	Increased velocity
Middle cerebral artery (MCA)	Perpendicular	35–60	Toward	Reduced velocity	No change
Posterior cerebral artery	Posterior	55–70	Toward	No change or increased velocity	No change

Reproduced from I.K. Moppett and R.P. Mahajan (2004), Transcranial Doppler ultrasonography in anaesthesia and intensive care, *British Journal of Anaesthesia*; 93: 710–724. By permission of Oxford University Press.

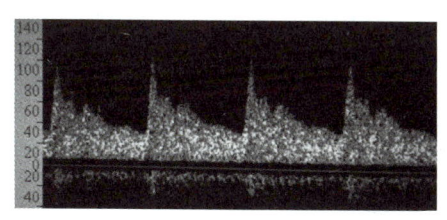

Fig. 3.6 A TCD trace from the middle cerebral artery of a normal subject.

Measured and derived values

Most modern equipment will measure systolic, diastolic and time-averaged FV. Other indices can be derived from these.

Flow velocity
- Quoted 'normal' values in the healthy adult population vary between 35–90 cm s^{-1}.
- This variability is mainly due to technical factors and inter-observer variability, rather than differences in blood flow per se.
- There is cyclical variation of around 10%.
- Side to side variation is usually <14%.

- Other factors influence FV including:
  - exercise
  - menstrual cycle
  - pregnancy
  - haematocrit
  - age (~24 cm s^{-1} at birth; 100 cm s^{-1} at 4–6 years; 40 cm s^{-1} > 60 years).

Derived indices

Vascular tone/resistance
Various methods have been described to quantify cerebrovascular resistance or vessel tone:
- Pulsatility index (PI) = (FVsyst—Fvdiast)/ Fvmean:
  - unaffected by angle of insonation
  - normal value = 0.6–1.1
  - may have paradoxical increase in PI with reduction in CPP.
- Ratio of FV to CPP (or MAP):
  - assumes direct relationship between FV and CBF.
- Zero flow pressure:
  - this is an estimate of the combined effect of ICP, CVP, and vascular tone on the downstream pressure of the cerebral circulation such that estimated CPP = MAP–ZFP
  - numerous methods described based on the premise that CPP = flow × resistance
  - trends more reliable than absolute values of eCPP or ZFP.

Vessel area
If vasospasm is present then changes in FV may not reflect changes in CBF.
- The ratio of MCA to internal carotid artery (ICA) FV can be used to help distinguish hyperaemia (normal MCA/ICA ratio (<3)) and vasospasm (increased MCA/ICA ratio).

Tests of regulatory capacity
The real-time, non-invasive nature of TCD allows it to be used for repeated or dynamic testing, in order to evaluate regulatory function of the cerebral circulation. Two aspects are commonly tested: pressure and carbon dioxide reactivity.

Pressure reactivity (autoregulation)
The response of the cerebral circulation to changes in perfusion pressure can be assessed in complementary ways.

Static autoregulation
The response of FV to pharmacologically induced, stable changes in MAP can be observed. In a normally autoregulating system, the change in FV will be small (though not zero).

Dynamic autoregulation
Transient reductions in cerebral perfusion pressure can be induced by various methods, most commonly deflation of thigh cuffs or compression of the ipsilateral carotid artery. Compensatory vasodilation should occur. Following thigh cuff release, the recovery profile of FV should be

faster than that of the MAP. Following carotid artery release, a temporary hyperaemic overshoot in FV should be seen.

Natural variation

Both of the above techniques induce relatively large, non-physiological changes in CPP. More recently, phase relationships have been described and quantified between MCA FV and the small, cyclical variations that naturally occur in MAP or CPP. If autoregulation is intact, then there should be little correlation between changes in CPP and FV. If autoregulation is impaired then FV becomes more dependent upon MAP.

Carbon dioxide reactivity

The diameter of the MCA does not change appreciably during changes in $PaCO_2$. The change in MCA FV in response to changes in $PaCO_2$ is, therefore, a reasonable estimate of the change in CBF. Within 1–2 kPa of the normal $PaCO_2$ this relationship is approximately linear.

Embolism

Emboli cause a characteristic distortion of the Doppler signal, heard as a 'chirruping' sound, and seen as signals of high intensity (bright) within a narrow frequency band.
- The sensitivity and specificity of embolus detection is dependent upon the operator and the processing software used.

Tips and pitfalls

- TCD provides an indirect measure of cerebral blood flow which is affected greatly by:
  - operator proficiency
  - angle of insonation
  - presence or absence of vasospasm.
- Trends or dynamic changes are probably more important that absolute values.

Multimodal monitoring

The goal of all neurocritical care therapies in brain injury is to ensure cerebral blood flow (CBF) is adequate to meet the oxygen and metabolic requirements of the brain, particularly in the penumbral areas of the brain around the site of the primary brain injury. The aim of monitoring brain injury is to prevent the development of secondary brain injury through early detection at a time when changes in management may provide benefit.

Standard ICU care should ensure the adequacy of oxygenation, ventilation, and perfusion, but will not assess the effects of these parameters on the brain itself. Multimodal monitoring describes the simultaneous use of several different kinds of monitors of brain function to follow the various physiological responses of the brain to changes in therapy. This allows therapy to be directed by the requirements of the individual patient's injured brain rather than those predicated by general theoretical physiological goals. For example, around 25% of patients with traumatic brain have impaired autoregulation. In such patients, simply using MAP targets in order to increase cerebral perfusion pressure (CPP) and thereby to improve CBF may result in an increase in cerebral oedema (by processes driving the classic Starling equilibrium). Intracranial pressure (ICP) would rise so that the CBF would fall rather than rise. Simultaneous monitoring of CBF or its surrogate markers would detect this and ensure that therapy aimed at reducing ICP rather than elevating CPP was initiated.

CBF is difficult to measure accurately and surrogate markers such as transcranial Doppler (TCD), brain tissue oxygenation by jugular venous bulb oxygenation, direct tissue oxygenation and brain metabolic changes by microdialysis aim to demonstrate the adequacy of CBF to meet the oxygenation and metabolic needs of the brain. There is some evidence that using this multimodal monitoring approach allows a protocolized response to changes in the measured parameters which may improve outcome.

Transcranial Doppler

TCD is described in detail elsewhere (see p. 82) but is included here as it is often used in multimodal monitoring as a measure of the adequacy of cerebral blood flow. It is generally applied to measure blood flow velocity in the middle cerebral artery (MCA).
- CBF = mean flow velocity × area of MCA × cosine of angle of insonation
- This relationship is linear if the vessel diameter and angle of insonation is constant during the examination
- When this occurs, CBF is adequate if MCA flow velocity is between 35–70 cm s^{-1}.

Tips and pitfalls

- Not every patient has a temporal bony window to allow insonation of the MCA.
- Accuracy is dependent on the skill of the individual applying the probe.
- Snapshot readings—it is difficult to prevent movement of the probe thereby changing the angle of insonation.
- Vasospasm results in greater flow velocity for the same CBF.
- Flow velocity also changes with altered haemorheology.

Jugular venous bulb oxygenation (SjO$_2$)

If the cerebral metabolic rate for oxygen (CMRO$_2$) remains constant despite any changes in cerebral blood flow, then the SjO$_2$ or arterio-jugular oxygen content difference (AJDO$_2$) may be used to determine the adequacy of CBF to meet the oxygen requirements of the brain.
- The normal range of SjO$_2$ is 50–75%.
- If the SjO$_2$ <50% then not enough oxygen is reaching the brain to meet its needs.
- If the SjO$_2$ is >75% (luxury perfusion) then either too much oxygen is being delivered, or the metabolic need is low or the brain has died.

SjO$_2$ catheters have a fibre-optic channel which allows the oxygen saturation of the blood at its tip to be measured in a manner similar to peripheral pulse oximetry. They also have a central lumen to allow samples to be taken from the tip of the catheter for blood gas analysis.

Catheter placement
- Locate right internal jugular vein (IJV) as for central venous cannula placement.
- Direct the cannula in a cephalic rather than caudal direction.
- Thread the fibreoptic catheter through cannula until resistance is felt.
- The catheter tip should lie at the inferior border of the jugular venous bulb:
  - This can be confirmed by lateral C-spine X-ray; the tip should be level with the inferior border of the first cervical vertebral body
  - The catheter tip must be above the junction of the facial vein with the internal jugular vein to avoid contamination with extracranial blood
- Ensure blood can be aspirated, flush and connect to continuous oximeter.

Tips and pitfalls
- Use assumes measurement from one jugular bulb reflects global rather than hemispherical CBF.
- The right jugular bulb generally has the dominant cerebral venous drainage—around 60% of the total.
- The dominant side may be detected by compressing each IJV in turn and observing the effect on the ICP. Compressing the side with the dominant drainage should cause a more marked elevation of ICP.
- Continuous fibreoptic measurement is often subject to 'wall artefact' (reflectance from the vessel wall) which gives a falsely high reading.
- When high readings are obtained take a sample for blood gas analysis and recalibrate the oximeter if required.
- Withdraw samples slowly otherwise venous admixture from facial vein drainage will occur and give a falsely high reading.
- Limited sensitivity for regional hypoxaemia/ischaemia so a large area of brain tissue may be hypoxaemic before changes in SjO$_2$ occur.

Focal tissue oxygen tension (PbrO$_2$)

Direct measurement of brain tissue oxygen partial pressure is possible using a very small Clarke oxygen electrode inserted into the brain tissue. Combined ICP and PbrO$_2$ devices are available. They may be placed in

the penumbral areas around the primary brain injury so that early detection of hypoxaemia and ischaemia may be detected and efforts made to increase the cerebral blood flow to these areas. Not all sites of injury are accessible and the majority of neurosurgeons place electrodes in non-damaged brain on the opposite side to the injury.
- In traumatic brain injury, low PbrO$_2$ is seen in around 50% of cases in the first 24 h; the severity and duration of the hypoxaemia in this period are independent predictors of adverse outcome.
- The lower limit of normal is around 1–2 kPa.
- Hyperventilation decreases PbrO$_2$ and this may be used to determine the acceptable PaCO$_2$ for the individual patient.
- Tissue oxygen response (TOR) can be calculated from the change in PbrO$_2$ following a change in F$_i$O$_2$:

    (ΔPbrO$_2$ /ΔPaO$_2$) × (1/PbrO$_2$ at baseline)

    - higher TOR predicts worse outcome and may be related to loss of autoregulation to oxygen.

Tips and pitfalls
- The volume of brain tissue that is monitored is limited to a few mm^3 around the tip of the probe.
- The electrode has little signal drift and the proportion of time of good data quality is reported to be around 95%.
- Initial signal stabilization may take 30 min to 2 h.
- Small haematomas at the catheter tip will decrease the signal to the extent that even large increases in oxygen will not be detected. This should be suspected if raising the arterial PaO$_2$ does not cause an immediate rise in PbrO$_2$.
- The measured value is also influenced by proximity to cerebral vasculature and whether the probe is positioned in white or grey matter.
- Hypothermia has been reported to both decrease and increase PbrO$_2$.
- SjvO$_2$ and Pbro$_2$ appear to correlate well when CPP falls below 60 mmHg but not on CO$_2$ reactivity testing.

Cerebral microdialysis
Cerebral microdialysis (CM) allows changes in the biochemical make up of the cerebral extracellular fluid (ECF) to be measured. Primary brain injury triggers a cascade of intracellular changes which increase the cells susceptibility to secondary insults such as hypoxaemia, hypotension or hypo- and hyperthermia. As cellular damage continues the cells release various biochemical markers that leak into to the ECF and the concentration of these markers reflect the development of the injury. Detection of increases in the level of such markers in areas of the brain 'at-risk' but not irretrievably damaged, such those in the penumbral areas around focal primary brain damage, may allow an early warning of worsening brain injury that may be modified by changes in therapy.

Markers and cause of secondary brain injury
The markers currently measured are glucose, lactate, pyruvate, lactate:pyruvate ratio (LPR), glycerol and glutamate.
- ↓ glucose: hypoxaemia, ischaemia, hypoglycaemia, cerebral hyperglycolysis.

- ↑ LPR—the most sensitive marker of ischaemia/hypoxaemia, cerebral hypoglycaemia, mitochondrial dysfunction.
- ↑ glycerol: hypoxaemia/ischaemia, cell membrane destruction, glucose to glycerol synthesis.
- ↑ glutamate: hypoxaemia/ischaemia, excitatory amino acid formation

The technique requires the insertion of a fine double-lumen catheter into the area of brain tissue to be monitored. The outer lumen of the catheter is slowly perfused (0.3 μl min^{-1}) with a solution that is isotonic to brain ECF. When biochemical markers accumulate in the ECF to levels higher than normal they diffuse across the semipermeable membrane at the tip of the catheter into the perfusate and this microdialysate is then collected from the inner lumen of the catheter for analysis. The concentration of the recovered microdialysate depends upon:

- pore size:
  - semipermeable membranes with a pore size of either 20 or 100 kDa are available.
- membrane area
- flow rate of the perfusate
- molecular weight of the marker concerned.

Tips and pitfalls

- Must be positioned close to site of brain injury to allow early detection of increased markers. No change in marker levels if placed at a distance from the penumbral area of damage.
- Location of catheter tip position should be verified by direct vision or CT.
- Published range of 'normal' marker concentrations derived from neurosurgical patients, not completely normal subjects.
- Glutamate levels very variable between patients and may not reflect excitatory toxicity.
- All marker levels vary with time and trend towards poor outcome rather than detect acute deterioration.

Near infra-red spectroscopy (NIRS)

NIRS is based on the non-invasive determination of the level of oxygenation of haemoglobin (and other chromophores such as cytochrome and myoglobin) by applying the modified Beer–Lambert Law whereby the absorption of two different wavelengths of near infra-red (NIR) light allow detection of oxygenated haemoglobin (HbO$_2$ at 850 nm) or de-oxygenated haemoglobin (Hb at 760 nm). NIR wavelengths of light can cross bone and be reflected back from the oxygenated blood flowing in the brain blood vessels.

- Two optodes, an emitter and detector, are placed on the forehead away from the midline, venous sinuses and temporalis muscle. Should the level of oxygenated haemoglobin fall as a consequence of hypoxaemia or ischaemia there will be a fall in the reflectance of the near infra-red wavelength for HbO$_2$.

- The normal range of HbO_2 is around 60–80% and ischaemia is associated with levels <50%.

Tips and pitfalls
- Reflectance measurement is greatly influenced by changes in blood flow of the extracranial tissues.
- Inter-optode distance of <4cm reflects flow in predominantly extracranial circulation.
- Limited to monitoring changes in a small area of the forebrain because of the need to avoid venous sinuses and muscular areas of scalp.
- Sequestered venous blood in areas of complete ischaemia may still give a normal value.

Regional cerebral blood flow

Cerebral blood flow is not homogenous in normal or pathological brain. There are differences in blood flow and metabolism between various areas of the brain, and the response of regional CBF (rCBF) to drugs, pathology, and interventions is variable. As a result, regional variations in autoregulation and responses to therapeutic interventions can occur. Certain pathologies are associated with regional cerebral vasoconstriction. Alterations in rCBF often precede structural changes seen on CT and MRI scan. Therapies that are beneficial to one region may even be harmful to another. For these reasons, the ability to monitor regional CBF may be extremely useful. As yet the benefits are unproven.

Indications for rCBF monitoring
- Detection of regional hypo- or hyperperfusion:
  - cerebral vasospasm following subarachnoid haemorrhage (SAH) or traumatic brain injury (TBI)
  - hyperperfusion or loss of autoregulation following brain injury
  - regional responses to global interventions.
- Intra- and postoperative monitoring of CBF in a region of interest (e.g. aneurysm clipping, large tumour resection).
- Detection of abnormalities not (yet) visible on structural imaging.
- Research into differential effects of pathology and treatments.
- To predict outcome.

Modalities
The main methods of measuring rCBF can be broadly divided into localized and continuous (thermal diffusion flowmetry, laser Doppler flowmetry) or widespread and discontinuous (CT, positron emission tomography [PET] and MRI). There are advantages and disadvantages to each method.

Thermal diffusion flowmetry
- Measures CBF across a small area of the cerebral cortex.
- Based on the principle that heat dissipation is affected by rCBF.
- A thermocouple, placed at craniotomy or through a burr hole, measures the dissipation of heat and thus CBF across a small volume of the cerebral cortex.

Advantages
- Allows continuous bedside monitoring.

Disadvantages
- Measures CBF only in a localized area determined by position of burr hole
- No information about subcortical CBF
- Inaccurate if placed near a large blood vessel
- Invasive.

Specific uses
- Following surgery for SAH

- TBI (detect hyperaemia; normalizing values associated with better outcome)
- Epilepsy (to localize seizures).

Laser Doppler flowmetry
- Measures cortical microcirculatory CBF flow in a 1 mm^3 volume.
- A burr hole is required for placement of the probe (can be placed at the same time as an ICP bolt).

Advantages
- Allows continuous bedside monitoring
- May be used as part of a multimodal monitoring approach.

Disadvantages
- Measures CBF only in a localized area determined by position of burr hole
- No information about subcortical CBF
- Results are not quantitative and are expressed in arbitrary units
- Invasive.

Specific uses
- Intra-operatively: placed over an area of interest, e.g. during aneurysm clipping
- Postoperatively, to detect ischaemia following SAH.

^{133}Xenon
- Measures CBF. Can be combined with induced hypercapnia or hypotension to assess regional autoregulation.
- ^{133}Xe is an inert radioisotope administered by inhalation. CBF is calculated using 5–8 stationary scintillation counters placed over the scalp.

Advantages
- Bedside test
- Not metabolized and rapidly cleared so can be repeated within 30 min.

Disadvantages
- Inaccurate
- Does not give information about subcortical blood flow.

Specific uses
- Acute phase of TBI or SAH, carotid endarterectomy surgery.

Xenon-enhanced CT scan
- Measures cerebral perfusion, CBF, cerebral blood volume and mean transit time.
- Baseline CT scan followed by a sequence of high resolution serial CT scan slices after inhaled 28% ^{131}Xe (non-radioactive) in oxygen.
- Based on a modified Fick principle and the fact that ^{131}Xe readily crosses the blood–brain barrier.
- Brain tissue ^{131}Xe uptake and enhancement on CT scan are proportional to CBF.

Advantages
- Due to the short half-life of inhaled xenon, the studies can be repeated after a short time to assess response to therapy

- Uses technology readily available in most centres
- Provides a structural scan.

Disadvantages
- Xenon can increase CBF and ICP although not significant at the dose and duration required for scan
- Anaesthetic effect of 28% xenon in awake patients can cause movement artefacts
- Results are affected by lung pathology as end-tidal xenon is assumed to be equal to arterial xenon concentrations.

Specific uses
- Acute phase of TBI

SPECT (single photon emission computed tomography)
- Measures cerebral perfusion and demonstrates areas of hypoperfusion.
- Tomographic images of injected radio-isotopes (^{133}Xe or technetium-99) which emit single photons.

Advantages
- Simple and relatively cheap.

Disadvantages
- Images are low resolution and non-quantitative.

Specific uses
- Imaging of infarction and ischaemia.

PET
- More expensive and complex than SPECT, but with wider applications.
- Measures regional CBF, CBV, $CMRO_2$, O_2 extraction fraction (OEF) and cerebral glucose metabolism (depending on the isotope used).
- Tomographic images of injected (18-fluorodeoxyglucose) or inhaled ($^{15}O_2$) positron-emitting isotopes. These isotopes can also be further combined with markers for specific neuronal injury.

Advantages
- Repeat studies to show effect of intervention
- Calculate OEF and derive information about ischaemic brain volume.

Disadvantages
- Limited to use as a research tool due to the need for a cyclotron
- Expensive, not universally available
- Requires patient transfer to scanner
- Not continuous.

Specific uses
- Can be used early to predict outcome—a decrease in cerebral perfusion correlates with a poor outcome (even when ICP still normal)
- Research studies have demonstrated increases in ischaemic brain volume in response to hyperventilation, despite 'improvements' in global parameters.

Perfusion CT
- Regional CBF is determined by measuring the first pass of an injected iodinated contrast agent through the brain.
- Requires high-speed helical CT scanner and special software.

Advantages
- Provides a structural scan.

Disadvantages
- The size of the volume that can be studied is limited by the total dose of radiation
- The volume of contrast used limits repeat imaging.

Specific uses
- Can detect areas of normal perfusion, hyperaemia and oligaemia
- May be able to detect areas of secondary ischaemic changes in TBI.

Functional MRI (fMRI)
- Maps CBF and neuronal activation.
- Most fMRIs are based on the BOLD (blood oxygen level-dependent) method. This measures the regional changes in the de-oxyhaemoglobin to oxyhaemoglobin ratio after performing a particular cognitive task.

Advantages
- Combines the structural accuracy of a conventional MRI with functional information
- Does not require exposure to ionizing radiation and can therefore be repeated multiple times.

Disadvantages
- Time-consuming
- Requires specific MRI-compatible equipment
- Requires transfer to MRI suite.

Specific uses
- Can be used to predict outcome after TBI in patients in vegetative state
- Best used in the chronic phase of TBI when patients are able to cooperate.

Diffusion weighted imaging (DWI) MRI
- DWI MRI can be used to demonstrate any regional perfusion delay.
- Primarily used to detect cytotoxic or vasogenic cerebral oedema.

Perfusion MRI
- Measures CBV and CBF following injection of paramagnetic contrast (Gadolinium-chelate).
- Demonstrates reduced CBV in areas of focal pathology but results are difficult to quantify and is of little use in the acute setting.

MRI angiography
- A simultaneous mapping of entire intracranial circulation, although image quality is not sharp.

Tips and pitfalls
- The usefulness of regional CBF monitoring is limited by the fact that most therapeutic interventions have a global effect.
- Most of the current techniques require moving the patient to a scanner; this is not without its risks, particularly in the unstable TBI patient.
- Few of the modalities available for measuring regional CBF are continuous and can be used at the bedside.
- None of the modalities have been shown to improve outcome.

Glasgow Coma Scale

The first description of the Glasgow Coma Scale (GCS) was published in 1974. It is a reproducible and easily performed measure of consciousness—particularly after traumatic brain injury. The GCS can also be used to predict outcome in head-injured patients. There is a low rate of interobserver variability. However, the GCS is poor at discriminating between mild disturbances of consciousness.

Other factors apart from head injury may alter the level of consciousness such as shock, alcohol and metabolic disturbances, and these may be present in combination. However, it is the end result—depression of consciousness—that is important.

The absolute score may be less important than a change in the score. Any reduction in the score may herald a worsening condition of the brain (or brainstem) and warrants further action—diagnostic and/or therapeutic. A score ≤8 is considered to be 'coma'. To monitor progress after an acute injury, the first GCS should be determined as soon as possible. The best time to assess GCS for prognostic purposes is after initial resuscitation and stabilization.

Using the GCS

- If the eyes are closed due to swelling, this should be recorded (as E_C) and the E part of the score is invalid.
- The best response from either upper limb is recorded. If the patient will not respond to verbal command, a painful stimulus is applied to the nail bed, and if still no response is elicited, a painful stimulus is applied centrally via the supraorbital nerve or the angle of the jaw.
- If speech is impossible, for example the patient's trachea is intubated, this is recorded V_T, and if the patient dysphasic, V_D. The V part of the score is then invalid.
- The score most poorly understood is the motor score and particularly differentiating between:
  - localizing to pain (e.g. the limb moves towards the painful stimulus)
  - withdrawing the limb away from pain (normal flexion at the knee or elbow)
  - abnormal flexion (decorticate posturing with slow withdrawal associated with pronation of the wrist and adduction of the shoulder).
- The GCS should always be recorded as three individual responses, not as a total score. For example, GCS E_3 V_5 M_6, and not GCS 14.
- If the eyes are closed the GCS may be: E_C V_3 M_3, and if the patient's trachea is intubated, E_1 V_T M_4.

Table 3.4 Adult Glasgow Coma Scale

Eye opening:	Spontaneous	4
	To speech	3
	To pain	2
	None	1
Best motor response:	Obeys commands	6
	Localizes to pain	5
	Withdraws to pain	4
	Abnormal flexion	3
	Extension	2
	No movement	1
Best verbal response:	Orientated	5
	Confused	4
	Inappropriate words	3
	Incomprehensible sounds	2
	None	1

Maximum score = 15, minimum score = 3. Coma is usually defined as a GCS score of ≤ 8.

Other physical signs used in head injured or comatose patients

The GCS is usually combined with the pupillary size and reactivity to light, and evidence of asymmetrical limb weakness. A difference in pupil size of more than 1 mm is significant (although in some people this is a normal variant—anisocoria). An expanding supratentorial lesion causes an ipsilateral fixed, dilated pupil (due to compression of the IIIrd (oculomotor) cranial nerve) and contralateral limb weakness due to compression of the brainstem and corticospinal tracts.

Use in children

A number of modifications of the GCS are used for children. Examples are given in Tables 3.5 and 3.6.

Table 3.5 Paediatric Glasgow Coma Scale (ages 2–5)

Eye opening:	Spontaneous	4
	To speech	3
	To pain	2
	None	1
Best motor response:	Obeys commands	5
	Localizes to pain	4
	Flexes to pain	3
	Extends to pain	2
	No movement	1
Best verbal response:	Appropriate words, phrases	5
	Inappropriate words, monosyllables	4
	Cries, screams	3
	Grunts	2
	None	1

Maximum score = 14, minimum score = 3

Table 3.6 Paediatric Glasgow Coma Scale (age <2)

Eye opening:	Spontaneous	4
	To speech	3
	To pain	2
	None	1
Best motor response:	Normal spontaneous movements	5
	Localizes to pain	4
	Flexes to pain	3
	Extends to pain	2
	No movement	1
Best verbal response:	Appropriate smile, coos	5
	Cries	4
	Inappropriate cries, screams	3
	Grunts	2
	None	1

Maximum = 14, minimum = 3

Tips and pitfalls
- The absolute score is less important than a change in score. A deterioration in the score warrants reassessment of the patient.
- When determining the GCS the observer looks for the best motor score; when examining the patient for lateralizing signs in the limbs the observer measures the worst motor response.
- Always try to determine what has led to the depression of consciousness.

Chapter 4

General principles of neuroanaesthesia

Pre-operative assessment *104*
General principles of neuroanaesthesia *110*
Paediatric neuroanaesthesia *120*
Cerebral protection *130*
TIVA or volatile-based anaesthesia *134*
Intra-operative temperature control *136*
Management of intra-operative brain swelling *140*
Air embolism *142*
Blood loss and cell salvage *146*
Glycaemic control *150*
Thromboprophylaxis *152*
Pregnancy *156*

Pre-operative assessment

Appropriate assessment of the neurosurgical patient is essential. Many aspects are common to all patients undergoing surgery or interventional procedures, but some require specific or more detailed assessment in this patient group. The generic aspects of anaesthetic assessment common to all patients presenting for surgery will not be covered here, only issues of importance to neurosurgical patients. This chapter is weighted towards the elective patient; the same principles apply to the assessment of the urgent and emergency patient, though time pressure will necessitate some changes. Issues of special relevance to particular conditions are discussed in Chapters 6–10.

Purpose of pre-operative assessment

Pre-operative assessment of the neurosurgical patient has five overlapping roles:
- identification of the urgency of surgery
- timely identification of medical and surgical conditions and drug therapy that may affect anaesthetic and surgical technique
- identification of patients who may benefit from optimization of co-existing medical conditions before proceeding to surgery
- identification of patients who may benefit from high level care postoperatively
- counselling of patients about the benefits and risks of the proposed anaesthetic technique, analgesia and postoperative care.

Although these aspects are more straightforward to organize for elective patients, the same principles apply to urgent and emergency surgery.

Organization of pre-operative assessment

How the pre-operative assessment process is organized is dependent upon many factors which will be specific to individual units. However the key features are:

Timeliness
Sufficient time should be allowed between assessment and planned date of surgery to allow completion and review of investigations so that problems can be resolved in good time. Conversely, an excessive time interval between assessment and surgery may cause concern over progression of neurological symptoms.

Multiprofessional
The pre-operative assessment should cover not just medical issues but also areas traditionally covered by nursing assessment, such as social support, discharge needs, fears and anxieties related to illness and surgery. The needs of the surgeon are not necessarily the same as of the anaesthetist, so both professions will need to be involved in the process. Units may choose to use specially trained nurses to perform all the nursing, surgical, and anaesthetic roles. Alternatively a more traditional clerking by a trainee doctor may be used with a variable degree of anaesthetic involvement.

Robust processes

Documentation must be clear and unambiguous. A system must be in place which always identifies patients early with significant past medical history or abnormal investigations. Agreed guidelines should be in place regarding venous thrombo-embolism prophylaxis, use of appropriate investigations, continuation (or discontinuation) of certain drugs (e.g. aspirin, clopidogrel, NSAIDs, warfarin).

History and examination

Regardless of who performs the pre-operative assessment, there are key features that should be sought of particular relevance to neuroanaesthetic practice.

Airway

A history of difficult intubation is clearly important. Patients with degenerative disease of the lower spine may also have disease in their cervical spine which may limit movement, or be associated with myelopathic symptoms on movement. Previous cervical spine fusion may result in patients with their neck fixed in a position which makes direct laryngoscopy impossible. More details on assessment of the injured or diseased cervical spine are found in Chapter 9.

A high proportion of patients with traumatic brain injury have an associated cervical spine injury.

A large proportion of patients with acromegaly are reported to have a degree of obstructive sleep apnoea (OSA) and a subset may also have central sleep apnoea. Treatment of acromegaly does not necessarily reverse the anatomic changes predisposing to OSA.

Respiratory system

Patients presenting with high cervical myelopathy due to intrinsic or extrinsic cord compression may have significant respiratory embarrassment. This may be difficult to assess because of limited walking distance as a consequence of their neurology.

Patients with bulbar involvement of their neurological disease (cerebellopontine angle tumours, multiple sclerosis, syringomyelia/bulbia) or reduced conscious level are at risk of aspiration, which can often be elicited by a careful history and examination.

Cardiovascular system

Hypertension is common in the neurosurgical population. Most often this is essential hypertension, but occasionally it will be a consequence of the neurosurgical condition itself or its treatment, e.g. acutely raised intracranial pressure, acromegaly, hyper- or hypothyroidism, corticosteroid treatment. Peri-operative hypertension is a risk factor for intracranial bleeding after craniotomy, so if time permits, control of blood pressure should be aimed for. Neurosurgical emergencies such as intracranial haematoma, traumatic brain injury, subarachnoid haemorrhage, and spinal cord injury can all be associated with dramatic cardiovascular instability. These are discussed separately in their respective chapters.

Neurological system

A full record of the patient's current neurological state should be made prior to anaesthesia, mainly to inform postoperative assessment. This should include mental state. If patients are confused a corroborating history from family, friends or GP is useful. Symptoms of raised intracranial pressure include a postural headache, worse in the morning or with coughing and sneezing, and vomiting. Signs include papilloedema, unilateral or bilateral papillary dilatation, IIIrd or VIth nerve palsy, absent brainstem reflexes and, when severe, systemic hypertension, bradycardia and abnormal respiration (Cushing's triad). The Glasgow Coma Scale score (see p.98) should be noted.

Frequency and type of seizures should also be documented, along with known precipitating factors.

Endocrine system

Many patients will have type II diabetes, and the level of glycaemic control should be recorded, particularly in patients recently started on corticosteroids. Assessment of pituitary function is important for patients undergoing pituitary surgery and is discussed in Chapter 6.

Haematological system

A personal or family history of easy bruising, prolonged bleeding and other stigmata of bleeding disorders should be sought. Liver disease is a risk factor for coagulopathy. Similarly, risk factors for venous thrombo-embolism should be documented and acted upon.

Drugs

The drugs of special interest in the neurosurgical patient are those affecting blood pressure, glycaemic control, coagulation and platelet function, renal function and electrolytes, steroids, anticonvulsants, analgesics and analgesic adjuvants. Units should have locally agreed protocols guiding the continuation or discontinuation of common classes of drugs.

Most *antihypertensive medication* should be continued pre- and postoperatively. Some units stop ACE inhibitors and angiotensin II antagonists because of the risk of peri-operative hypotension.

Oral hypoglycaemics should be stopped in accordance with local protocols and many diabetic patients will need some form of insulin-based therapy peri-operatively.

Aspirin therapy is a matter of debate. The risks of stopping it (markedly increased risk of peri-operative myocardial infarction (MI)) should be balanced against the small, but potentially catastrophic risk of postoperative haematoma in a confined site.

Clopidogrel therapy is associated with significant risk of bleeding but stopping it is associated with significant risk also. Patients with bare metal coronary stents have a risk of up to 20% of stent occlusion in the peri-operative period if clopidogrel is stopped prior to surgery. If possible surgery should be delayed until clopidogrel is no longer needed. Direct discussion between surgeon, anaesthetist, and cardiologist is advised if urgent surgery is required. Most units stop clopidogrel in patients prior to intracranial or spinal intramedullary surgery.

Warfarin can safely be stopped in most patients. The risk of thrombotic stroke associated with AF or of venous thrombo-embolism is smaller than the risk of neurological injury caused by bleeding. Even for patients with mechanical valves, the risk:benefit ratio is in favour of stopping warfarin, though clearly there is a risk of valve occlusion which should be discussed with the patient. Some units favour continuing heparin infusion until 6–8 h before elective surgery.

Anticonvulsants should be continued peri-operatively. The anaesthetist should be aware of the potential changes in pharmacokinetics and pharmacodynamics of anaesthetic drugs due to alterations in hepatic metabolism and sensitivity to sedative effects. Patients on long term anticonvulsants are at greater risk of intra-operative awareness.

Investigations

In common with all other patients, the investigations ordered should be those where abnormalities are common and where knowledge of an abnormal result will change management. Units should have locally agreed protocols guiding the use of routine investigations.

Blood tests

Full blood count
The risk of bleeding with almost every neurosurgical procedure is such that it is prudent to document the full blood count before surgery in all but the most minor of cases.

Urea and electrolytes (U&Es)
Electrolyte derangement is common in the neurosurgical population both as a consequence of their age and medical comorbidity, but also due to the effects of disease (e.g. pituitary disease, intracranial tumours) and treatment (e.g. diuretics for intracranial hypertension, steroids for tumours). Patients without risk factors for renal/electrolyte disturbance do not need routine U&Es performed. Emergency patients almost always have a risk factor for deranged U&Es.

Coagulation
Coagulation tests were not designed as screening tools for coagulopathy and are not a substitute for a properly taken bleeding history. There is no evidence to support the use of routine coagulation tests prior to neurosurgery. However, any patient with a positive bleeding history, including possible liver disease or drugs that affect coagulation, should have a coagulation screen. Subarachnoid haemorrhage may affect coagulation so these patients should undergo formal coagulation testing prior to surgery.

Blood glucose
This should be recorded for all patients undergoing intracranial or major spinal procedures.

Electrocardiogram (ECG)

This should be performed according to local guidance with respect to comorbidity, smoking and age. Patients with subarachnoid haemorrhage have a high (50%) incidence of ECG changes following the bleed. It is not clear whether the presence of these changes should alter anaesthetic management though their presence is associated with left ventricular dysfunction.

Chest X-ray (CXR)
Many patients with intracranial tumours will have had CT or plain X-ray of their chest as part an oncology work up. These do not need repeating. Stable respiratory disease is not an indication for CXR. There is no good evidence that an abnormal chest X-ray makes any difference to patient management or outcome beyond the details elicited from a careful history. Some units may have local guidelines suggesting CXR for patients planned for postoperative critical care.

Echocardiography
Patients with subarachnoid haemorrhage have a high incidence of regional or global ventricular dysfunction following the bleed which can be detected by echocardiography. There is no evidence to suggest that routine use of this investigation results in improved patient outcome.

The investigation of cardiac murmurs and heart failure should follow local guidelines.

Arterial blood gases (ABG)
Arterial blood gases may be an important part of critical care management where control of $PaCO_2$ is important. In the elective patient there is little evidence to support the use of pre-operative ABG. Although they may be used to document the degree of hypoxia or hypercapnia in patients with respiratory compromise, there is no evidence that outcome is changed by knowing the results. The patient's exercise tolerance, regardless of underlying pathology, is probably a better marker.

Pulmonary function tests (PFT)
As with ABGs, PFTs do not offer information that is likely to particularly alter management, beyond that obtained from the history. For patients with high cervical cord lesions PFTs may help to define how much respiratory involvement there is. Some units may have local guidance suggesting that PFTs or ABGs are performed on patients planned for postoperative critical care.

Neurosurgical imaging
It is good practice to review the imaging that has been ordered by the neurosurgeons as this will inform the anaesthetist of the likely surgical approach, magnitude of surgery, risk of bleeding etc.

Postoperative care
Some units routinely send every neurosurgical patient to a high-level care area; others routinely send every patient back to a specialist neurosurgical ward. Most have a practice which falls between the two. Deciding who should have high dependency or intensive care postoperatively is notoriously difficult and largely comes down to individual judgement and experience.

Patient counselling

Pre-operative assessment is a two-way process and patients should be given appropriate information about the choices available to them for anaesthesia and postoperative management. An honest appraisal of the risks and benefits pertaining to anaesthesia should always be given at a level appropriate to the patient. Written information is a useful adjunct for this. Given that many neurosurgical procedures are high risk it is prudent to discuss risks and benefits with family members if the patient is in agreement. All discussions should be clearly documented in the patient record.

Tips and pitfalls

- Pre-operative assessment of the neurosurgical patient is not markedly different to any other patient, but certain conditions are more likely to be present.
- Emergency patients are likely to need more investigation than elective patients due to either lack of history or the conditions that require urgent treatment.
- There is very little point in requesting a test unless the result is going to influence management.
- Close cooperation between all the professional teams involved with the patient is likely to lead to a more robust and logical system of preoperative assessment.
- Locally agreed policies and guidelines should be in place for common problems such as routine investigations, antiplatelet drugs and postoperative care.
- If possible review the neurosurgical scans, and use the formal reports to help interpret them.

General principles of neuroanaesthesia

The basic principles of neuroanaesthesia are the same as for any other branch of anaesthesia. The anaesthetist is concerned with patient safety, providing optimal operating conditions and patient comfort, and facilitating prompt, safe recovery. The challenge for the neuroanaesthetist is to achieve all of this during procedures which risk significant injury to neural tissue. This section does not provide a recipe for every case, but is intended to give a guide to the general conduct of a 'standard' neuroanaesthetic.

Pre-operative issues

Pre-operative assessment

Pre-operative assessment is covered elsewhere (Pre-operative assessment, p.104). The pre-operative visit includes the anaesthetist introducing themselves to the patient, providing information to enable informed consent and establishing, prior to surgery, the patient's level of consciousness and understanding of the proposed procedure.

As with any major surgery, patients may be frightened about the proposed surgical procedure, the anaesthetic technique, the recovery from surgery, or the results of biopsies or samples taken during surgery. Establishing a rapport with the patient is important for all patients and particularly so if an awake procedure is planned (Awake craniotomy, p.242).

The pre-operative GCS and any other neurological deficit should be recorded.

Consent

Valid consent from the patient can only be given after a description of the proposed anaesthetic technique (and offering a choice if appropriate). This will include an explanation of the risks, the use of analgesia, and the potential for a blood transfusion (although blood is rarely used for most neurosurgical or neuroradiology procedures).

Anaesthetic consent in the UK is usually verbal (this is just as valid and as important as formal, written consent) and should be documented on the anaesthetic chart. For most neurosurgical procedures there is no realistic alternative to general anaesthesia. However, the broad outline of the technique should be described, including the use of invasive monitoring, urinary catheters and central lines (if appropriate). Plans for analgesia and postoperative care, including the use of a high dependency unit (HDU) or ICU if either is planned or possible should be explained.

An incapable patient may not be able to give consent. In the UK, consent from a relative or other next-of-kin is not valid, unless they have been granted Lasting Power of Attorney or have been appointed as a proxy decision maker under the terms of the Mental Capacity Act (2005). However good practice suggests that relatives should be informed of the procedure and be given an opportunity to ask questions. In an emergency, action taken in the patient's best interest will usually be supported by the Courts.

Premedication

Premedication is rarely used in modern anaesthetic practice, and sedative premedication has been avoided in neuroanaesthesia for many years except in very anxious patients who are otherwise neurologically intact, i.e. GCS 15.

The patient's normal medication is usually given on the day of surgery, with the exception of ACE inhibitors and angiotension II antagonists. Occasionally an H_2 antagonist or proton pump inhibitor will be given patients at risk of aspiration, although there is no evidence this reduces the frequency or severity of aspiration pneumonitis. Patients due to undergo awake fibreoptic intubation may be given an antisialogogue, e.g. hyoscine or glycopyrrolate.

Induction of anaesthesia

Monitoring

The minimum standard for intra-operative monitoring in the UK is detailed in the Association of Anaesthetists of Great Britain and Ireland publication *Recommendations for standards of monitoring during anaesthesia and recovery* (http://www.aagbi.org). Other specialist monitors such as transcranial Doppler, jugular bulb saturation monitoring, ICP bolts, EEG and BIS are covered in Chapter 3.

Alarms

Alarms are only useful if set to appropriate values. This includes alarm limits on infusion devices, anaesthetic agent monitors and ventilators.

Intra-arterial blood pressure monitoring

All but the most minor neurosurgical procedures will require invasive blood pressure monitoring. In addition to allowing accurate manipulation of blood pressure and calibration of end-tidal carbon dioxide ($ETCO_2$) levels, beat-to-beat arterial pressure monitoring provides some warning about neurological damage due to surgical traction or compression of nervous tissue.

Peripheral nerve stimulator

A peripheral nerve stimulator is used to measure depth of neuromuscular blockade and should be used whenever muscle relaxants are used. The motor response to electrical stimulation is usually made by a subjective, visual assessment of 'train-of-four'. In neuroanaesthesia, peripheral nerve stimulators are used in three main ways:
- at tracheal intubation of the trachea—to avoid increases in ICP caused by inadequate paralysis of the vocal cords
- intra-operative monitoring when an infusion of neuromuscular blocking drug is used
- prior to extubation to guide the administration of neuromuscular blockade 'reversal' (neostigmine or sugammadex).

Temperature monitoring

Bladder, oesophageal, and tympanic measuring devices all produce readings that are consistent with brain temperature over a normal clinical range. Rectal temperature readings show poorer correlation. Due to the deleterious effects of hyperthermia on the brain, a patient's core temperature should be measured whenever warming devices are being used.

Central venous pressure monitoring
There are no absolute indications in neuroanaesthesia. Situations where CVP catheters are commonly sited include:
- Cases where VAE is a risk, e.g. the sitting position.
- Significant intra-operative risk of major haemorrhage.
- Intracranial aneurysm clipping—when intravascular fluid depletion may exacerbate hypoperfusion secondary to vasospasm.
- To measure central venous pressures as a guide to peri-operative fluid administration in patients with cardiac comorbidities.
- Administration of drugs that may only be delivered via a central vein.
- Long-term intravenous access, e.g. for antibiotic therapy.

Cardiac output monitoring
Over the past 10 years the use of pulmonary artery flotation catheters has declined in UK practice, with the focus shifting to more non-invasive cardiac output measurement devices. Arterial pulse wave analysis and transoesophageal Doppler have both been used to guide intravenous fluid administration in neurosurgery and may be of value in patients with significant cardiac comorbidity. However, their use is exceptional, rather than routine.

Precordial Doppler ultrasound
This is the most sensitive monitor for the detection of VAE. It will detect VAE before cardiopulmonary changes become manifest on other monitoring devices (e.g. oesophageal stethoscope, $ETCO_2$, IABP or CVP).

Induction agents

Induction of anaesthesia is usually with intravenous drugs. While inhalational induction may be used occasionally in uncooperative or anxious children (see Paediatric neuroanaesthesia, p.120) there are no absolute indications in adult practice. Wide bore intravenous access (minimum 16G) should be placed.
- The most commonly used intravenous agents are propofol and thiopental.
- Etomidate is usually avoided due to concerns about its effects on cerebral blood flow.
- Ketamine has no place in neuroanaesthesia, due to changes in cerebral blood flow and ICP (although its use a neuroprotective agent is being studied).
- A co-induction technique with an opioid is used for major intracranial surgery.
- Remifentanil is the commonest opioid (although there is no evidence for a better outcome than after fentanyl or alfentanil). Remifentanil is usually given as a bolus followed by an infusion, or by TCI infusion.
- For more minor intracranial surgery and most spinal surgery, boluses of fentanyl are an alternative.

While it is important to ensure adequate depth of anaesthesia, patients with raised ICP are at risk of brain hypoperfusion if the systemic blood pressure falls. In particular acute brain-injured patients (especially those with other major injuries) are very sensitive to these agents, which should be used with great care. Agents should be prepared for urgent manipulation of blood pressure.

Airway management

Nearly all neurosurgical procedures are performed with a tracheal tube in place and with mechanical lung ventilation. This is because of the need to control $PaCO_2$ carefully, the use of positions other than supine, and the lack of access to the airway once surgical drapes are in place.

- Tracheal intubation is undertaken with neuromuscular blockade.
- In patients at risk of raised ICP, care should be taken to avoid laryngoscopy and tracheal intubation before full muscle relaxation is in place.
- The airway is maintained with a face mask and oral airway (if needed) until TOF stimulation shows complete relaxation.
- In patients with a potentially full stomach a rapid sequence induction may be used.
- Rapid sequence induction (RSI) with just thiopental and suxamethonium is associated with large swings in blood pressure. A 'modified' induction with use of an opioid or high-dose rocuronium in addition to the intravenous induction agent is commonly used.
- Other drugs may be given before laryngoscopy to obtund the pressor response such as a second dose of induction agent, opioids and β-blockers.

Tracheal tube

Normal practice is to use a reinforced (spiral wound) tracheal tube though some centres use pre-formed 'RAE' tubes or similar.

- Reinforced tubes cannot be cut to length and are easily placed too far into the trachea. Most have a marker line (or lines) which guide the user to the correct insertion length. Tube position must be checked after final taping to ensure it has not slipped in too far.
- If a patient already has a tracheal tube in place, for example having been transferred from another hospital, the anaesthetist should consider changing it over a bougie for a reinforced tube prior to surgery.
- Reinforced tubes are used as they resist kinking better than standard plastic tubes after they reach body temperature.
- The tracheal tube must be secured in place. Tube ties are not used as these impede venous drainage from the head. Most units have their own technique to secure the tracheal tube; typically this includes a combination of fabric Elastoplast and other sticky tape.
- A laryngeal mask airway is occasionally used for starved patients if close control of $PaCO_2$ is not required.
- With use of copious skin preparation solutions some may seep onto the face, and attempts should be made to waterproof the tube securing tape and protect the eyes as much as possible (see below).

Eye protection

The eyes are at risk during neurosurgical procedures for three reasons: they are inaccessible; they are prone to pressure from instruments, supports or staff; and skin prep, blood, CSF and wash can all seep over or collect around the eyes.

CHAPTER 4 General principles of neuroanaesthesia

- The most important protection for the eyes is to ensure that they are closed.
- The closed eyelids are covered with paraffin gauze and the eyes are usually covered and made watertight with sticky tape.
- It is imperative that there is no pressure on the eye from the taping, the face and head supports in prone or laterally positioned patients, or from surgical instruments or the arms of surgical staff.
- Commercial eyeshields are available, but injuries have been reported with these as well.

Throat pack
The use of throat packs in all neurosurgical patients has become standard practice, even though there are few operations in which there is a risk of contamination of the larynx or trachea with blood (one is transphenoidal hypophysectomy).
- The reasons to place a throat pack are to:
  - stabilize the tracheal tube
  - to soak up secretions, particularly in patients who are prone.
- Throat packs are not without risk. They cause postoperative sore throat, they may be associated with oral/laryngeal trauma, and there are numerous reports of failure to remove the throat pack at the end of the procedure.
- Good practice is that part of the pack is left out of the mouth and attached to the tracheal tube so that the tube cannot be removed while the pack remains throat pack is still in place. If placed, its use must be recorded on the anaesthetic chart and its removal witnessed by another member of the team. Specific guidance for UK practice is available from the NPSA.

Asleep or awake (fibre-optic) intubation
There are few indications for elective awake intubation in neuroanaesthesia. Even patients with cervical spine disease are usually easy to intubate with a standard laryngoscope. Some patients with widespread osteoarthritis of the spine will be more difficult. Patients with acromegaly may have increased soft tissue around the airway but are still easy to intubate. Patients with some specific cervical spine diseases such as ankylosing spondylitis or severe rheumatoid arthritis leading to atlanto-axial subluxation may be more difficult and planned awake intubation is a suitable technique to offer the patient.

The anaesthetist may elect to perform awake intubation in a patient whose neurology alters with head and neck movement. Their neurology can then be reassessed following intubation prior to general anaesthesia.

Urinary catheterization
This is necessary for prolonged procedures, patients with raised intracranial pressure who may require osmotic diuresis with mannitol, and patients who are expected to remain unconscious postoperatively. Urine output is a good surrogate for volaemic status providing a diuretic has not been given.

GENERAL PRINCIPLES OF NEUROANAESTHESIA

Positioning

This is covered in Chapter 5. Care should be taken when positioning the patient as this is a time when attention may be drawn away from the patient, and often monitoring is partially interrupted to allow turning or transfer from the trolley to operating table.

Maintenance of anaesthesia

Nitrous oxide is avoided for intracranial procedures. Overall, there is little objective evidence to help choose between TIVA (with propofol) or inhalational anaesthesia (usually with sevoflurane; see Chapter 4). For major intracranial surgery a remifentanil infusion is used and reduces the requirement for either propofol or sevoflurane.

Anaesthesia depth can be titrated against either clinical signs or with a depth of anaesthesia monitor. Good communication between the surgical and anaesthetic teams is vital in order for surgical stimulation to be adequately covered with appropriate analgesia, for example prior to the insertion of head pins and 'knife to skin'. Once the brain substance is exposed (after the craniotomy and opening of the dura) there is often little surgical stimulation, as the brain contains no sensory pain nerve endings. It is important to maintain an adequate perfusion pressure (see below) so little anaesthesia may be needed; there may be concern that anaesthesia is too light. Use of sympathomimetic and vasopressor agents has become routine—with ephedrine and metaraminol being most commonly used.

Spinal surgery is often undertaken with fentanyl boluses followed by long-acting opioids such as morphine. There is less risk from the use of nitrous oxide for extradural operations.

Blood pressure control

In the absence of other indications the blood pressure is usually maintained with a MAP ~70–80 mmHg. The range of acceptable blood pressure will need to take into account the patient's age, their pre-morbid blood pressure, and their overall cardiac status.

Hypotension

Some authorities state that a fall in blood pressure greater than a certain percentage (e.g. a fall of >20% from baseline) should be treated. The problem with such a strategy is deciding which baseline pressure to use.

Induced hypotension is rarely used because it is believed that areas of the brain affected by, or near to, pathological lesions may not autoregulate normally and any falls in blood pressure may be associated with hypoperfusion. Furthermore, after subarachnoid haemorrhage, vasospasm may result in flow through affected arteries being pressure dependent. Evidence from jugular bulb venous catheters has shown that falls in blood pressure are associated with increased oxygen extraction suggesting relative hypoperfusion. Finally, evidence from head-injured patients has shown that episodes of hypotension (early, post-resuscitation and intraoperative) are associated with a poor outcome. Generally, hypotension should be avoided and, if it occurs, should be corrected.

The use of fluid loading (see below), vasopressors (such as metaraminol) or sympathomimetic agents (such as ephedrine) is common (see Chapter 2).

Noradrenaline is used in ICU to maintain blood pressure in some head injury patients (see Chapter 11).

Hypovolaemia is often a contributing factor for intra-operative (and postoperative) hypotension. The risk of creating (or worsening) cerebral oedema has been overstated in the past, and providing isotonic fluids are used, some fluid loading (for example 250–500 ml of isotonic fluid over 10–15 min) is safe in most patients. Long procedures combined with slow but continuous blood loss may result in a large total blood loss over several hours.

Hypertension

Diagnosing hypertension poses an equally difficult question as deciding the lower limit of acceptable pressure; in SAH patients the upper limit is set higher than in most other patients due to the risk of vasospasm. In general a MAP >100 mmHg usually warrants treatment. As with all other anaesthetics, it is essential to first make sure that patient is anaesthetized to an adequate depth. Even if this is so, an increase in anaesthesia is used as the first line treatment (providing the dose of volatile is not above that which lead to disruption of autoregulation i.e. 1.2 MAC for sevoflurane), for example, by increasing the infusion rate of remifantanil. If further agents are required the commonest agents are beta-blockers such as esmolol or labetalol (see Chapter 2). Vasodilators are avoided, if possible, because of the risk of arterial and venous vasodilatation contributing to an increase in ICP.

Carbon dioxide control

Due to the unpredictable difference between arterial and end-tidal CO_2 tensions, an arterial blood gas sample should be analysed in all patients where the brain is 'tight' or when undergoing prolonged surgery. The difference can vary from 0.5 kPa to 1.5 kPa.

There is no indication for routine hyperventilation to provide a 'slack' brain for the surgeon. Marked hyperventilation risks hypoperfusion secondary to vasoconstriction, therefore only mild hyperventilation, aiming for a CO_2 at the lower end of the normal range should be used (arterial CO_2 ~4.5 kPa). The only indication to aim for a lower CO_2 is in extremis, when brain swelling is so marked that the operation cannot continue and the brain is protruding through the craniotomy. For more details on the management of intra-operative brain swelling see Chapter 4.

Intra-operative fluids

As described above, blood loss in long duration operations may be greater than realized or measured. As hypotension is poorly tolerated, a euvolaemic state is maintained with isotonic fluids. As with other organs, the brain can tolerate a modest fall in haematocrit, and 'lost' blood should not be replaced immediately. Due to concerns regarding hyperchloraemic acidosis, Hartmann's solution (compound sodium lactate) is used initially, in preference to 0.9% saline. Colloid solutions are used, although there is a risk of dilutional coagulopathy if large amounts are given.

As postoperative bleeding is such a feared complication, it is important to ensure clotting is kept normal by transfusion of adequate clotting factors and platelets if blood loss has been significant. In head injured patients, disseminated intravascular coagulation (DIC) is common.

Transfusion triggers for red cells administration are identical to those in usual anaesthetic/ICU practice.

Temperature control
Body temperature has a direct effect upon the normal and the ischaemic brain and thus the control of a patient's temperature is of great importance. Induced hypothermia has not been shown to improve outcome after neurosurgery and is associated with deleterious effects. Hyperthermia is associated with an increase in mortality after ischaemic and traumatic brain injury and should be aggressively treated. 📖 For full details see Chapter 4.

Other peroperative drugs
📖 The pharmacology of drugs relevant to neuroanaesthesia is discussed more fully in Chapter 2.

Antibiotics
These are given at surgical discretion. There is little evidence of benefit for routine use for intracranial or spinal surgery unless there is pre-existing infection, use of surgical access through an airspace or nose, or if an implant is to be placed. It recommended that antibiotics should be administered up to 60 min prior to 'knife to skin'.

Steroids
Patients with presumed tumours will often been started on oral steroids (usually dexamethasone). A further bolus dose should be given after induction, although the optimal dose is unclear. If there is a suspicion of intracranial lymphoma, steroids are withheld as they may obscure the histological picture. If in doubt, check with the surgeon.

There is no evidence to support the use of steroids in other situations (except as replacement therapy for patients with pituitary disease) or as prophylaxis for PONV. In particular, their use for head injuries has been abandoned.

DVT prophylaxis
Neurosurgical patients are at risk of deep vein thrombosis (DVT) and pulmonary embolism (PE), but the role of heparin prophylaxis is unclear and the risk of postoperative haemorrhage may outweigh the benefit. Mechanical methods of DVT prevention such as compression stockings or pneumatic compression devices may be used intra- and postoperatively, and early mobilization is encouraged whenever possible.

Mannitol
Mannitol is given intra-operatively if there is evidence of acute brain swelling (📖 see Chapter 4). There is no role for routine use for elective surgery.

Emergence
Emergence from anaesthesia is as important as induction. The risks to the brain from hypoperfusion, surges in arterial pressure or ICP and hypoxia may be easily overlooked while the patient is 'awakening'. There are many distractions such as arrival of the patient's bed in theatre, surgeons and theatre staff clearing away used instruments and equipment and the imminent arrival of the next patient.

While a smooth emergence and tracheal extubation are ideal, there are conflicting requirements for the patient to be as awake as possible, with a clear airway. Some neurosurgical procedures are more painful, such as major spinal surgery and temporo-parietal craniotomy. Suitable analgesia with simple and opioid-based agents will help smooth emergence. Many anaesthetists try to maintain a calm atmosphere and an undisturbed patient during emergence. Preventing excess stimulation from hair washing, movement from the operating table to bed, and premature attempts to produce spontaneous ventilation and eye opening will assist.

Many pharmacological agents have been used to obtund the hypertensive and coughing response to extubation including beta-blockers and small boluses of intravenous induction agents. Most UK practitioners use an opioid such as a low-dose remifentanil infusion until extubation is complete.

The airway should be immediately assessed and failure to maintain a good airway with adequate ventilation and oxygenation should precipitate urgent action including, if necessary, re-intubation.

The level of consciousness is also assessed. Not withstanding the presence of opioids for analgesia and residual anaesthetic agents, the patient's GCS should be at, or very near the pre-operative level. In some situations it should be better—for example after draining of intracranial blood collections such as subdural and extradural haematomas or after shunts and external ventricular drains (EVDs) for hydrocephalus. Failure to achieve this degree of recovery should lead to urgent neurological assessment and imaging. The most feared complication of anaesthesia and surgery is an intracranial haemorrhage (see below).

Postoperative management

Analgesia

Pain after neurosurgical procedures is common and may be severe. 📖 Postoperative analgesia is covered in Chapter 12.

Postoperative care

There is no convincing evidence that where patients are managed postoperatively alters outcome and different neurosurgical units have different policies regarding where and how postoperative patients are managed. 📖 Factors which may suggest a need for postoperative care in a HDU/ICU environment are discussed in Chapter 12.

Postoperative complications

Bleeding

Postoperative bleeding after intracranial procedures (or intradural spinal surgery) is feared as the rigid skull does not allow any degree of compensation.

- The surgeon will ensure that all active bleeding points are stopped and the anaesthetist can contribute by ensuring that clotting is normal.
- NSAIDs are usually avoided after intracranial surgery although the evidence that they contribute to postoperative bleeding is slight.
- There is no evidence that raising the blood pressure intra-operatively provides better clues to the site of likely bleeding points.
- However, avoiding hypertension during emergence and the initial postoperative period, is considered good practice.

GENERAL PRINCIPLES OF NEUROANAESTHESIA

Failure to recover consciousness
Failure to recover to a conscious level at or near to the pre-operative state within a few minutes of emergence warrants investigation: a full neurological assessment including GCS; pupillary responses; and evidence of motor lateralizing signs. If a haematoma is suspected then a CT scan is performed.

Seizures
Anti-epileptics are not used routinely after straightforward craniotomy. If seizures occur, they are managed with a loading dose of phenytoin. If this is unsuccessful, then either benzodiazepines or, if necessary, intravenous induction agents are used (see Chapter 12). Status epilepticus, including non-convulsive (when no fitting is observed), is one cause of failure to regain consciousness.

Hypotension
Postoperative hypotension is due to hypovolaemia in most cases. This may be accentuated by warming leading to peripheral vasodilation. Intracranial bleeding is very unlikely to cause hypovolaemia. However, bleeding from skin edges or after spinal surgery can be significant. As described above, hypotension is poorly tolerated. Initial treatment will include assessment of the cause, a fluid bolus and management of other factors. Persistent hypotension requires more extensive investigation, for example for a cardiac cause.

Hypertension
Postoperative hypertension is most often due to pain or a rebound/protective mechanism (i.e. a Cushing's-type response). The exact pressure that can be safely tolerated is dependent on many factors, and sudden falls in blood pressure from previously high levels may also be harmful. Pain should be treated. If a Cushing's response is suspected the cause should be sought—perform a neurological examination for evidence of a mass lesion. There is an association between systolic pressures >160 mmHg and postoperative intracranial haemorrhage. Emergence and postoperative care should be tailored to minimize the occurrence and duration of hypertension. If hypertension does occur, it is a matter of clinical judgement regarding how aggressively to treat it. Vasodilators are usually avoided because of their effects on the cerebral vessels.

Tips and pitfalls

- The art of neurosurgical anaesthesia is the ability to maintain the normal in the face of numerous abnormal physiological insults.
- Sudden surges in arterial blood pressure may suggest irritation or damage to nervous tissue.
- Despite numerous advances in technology, the best monitoring device remains the observant anaesthetist.
- Emergence is just as an important/risky part of neuroanaesthesia as induction.
- Smooth induction and emergence are an art, based on science. Most anaesthetists have been trying to perfect their techniques for many years. Blindly copying a senior colleague's technique is likely to result in less than ideal conditions.

Paediatric neuroanaesthesia

Optimal anaesthetic care requires an understanding of paediatric neurophysiology and pathophysiology, supported by the knowledge and skills of paediatric anaesthesia.

Central nervous system development
The neonate is neurologically immature.
- The blood–brain barrier (BBB) is structurally and functionally incomplete.
- Significant CNS development (myelination and dendritic proliferation) continues after birth, and for the first year of life.
- The newborn brain weighs about 335 g and comprises 10–15% of total body weight. Brain mass doubles by 6 months, is 900 g at 1 year, and reaches adult size (1200–1400 g) by the age of 12 years (1–2% total body weight).
- At birth fibrous sutures and the posterior and anterior fontanelles separate the ossified plates of the calvarium.
  - The posterior and anterior fontanelles close at 2–3 months and 10–18 months of age, respectively, though ossification is not complete until adolescence.
  - Expansion of the fontanelles and separation of the fibrous sutures allow slow increases in intracranial volume to be accommodated in young children.
  - Until it closes gross changes in ICP may be estimated by palpation of the anterior fontanelle.
- Differential growth of the spinal cord and vertebral canal cause increasingly cephalad termination of the spinal cord.
  - At 28 weeks post-conception it terminates at the level of S1; in the term baby it is at L3; it reaches its adult position of L1–2 by 8 years.

Neurophysiology
The extent of understanding of paediatric neurophysiology is incomplete compared with adults, but there are some known, important differences to consider.

Cerebral blood flow
As in adults CBF depends upon cerebral metabolic rate, cerebral perfusion pressure, $PaCO_2$, and PaO_2, and blood viscosity. The metabolic demands of the young brain vary with age, and are higher than in adults.
- At 6 years $CMRO_2$ is 5.8 ml min^{-1} 100 g^{-1} and glucose requirements are 6.8 mg min^{-1} 100 g^{-1}, compared with 3.5 ml min^{-1} 100 g^{-1} and 5.5 mg min^{-1} 100 g^{-1} in adults.
- In neonates global cerebral blood flow is around 40 ml min^{-1} 100 g^{-1}. This is similar to the adult CBF of around 50 ml min^{-1} 100 g^{-1}.
  - During the period of rapid neurological growth CBF increases, and is 90 ml min^{-1} 100 g^{-1} at 6 months.
  - CBF peaks at 3–4 years at 100–110 ml min^{-1} 100 g^{-1}, then declines to 80 ml min^{-1} 100 g^{-1} at 9 years.

- The cerebrovascular response to changes in $PaCO_2$ is immature at birth.
  - The neonatal cerebral circulation is relatively insensitive to moderate hypocapnia, but is more responsive to small decreases in PaO_2 than the adult brain.
- The limits of autoregulation of CBF in infants and children are incompletely defined.
  - As in adults, autoregulation is impaired in the injured or diseased brain. In areas of focal pathology autoregulation may be absent and perfusion becomes pressure-dependent.
  - Critically ill neonates have altered autoregulation and are at risk of intraventricular haemorrhage.

Intracranial pressure

Normal ICP in neonates and infants is 2–4 mmHg, lower than in adults and older children (8–18 mmHg). ICP is positive at birth, but becomes negative in the first few days of life as salt and water are lost and cerebral volume decreases. This may contribute to the vulnerability of premature neonates to intraventricular haemorrhage.

- Slow rises in intracranial volume may be accommodated in children with open fontanelles and fibrous sutures.
- In older children, or if change is acute, the cranium behaves as a rigid box, as in adults.
  - The pressure volume index, a measure of intracranial elastance, is higher in children than in adults. Rapid increases in intracranial volume will therefore cause rapid neurological deterioration.

Hydrocephalus

Hydrocephalus occurs when CSF volume increases within the ventricular system. This is usually secondary to obstruction of CSF circulation, or due to reduced CSF absorption.

- ICP may be raised or normal.
- Tumours are the commonest cause of childhood hydrocephalus.
- In neonates causes of hydrocephalus include intraventricular haemorrhage, neural tube defects and the Arnold–Chiari malformation in which anatomical abnormalities cause downward displacement of the brainstem and compression of the fourth ventricle.

Neuropharmacology

The sensitivity of children to anaesthetic drugs varies with age. Neonates and premature infants have lower anaesthetic requirements than older children and are more sensitive to opioid and barbiturate drugs (due to an immature CNS and BBB). The CNS depressant effects of anaesthetic agents may be compounded by sudden changes in intracranial volume (e.g. following shunts) in pre-term and ex-preterm infants, increasing the risk of postoperative apnoea. Neurophysiological effects of commonly used anaesthetic drugs are similar in children and adults.

- Volatile anaesthetic agents increase CBF, but autoregulation and CO_2 responsiveness are preserved during isoflurane or sevoflurane anaesthesia at 0.5–1.0 MAC.
- N_2O is a cerebral vasodilator and, in contrast to volatile agents, has been shown to increase $CMRO_2$. It may be used during gaseous induction of anaesthesia, although it is more usual to use an oxygen/air mixture if there are concerns regarding cerebral perfusion or raised ICP.
- With the exception of ketamine, intravenous agents reduce both CBF and $CMRO_2$.
- Total intravenous anaesthesia (TIVA), using propofol and remifentanil, has theoretical advantages for intracranial surgery.
  - TCI algorithms and programmable pumps facilitate the use of propofol for intravenous anaesthesia. The alogorithms account for the high central volume of distribution and more rapid clearance in children compared with adults.
  - TIVA is usually only used with specific indications such as during procedures where the motor evoked potentials are to be monitored.
  - Propofol infusion syndrome is a potentially fatal complication of propofol infusion and has been reported more commonly in children than in adults. It is related to both dose and duration of infusion. It is rare when infusions are used for less than 48 h and when the dose is <5 mg kg^{-1} h^{-1}.

Anaesthesia

Pre-operative assessment

The emphasis is on assessment of neurological status. In addition to routine history and examination, the degree of neurological deficit should be assessed. Clinical presentation of intracranial hypertension varies according to the time course of illness and age of patient. Younger children and infants may present non-specifically with lethargy, reduced appetite and loss of developmental milestones. An increase in head circumference, or a bulging fontanelle may also be found. Older children present with more classical symptoms: headache; visual disturbance; nausea and vomiting; and an altered level of consciousness. An age-specific GCS is useful if conscious level is reduced (see p.98). Measures to control intracranial pressure may be required before proceeding to definitive surgery.

Aspiration risk is assessed. Raised ICP may cause delayed gastric emptying. Brainstem lesions may be associated with bulbar palsies and loss of airway protective reflexes.

Vomiting and anorexia, and administration of diuretics may lead to dehydration and biochemical abnormalities. Fluid losses are replaced pre-operatively, and renal profile should be checked and corrected as necessary. Endocrine abnormalities, diabetes insipidus, syndrome of inappropriate antidiuretic hormone hypersecretion (SIADH) and seizure control are optimized pre-operatively.

A baseline full blood count and group and save samples are taken. For major intracranial surgery, e.g. tumour resection or craniofacial reconstruction, blood is cross-matched. Around 10–15 ml kg^{-1} of packed cells should be available. For neonates a single donor unit may be split into paediatric packs. This helps to reduce exposure to different donors should multiple transfusions be required.

Neuroradiological images should be reviewed to confirm the site and extent of intracranial pathology.

Cardiovascular disease is rare in children. ECG and echocardiography should be considered in children with congenital syndromes associated with cardiac abnormalities. Brainstem lesions occasionally cause dysrhythmias which require investigation to exclude intrinsic cardiac disease prior to surgery. Short-acting agents are recommended if medical treatment is required, as the effects of surgery are unpredictable.

Anaesthetic consent

The pre-operative visit is an opportunity to establish a rapport with the patient and his/her parents. The nature of the surgery and relevant anaesthetic risks should be discussed. In particular, positioning of the patient, the need for invasive monitoring, the potential use of blood and blood products, and location and type of planned postoperative care are addressed.

Premedication

Routine use of sedative premedication is avoided because of the risk of respiratory depression and hypercapnia in patients with raised ICP. However, in very anxious or uncooperative patients with normal ICP, oral premedication is acceptable, e.g. midazolam 0.5 mg kg^{-1} (max 15 mg).

Induction and tracheal intubation

A compromise is reached between theoretical neuroanaesthetic principles and the realities of anaesthetizing children.

- Intravenous induction is preferred (propofol 2–4 mg kg^{-1} or thiopentone 4–7 mg kg^{-1}), but a smooth inhalation induction with sevoflurane in oxygen or a 50/50 mix oxygen/nitrous oxide is superior to fraught attempts at cannulation.
- A neuromuscular blocking drug (e.g. rocuronium 0.6 mg kg^{-1} or atracurium 0.5 mg kg^{-1}) is given to facilitate tracheal intubation.
- Short-acting opioids will obtund the CVS response to laryngoscopy.
- If there is a risk of aspiration, RSI and the use of cricoid pressure should be considered.
  - Emergent situations, e.g. head trauma, are usually managed with classic RSI, using an intravenous induction agent and succinylcholine 1–2 mg kg^{-1}. In other situations a modified technique, using rocuronium 0.8–1 mg kg^{-1}, may be used.

- Reinforced tracheal tubes, placed orally, are suitable for most procedures.
  - An internal diameter half a size (0.5 mm) smaller than predicted maybe needed to compensate for the greater external diameter of these tubes compared with standard tracheal tubes.
- Nasal intubation facilitates stable fixation of the tracheal tube.
  - Nasal intubation may be the preferred choice for neonates and infants, particularly for prone positioning.
- Bilateral lung ventilation is confirmed with the head in neutral and operative positions, and the tube secured.

Maintenance of anaesthesia

Balanced anaesthesia using sevoflurane in oxygen/air allows hyperventilation to a low-normal $PaCO_2$ for control of ICP. Nitrous oxide may be used for short procedures in young children, if ICP is normal, and there is minimal venous air embolism (VAE) risk. In children with intracranial mass lesions, or raised ICP, nitrous oxide is contra-indicated. Intra-operative analgesia is provided using fentanyl 2–5 µg kg^{-1} for short procedures, or a remifentanil infusion, titrated to surgical stimulus for more complex surgery. Target-controlled infusions of remifentanil can be used for children >12 years and >30 kg.

Neuromuscular blockade is maintained either by intermittent bolus or by continuous infusion.

Positioning

As with adult surgery, positioning varies according to surgical site and local preference. The aim is to protect the patient, provide good surgical access, and optimize operating conditions. The operating field is compromised, and blood loss increased, if venous drainage is obstructed. Therefore, the tracheal tube is taped, not tied. Extra care is needed when rotating the head, or flexing the neck to expose the operating site. A 10° head-up tilt improves cerebral venous return.

Bony prominences are padded and limbs supported in a neutral position to prevent stretching or compression of peripheral nerves.

The eyes are closed and padded to protect against corneal injury or globe compression.

For intracranial procedures the head may be supported on a horseshoe rest, or held in pins. In children <3 years the use of pins may cause bony injury, intracranial haemorrhage or a dural tear and is generally avoided.

Supine position

Used for most supratentorial surgery. The head is turned to the side to expose the surgical site. Rotation of the torso with a sandbag under the shoulder along with the head and neck avoids venous obstruction.

Prone positioning.

Used for spinal surgery, correction of neural tube defects and for posterior fossa surgery. The patient must be supported on bolsters placed under the iliac crests, or a specialized frame, to allow free abdominal movement and facilitate intermittent positive pressure ventilation (IPPV).

Sitting position

In some centres this is preferred for posterior fossa surgery. The main reasons are to improve surgical access and orientation, reduce blood loss, lower intracranial pressures, reduce risk of cranial nerve injury, and improve postoperative recovery. There are two main concerns:

- *Cardiovascular instability:* reduced venous return during movement from supine to upright position causes postural hypotension. Strategies to attenuate pressure drop include slow-staged positioning, with continuous arterial pressure monitoring, infusion of crystalloid fluid 5–10 ml kg^{-1}, inflatable anti-shock trousers, or compression bandaging of legs and limiting volatile anaesthesia to ≤ 1 MAC at the time of positioning.
- *Venous air embolism* (VAE) and the risk of paradoxical air embolism (PAE). The reported incidence in children undergoing surgery in the sitting position varies according to the method used for detection. A large retrospective UK series, using capnography to detect a fall in end-tidal CO_2, found an incidence of 9.3%, with 20% of cases associated with arterial hypotension, and <5% associated with long term sequelae. Transoesophageal echocardiography (TOE) and precordial Doppler ultrasound are sensitive monitors. However, TOE is invasive and difficult to place in children <10 kg, while interference from diathermy limits the usefulness of Doppler ultrasound. A sudden drop in end-tidal CO_2 is highly suggestive of VAE, and this, together with a high index of suspicion, is the most commonly employed monitor. Prevention and management are as for adult patients.

Monitoring

Standard monitoring during maintenance of anaesthesia includes pulse oximeter, non-invasive blood pressure monitor (cuff width should cover approximately 2/3 of the upper arm, or other limb portion), ECG, airway gas analysis, and an airway pressure monitor. A pragmatic approach is taken to the timing of application. Application of monitoring prior to induction of anaesthesia is the 'gold standard'. The young or anxious child may not cooperate with this and it may not be possible to establish full monitoring until immediately after induction. Core temperature (oesophageal or rectal) is monitored in any child when the anticipated procedure time is >30 min. A nerve stimulator is used to monitor neuromuscular blockade.

Direct arterial pressure monitoring

This is indicated in children who are expected to have haemodynamic instability, e.g. some neuro-endoscopic procedures, procedures associated with large potential blood loss such as craniotomies for tumour excision, and major craniofacial surgery. The radial artery is generally preferred, but other peripheral arteries or the femoral artery maybe used. Central venous catheters are used less frequently. Indications include inadequate peripheral venous access, anticipated massive blood loss, planned infusion of drugs that require central administration, and surgery with a high risk of VAE. The choice of site depends on operator experience and the indication. Internal jugular vein cannulation in small children may result in venous obstruction.

Urine output
Monitored in children undergoing surgery associated with large intra-operative blood loss or if mannitol or other diuretics are given. Catherization is indicated for surgery involving the spinal cord and should be considered for procedures close to the hypothalamus and pituitary when diabetes insipidus may occur.

Fluid management

As for adult patients, isotonic crystalloid or colloid solutions are the mainstay of fluid replacement. The Holliday and Segar 4–2–1 formula (see Table 4.1) is used to calculate hourly maintenance requirements of 0.9 % saline for children over 8 weeks of age.

- Neonates will usually receive maintenance fluids as 10% dextrose with electrolytes added based on serum Na^+/K^+ prescribed individually.
- Older children do not require intra-operative dextrose and can receive all fluids as isotonic fluids (e.g. 0.9% NaCl, Hartmann's).
- Solutions such as 0.45% saline with 5% dextrose are contraindicated.
  - If inadvertently used at greater than maintenance amounts iatrogenic cerebral oedema (with associated mortality) may occur.
- The only indication for hypotonic fluids in neuroanaesthesia is the management of established diabetes insipidus.

Intra-operative blood loss

Tumour surgery, craniofacial reconstructive surgery and surgery for large neural tube defects may result in substantial blood loss. Measurement of loss is difficult as blood may be concealed in surgical drapes and diluted with irrigation fluids. However, swabs are weighed and small volume suction canisters (50–250 ml) used to collect and measure losses. The volume of irrigation fluid used is recorded. Blood loss may be slow and steady (craniofacial surgery) or swift and unexpected if a large vessel is injured.

Prior to starting surgery the allowable operative blood loss (ABL) can be estimated using the formula:

$$ABL = [HB_O]-[HB_L]/[HB_O] \times CBV$$

where CBV is the circulating blood volume, estimated according to age and weight of child (see Table 4.2), $[HB_O]$ is the pre-operative haemoglobin concentration and $[HB_L]$ is lowest acceptable peri-operative haemoglobin concentration, usually 7–8 g dl^{-1} in children with normal cardiovascular and respiratory physiology. Together with clinical assessment (e.g. capillary refill time), information from invasive monitoring, arterial blood gas analysis and peri-operative haematocrit measurement, ABL is used to guide transfusion. Once ABL is exceeded, on-going loss should be replaced with a mixture of packed red blood cells (PRBC) and colloid solutions to maintain the haematocrit around (Hb_L). This strategy will tend to minimize the number of donor units to which the child is exposed. In the absence of ongoing blood loss, to raise the measured haemoglobin $[HB_M]$ to a target concentration $[HB_T]$ using PRBC the following formula may be employed:

$$PRBC\ (ml) = [HB_T]—[HB_M] \times weight\ (kg) \times 3$$

Assuming normal pre-operative clotting and platelets:
- Clotting factors are likely to be required after approximately 1 blood volume loss. The need for clotting factors should be anticipated before this.
- Platelet counts are likely to fall below 100×10^9 ml^{-1} at between 1 and 2 blood volume loss. This should be anticipated (see Table 4.3).

Blood conservation strategies

The principles are same as for adult patients:
- Careful positioning
  - if prone ensure a free abdomen to prevent IVC obstruction
  - if supine use a head-up tilt to encourage drainage from neck veins
- Haemodilution.
- Hypotension.
- Cell salvage during non-tumour surgery.

Maintainance of temperature

- Minimize exposure.
- Ensure adequate ambient temperature. For neonatal surgery the theatre should be capable of warming to 28°C.
- Overhead radiant heaters may be used to prevent hypothermia during line insertion and positioning when small babies are exposed.
- Forced air blowers.
- Warmed fluids.
- Warm humidified gases.

Postoperative care

Consideration should be given to the level of postoperative care likely to be required during the pre-operative assessment. In the absence of pre-existing respiratory or cardiovascular disease few children require elective postoperative lung ventilation.

- All patients should be nursed on a specialist neurosciences ward postoperatively. For patients undergoing major or complex surgery the need for postoperative admission to critical care areas should be guided by local policy and the predicted need for critical care support postoperatively.
- Term neonates up to 50 weeks post-conceptual age and premature neonates up to 60 weeks post-conceptual age, neonates with anaemia of prematurity (Hb <10 g dl^{-1}) and neonates who experience large intracranial volume changes during surgery are at increased risk of postoperative apnoeas.
  - As a minimum, overnight apnoea and SpO_2 monitoring are required.

Postoperative analgesia

- Surgical infiltration of the wound with local anaesthetic is useful for some procedures, e.g. a ventriculoperitoneal (VP) shunt.
- At the end of surgery short-acting opioids are discontinued. If longer acting opioid-based analgesia is required, morphine 0.05–0.1 mg kg^{-1} may be used. The child is assessed in the recovery area, and further doses titrated as required.

- Regular paracetamol (oral or iv) is effective and has the advantage of being devoid of sedative side effects.
- NSAIDs are not usually used following intracranial procedures because of effects on platelet function. The concern is that even a small intracranial haematoma may have profound neurological impact. NSAIDs are used commonly after operations on the lumbar spine.
- Codeine phosphate is commonly used to manage mild to moderate pain.
- Intravenous opioids are indicated to provide analgesia after craniotomy. Depending on the nature of the surgery these may or may not need to be continued in the postoperative period.
- Key to the safe use of opioids for postoperative analgesia is careful titration and appropriate monitoring.
- Opioid analgesia is often no longer needed after 12 h, and rarely needed >36 h after surgery.

Tips and pitfalls
- Inadequate analgesia may result in postoperative hypertension and raised intracranial pressure, with consequent risks of neurological injury.
- Blood loss can be difficult to estimate in small infants. Measured losses may markedly underestimate the extent of bleeding.
- Anticipate the need for platelets or clotting factors early.
- Do not be afraid to ask for a surgical pause if you think you need time to catch up with fluids or clotting derangements.

Table 4.1 Maintenance fluid requirements for children using the Holliday and Segar formula

Weight of child	Hourly infusion rate
3–10 kg	4 mL kg^{-1} l^{-1}
11–20 kg	40 ml + 2 mL kg^{-1} l^{-1} for each kg >10 kg
>20 kg	60 ml + 1 mL kg^{-1} l^{-1} for each kg >20 kg

Table 4.2 Estimated circulating blood volume

Patient age	Blood volume (ml kg^{-1})
Premature neonate	90–100
Full term neonate	80–90
Infant (up to 1 year)	75–80
3–6 years	70–75
> 6 years	70

Table 4.3 Blood product replacement volumes

Component	Volume
Fresh frozen plasma	10–20 ml kg^{-1}
Platelets	10–20 ml kg^{-1}
Cryoprecipitate	5 ml kg^{-1}

Cerebral protection

Protecting the brain is of particular significance due to the delicate nature of nervous tissue itself, the risk of physical harm and the environment which the brain and other nervous tissue requires to survive.

- In general, nervous tissue does not regenerate once damaged (axons in peripheral nerves may re-grow).
- Substrate requirements, for oxygen and glucose in particular, mean that the brain is very sensitive to changes in its environment.
- It is often stated that the brain can only withstand four minutes of anoxia. Although the clinical situation is more complex, it is true that only very brief periods of abnormally low blood flow and substrate delivery can be tolerated.
- Cerebral protection involves ensuring the best possible environment for the brain, e.g. physical space, maintaining substrate delivery sufficient for metabolic needs and employing techniques which may protect the brain from the consequences of anoxia.
- Brain injury is not an all or none phenomenon; following injury some areas of neural tissue may be more vulnerable than others to insults.

Most cerebral protection is provided by avoidance of insults, rather than specific protective strategies *per se*. Adequate cerebral perfusion pressure and oxygen delivery are the mainstay of any cerebral protection strategy.

Specific neuroprotective strategies

If possible, protective strategies should be put in place before the ischaemic insult.

Hypothermia

Hypothermia has beneficial effects in experimental models of brain injury. The underlying mechanisms are incompletely understood. However, there is experimental evidence that hypothermia affects:

- Cerebral metabolic rate (reduced by 7% per °C fall in temperature).
- Metabolic processes such as adenosine triphosphate (ATP) depletion and calcium accumulation following injury.
- Immune and inflammatory responses to injury.
- Neurotransmitter release and their postsynaptic effects.
- Apoptosis (programmed cell death).

Hyperthermia is associated with a poor outcome after brain injury. However, well-conducted trials of mild hypothermia have failed to show a protective benefit when used after brain injury or during aneurysm surgery (when temporary clips may be applied).

There may be a role for hypothermia in comatose patients with return of circulation following cardiac arrest.

CEREBRAL PROTECTION

Glycaemic control
There is an association between poor outcome after brain injury and hyperglycaemia. Good practice suggests that blood glucose should be controlled to within normal levels.
- If known temporary insults are predicted (e.g. temporary clipping), the anaesthetist should ensure normoglycaemia beforehand.
- Insulin-induced hypoglycaemia must be avoided. (See p. 150.)

Intravenous anaesthetic agents
The commonly used intravenous anaesthetic agents such as thiopental, propofol, and etomidate all reduce cerebral metabolism by suppressing cerebral activity. This is thought to reduce the likelihood of exhausting ATP reserves during ischaemia.
- Such drug-induced coma (sometimes titrated against the EEG or CFAM until burst-suppression is achieved) will reduce the brain's requirements for metabolic substrates and oxygen.
- However, the benefit is limited. The pathophysiological processes involved in ischaemia–reperfusion injury are more complicated than just balancing function against metabolism. Other factors may obscure any benefit from these drugs.
- Drug-induced hypotension should be avoided.
- There is experimental evidence that the reduction in flow with etomidate is greater than the fall in metabolism and this agent should not be used for cerebral protection.

Inhalational agents
The inhaled anaesthetic agents such as sevoflurane, isoflurane, and desflurane reduce metabolism as well as preserving flow-metabolism coupling at low concentrations.

They may also induce a cellular protection similar to that seen with ischaemic preconditioning. This phenomenon is seen in all mammalian tissue, although patient benefit has only been shown in cardiac tissue at present. Opioids may have a similar effect.

Seizure control
Seizures dramatically increase the brain's requirement for oxygen and substrates. Seizures may be difficult to detect especially if the only sign of status epilepticus is failure to recover consciousness after surgery or during periods of neuromuscular blockade. Prompt control is essential. (See p. 374.)

Pharmacological agents
There is experimental evidence for benefit from many therapeutic agents including albumin, ketamine (and other NMDA antagonists) and magnesium, but evidence from *in vivo* studies is either absent or has failed to show any clinically significant benefit.

CHAPTER 4 General principles of neuroanaesthesia

Tips and pitfalls
- Prevention of secondary injury is an obvious cerebral protection strategy.
- Outcome data from brain-injured patients suggests that hypoxia and, in particular, hypotension are associated with a poor outcome after brain injury.
- Avoid anaesthetic techniques or procedures which reduce blood pressure precipitously.
- There is little clinical evidence in favour of any of the currently used techniques or drugs.
- Treat seizures promptly.

TIVA or volatile-based anaesthesia

The most common anaesthesia technique for neurosurgical and neuroradiological procedures is intravenous induction followed by balanced anaesthesia with either propofol-based TIVA or volatile-based anaesthesia. In the UK sevoflurane is most commonly used but isoflurane or desflurane can be substituted.

Role of nitrous oxide
Evidence of harm in elective neurosurgical patients from nitrous oxide is lacking. However, in patients at risk of brain ischaemia (or with actual ischaemia), there are theoretical reasons and some limited evidence that nitrous oxide may be harmful. (See p. 30.)

Whether a TIVA or volatile-based technique is planned, nitrous oxide is unnecessary and easily replaced by a remifentanil infusion.

TIVA
To most anaesthetists TIVA implies an infusion, either manually adjusted or TCI (target-controlled infusion) of propofol. Other agents have been used.
- Thiopental is still used to produce drug-induced coma and metabolic suppression in severe TBI with raised ICP.
- Etomidate has no place as an infusion and bolus doses have been associated with marked reduction in cerebral blood flow in animal models.
- Ketamine has been avoided in patients with head injuries because of its effect on ICP (increased). However, there is renewed interest in this agent as it may be a cerebral protectant due to its NMDA antagonist properties.
- Propofol possesses properties that make it close to an ideal agent:
  - suppression of cerebral metabolism
  - preserves autoregulation and carbon dioxide reactivity
  - rapid recovery.

With a TCI system, propofol can be titrated against a clinical effect such as blood pressure or used with a depth of anaesthesia monitor such as the BIS system.

Disadvantages of propofol TIVA
- Concerns about propofol and seizures seem unwarranted. Although subcortical electrical activity can be detected in some patients on induction, this is not epilepsy. Propofol can be used to manage status epilepticus.
- Overdosage of propofol can be associated with hypotension, as with most other anaesthetic agents.
- High-dose, longer-term infusions can be associated with propofol infusion syndrome.
- Risk of awareness if the administration system is disconnected or blocked.

Volatile anaesthesia
There are theoretical reasons to prefer sevoflurane over isoflurane or desflurane. Sevoflurane is the most commonly used volatile for

neuroanaesthesia in the UK. However, there are no good outcome data suggesting superiority of one agent over another.
- Both sevoflurane and desflurane have fast recovery profiles, even after prolonged procedures. Isoflurane may result in relatively slow recovery.
- Desflurane is associated with increases in MAP and MCA FV when inspired concentrations are changed. It is not clear how important this is in patients receiving remifentanil or β-blockade, both of which may obtund this response.
- Sevoflurane has less effect on cerebral blood vessels at clinical concentrations than isoflurane or desflurane—resulting in less vasodilation and better maintenance of autoregulation, particularly if the MAC is kept below 1.2.
- The dose of all the volatile agents can be titrated against clinical effects such as blood pressure, depth of anaesthesia monitors or using the end-tidal concentration as a guide.

Disadvantages of volatile based anaesthesia
- Some countries (but not the UK) restrict use of sevoflurane at low fresh gas flow rates for long-duration procedures due to theoretical concerns about the build-up of toxic breakdown products in circle systems.
- Overdosage of volatile agents can be associated with hypotension, as with most other anaesthetic agents.

TIVA or volatile
There are only a few clinical studies comparing these techniques.
- Most studies used surrogate (such as surgeon assessment of brain conditions) or minor endpoints (such as speed of recovery).
- Studies of the relative speed of recovery of TIVA vs. volatile-based anaesthesia are conflicting.
- The difficulty of undertaking studies using neurological function (or dysfunction) after surgery as the outcome means there are few proper comparisons.
- The studies that do exist show little benefit of one technique over the other.

Tips and pitfalls
- TIVA may be preferred if the ICP is very high as any vasodilation may be detrimental. However, keep a watchful eye on the blood pressure.
- Remifentanil combined with either TIVA or volatile anaesthesia may also lead to hypotension.
- All these agents should be used with care in a shocked patient with a head injury.
- TIVA is required for some patients (e.g. stereotactic biopsies) who require anaesthesia during transfer to or from the CT scanner.

Intra-operative temperature control

Body temperature has a direct effect upon the functioning of the normal and the ischaemic brain. The control of a patient's temperature is therefore of great importance both in the operating theatre and on the neuro-critical care unit. Normothermia is typically defined as a core temperature of 36.5–37.5°C.

Hypothermia (core temperature <36°C)
Systemic effects
- *CNS*: $CMRO_2$ decreases by approximately 7% per °C decrease in temperature, with the EEG becoming isoelectric at temperatures below 20°C; confusion occurs <35°C.
- *CVS*: reduced cardiac output; ventricular arrhythmias; higher incidence of unstable angina and myocardial infarction postoperatively.
- *RS*: decreased oxygen demand and CO_2 production (by 50% for every 2°C decrease).
- *Coagulation*: impairment of clotting cascade and inhibition of platelet function; increased intra-operative blood loss and transfusion requirements.
- *Infection*: increased rate of wound infections.
- *Drugs*: prolonged duration of action of muscle relaxants; elevated plasma concentrations of propofol during TIVA; reduction in MAC of volatiles (approximately 5% per °C decrease).
- *Endocrine*: increased incidence of hyperglycaemia.

Numerous small studies have suggested a beneficial effect of mild intra-operative hypothermia in patients with traumatic or ischaemic brain injury. The International Hypothermia for Aneurysm Surgery Trial (IHAST) showed that induced intraoperative hypothermia (to 33°C) was not associated with an improvement in neurological outcome, but did result in a higher incidence of postoperative bacteraemia. Induced hypothermia (33°C for a minimum of 12 h) in survivors of a cardiac arrest has been shown to produce improvements in neurological outcome.

National guidance in the UK now advises that the induction of anaesthesia in elective patients should not take place unless their temperature is ≥36°C.

Management
- Pre-operative patient warming will help minimize the risk of intra-operative hypothermia.
- It may take up to 2 h to increase core temperature from 35 to 36°C.
- The most effective warming method appears to be forced air warming devices (e.g. BairHugger®), which have been shown to superior to heated gel mattresses, warmed cotton blankets or foil blankets. They should be used for all cases anticipated to take >30 min.
- Fluid warmers are effective at helping minimize patient cooling and should be used if >500 ml of fluid or packed red cells are given.
- Patients transferred from other hospitals are often hypothermic and will require aggressive rewarming on arrival.

Hyperthermia (core temperature ≥38°C)
Systemic effects
- CNS: once core temperature is >37°C, both CBF and $CMRO_2$ increase; confusion and seizures may occur.
- CVS: decrease in SVR with raised CO; increase in heart rate (HR).
- RS: increase in oxygen demand and CO_2 production; tachypnoea.
- Drugs: increased enzyme activity resulting in more rapid drug metabolism.
- Coagulation: platelet inhibition; DIC in severe cases.
- Endocrine: metabolic acidosis; hypoglycaemia if severe.

Hyperthermia is associated with an increase in mortality after ischaemic and traumatic brain injury and should be aggressively treated.

Post-traumatic hyperthermia (PTH) (or neurogenic fever) occurs as result of hypothalamic damage and complicates ~5% of head injuries. Temperatures tend to be very high for long periods of time but show no diurnal variation and patients tend not to sweat. PTH does not respond to antipyretic medication.

Management
- Localized cooling of the head is not as effective at reducing brain temperature as whole body cooling techniques.
- Paracetamol is an excellent antipyretic and in particularly good at reducing brain temperature. NSAIDs are less effective and are associated with a risk of bleeding.
- There is insufficient evidence to allow one cooling technique to be recommended over others. Options include:
  - Evaporative cooling—spraying of tepid water over exposed patient in the presence of cooling fans (can achieve falls of up to 2.5°C h^{-1})
  - Ice packing around groin, axillae, neck, and chest (often done in conjunction with evaporative cooling)
  - Gastric or peritoneal lavage
  - Cooled intravenous fluids—can be instituted immediately but will not produce a sustained cooling effect (1–1.5°C h^{-1})
  - Convectional cold water cooling—cooled water is passed through specially designed pads or blankets placed directly onto the skin (1–1.5°C h^{-1})
  - Air circulating cooling blankets (0.18°C h^{-1})
  - Intravascular cooling systems—modified central venous catheters that have cooled water passed through intravascular balloons (1°C h^{-1})
  - Extracorporeal cooling– but anticoagulation will be necessary (3.5°C h^{-1}).
- Shivering is a common side effect of cooling and will increase ICP. Neuromuscular blockade may be necessary.

Tips and pitfalls
- It is impossible to control a patient's temperature if it is not monitored.
- Bladder, oesophageal, and tympanic measuring devices all produce readings that are consistent with brain temperature over a normal clinical range. There can be a significant difference in cases of profound hypothermia.
- All fevers produce hyperthermia, but not all cases of hyperthermia are caused by fever.
- Neuroleptic malignant syndrome, malignant hyperthermia and the serotonergic syndrome are all rare causes of hyperthermia.

Management of intra-operative brain swelling

Acute intra-operative brain swelling poses acute challenges to the neuroanaesthetist. At its most extreme it is potentially life-threatening with acute herniation of brain tissue; with milder degrees of swelling the issue may be one of providing brain relaxation to facilitate surgical access.

It is most commonly seen after evacuation of post-traumatic intracranial heamatoma, but may also occur during elective procedures secondary to acute haemorrhage. The underlying causative mechanisms are unclear, but acute cerebral hyperaemia or brain tissue oedema have been postulated.

Presentation

Usually first noted by the operating surgeon, but if the cause is occult haemorrhage that is not within the surgical field, cardiovascular changes such as hypertension and bradycardia may be observed by the neuroanaesthetist.

Management

The principles of ICP reduction are identical whether the cranium is closed or open (see also Chapter 11)
- Communicate with the surgeon:
  - is there acute bleeding or hydrocephalus?
  - where are the surgical retractors?
- Exclude venous engorgement:
  - has the head been positioned correctly?
  - are tube ties or a cervical hard collar still in place?
  - institute 15–20° of head-up tilt.
- Ensure adequate oxygenation
- Ensure a $PaCO_2$ of 4.5–5.0 kPa
  - if this is already achieved consider transient hyperventilation
  - check an arterial blood gas
- Minimize $CMRO_2$
  - ensure adequate muscle relaxation, analgesia and anaesthesia
  - consider a bolus of thiopentone or propofol
- Diuretics
  - mannitol 0.25–1g kg^{-1}
- Steroids
  - although of no proven benefit in patients with TBI, a (further) dose of dexamethasone will often be requested by surgeons during tumour resection. Steroids do not exert their effect rapidly enough to have an intra-operative effect on cerebral oedema.

MANAGEMENT OF INTRA-OPERATIVE BRAIN SWELLING

Tips and pitfalls
- Aggressive, acute swelling is caused by occult bleeding until proven otherwise. Therapies based on reduction of ICP will not stop haemorrhage.
- Reducing the MAP may reduce cerebral hyperaemia but will place a brain with an already compromised perfusion at further risk of ischaemia.
- Do not assume that the end-tidal CO_2 is representative of the arterial value. In acute brain swelling always check an arterial blood gas.

Air embolism

Venous air embolism (VAE) is the result of air drawn into an open vein at subatmospheric pressure. The rate and volume of air drawn into the circulation determines the severity of the response. Air can pass through the right side of the heart and collect in the pulmonary circulation and, with quantities, can lead to an increase in pulmonary vascular resistance and central venous pressure. Air bubbles can also get trapped in the right ventricle, and lead to disruption of the forward flow of blood and a drop in cardiac output. Well-known risk factors are the sitting position or a steep head-up tilt, as this leads to relative hypovolaemia at the site of the operation. Common points of air entry are venous sinuses, intra-osseus veins, veins within the cervical musculature and epidural veins. Nitrous oxide enlarges air bubbles and can worsen the outcome.

A patent foramen ovale can allow air to cross over to the arterial circulation leading to paradoxical air embolism. This can disrupt the perfusion of the brain and the heart and result in further morbidity and mortality.

Pre-operative assessment

Pre-operative imaging can show the proximity of tumours, especially meningiomas, to venous sinuses and can provide information about possible invasion of the tumour into the bone.

- Highly vascularized tumours place patients at risk of sudden and massive bleeding and, therefore, at risk of hypovolaemia and low venous pressure.
- Transoesophageal echocardiography can identify patients with a patent foramen ovale, who are at particular risk of the effects of air embolism. Some units use this investigation pre-operatively if the sitting position is to be used.

Patient population

Large air emboli are now less common as the sitting position is used less frequently than in the past. However, vigilance is necessary especially during posterior fossa and upper cervical spine operations, particularly during the initial incision and while the craniectomy is carried out.

Patients thought to be particularly at risk are:
- those requiring supratentorial procedures for meningioma in close proximity to a sinus
- those undergoing spinal procedures if epidural veins are opened
- those undergoing craniosynostosis surgery.

Presentation

- Disruption of the forward flow of blood leads to a rapid fall in the end-tidal CO_2 (due to the increase in physiological dead-space) and a drop in arterial oxygen saturation. Cardiac arrhythmias and hypotension can follow.
- Transoesophageal echocardiography is very sensitive and can demonstrate VAE in over 70% of patients undergoing posterior fossa

surgery in the sitting position. However, many of these patients will have no other symptoms or signs of VAE.
- The classic 'mill-wheel' murmur can be detected by auscultation with a precordial stethoscope if large quantities of air enter the circulation.
- Large amounts of air will lead to sudden cardiac arrest.

Treatment of air embolism
- Alert the surgeon who should flood the operative field with saline.
- Ventilate with 100% oxygen, turn off nitrous oxide if used. Adding positive end-expiratory pressure (PEEP) is frequently advocated. However, in a patient with a patent foramen ovale, PEEP may increase the risk of a paradoxical air embolus.
- If possible, patients should be positioned head down with a right side up tilt, to entrap air in the right side of the heart.
- Vasopressors may be required to support the circulation.
- Cardiovascular resuscitation according to standard guidelines needs to be initiated promptly in case of cardiovascular collapse.
- Treat hypovolaemia and replace blood loss if indicated.
- An attempt can be made to aspirate air through a right heart catheter.
  - Success of this method is not well documented, but complications of catheters placed in the right atrium are known.
  - Multiple orifice catheters (e.g. the Bunegin–Albin) have been specifically designed for this purpose but are not used routinely. (Some authors advocate the insertion of such lines for high-risk procedures).
  - For the catheter to be effective they should be positioned at the junction of the superior vena cava and right atrium.
  - Success may be limited due to the formation of a foam of blood and air as it mixes during its passage from dural veins to heart.

Monitoring
- The precordial Doppler is a sensitive method to detect air emboli, although not routinely employed in neuroanaesthesia.
- Transoesophageal echocardiography is very sensitive, and will detect microbubbles in the right atrium in most patients undergoing sitting position neurosurgery. Most of these microbubbles are of no clinical relevance.
- End-tidal CO_2 monitoring is the most sensitive of the methods used routinely to detect air emboli. An abrupt fall in $ETCO_2$ of >0.5 kPa is a commonly used threshold for diagnosis of VAE.

Postoperative care
A small air embolus will only cause transient effects and patients can be treated according to general principles. Intensive care treatment will be required postoperatively if the effect is more profound.

Prognosis
Patients suffering small air emboli usually make a complete recovery, while massive emboli are often fatal regardless of treatment. Paradoxical emboli may result in temporary or permanent symptoms of stroke or ischaemia in other organs.

Tips and pitfalls
- Patients at high risk should be carefully observed throughout surgery for signs of VAE.
- Set the alarms on the capnograph for 0.5 kPa below baseline $ETCO_2$, once a stable value has been achieved.
- If there is any suspicion of VAE inform the surgeon immediately.
- Prepare yourself, and your team, for resuscitation according to standard guidelines if there are marked cardiovascular changes.

Blood loss and cell salvage

Management of both anticipated and unanticipated major haemorrhage is a key part of neuroanaesthetic practice. Procedures with the potential for significant blood loss include decompressive spinal surgery, resection of intramedullary or large intracranial tumours (particularly meningiomas), vascular neurosurgery, and transphenoidal resection of the pituitary.

The morbidity associated with the use of allogeneic blood along with the high cost and decreasing pool of donors have resulted in an increase in the use of lower haemoglobin triggers, cell salvage, transfusion teams, and transfusion protocols.

Disadvantages of allogeneic transfusion

Infective
- Hepatitis B and C
- Human immunodeficiency virus (HIV) 1 and 2
- Human T-cell Lymphoma Virus (HTLV)
- Cytomegalovirus (CMV) in immunocompromised patients
- Bacteria
- Parasites
- Prions such as variant Creutzfeldt–Jakob (vCJD).

Immunological
- Potentially fatal reactions resulting from administration of incompatible blood
- Transfusion-related acute lung injury (TRALI).

Cost
- Currently ~£140 per unit of red cells.

Availability
- Decreasing donor pool.

Techniques to minimize blood loss

Optimal positioning
15–30° of head-up tilt is often used for intracranial surgery and cervical laminectomy to aid venous drainage and provide a clear surgical field. Blood loss in laminectomy correlates with the intra-osseous pressure rather than MAP, therefore great care should be taken particularly in the prone patient to ensure there is no increase in venous pressure from IVC compression. (See Chapter 5.)

Hypotension
Moderate hypotension to a MAP of 60 mmHg may be considered in healthy normotensive individuals for some surgery but is rarely used for intracranial procedures. Care should be taken using hypotension if the blood supply to the spinal cord is compromised. Hypotension may be achieved with a combination of volatile anaesthetic agent and a β-blocker such as labetalol. Carbon dioxide reactivity is diminished during hypotension and lost when MAP <50 mmHg. Care should be taken in patients in whom

autoregulation has been abolished as a result of tumour or subarachnoid haemorrhage or in those with raised intracranial pressure. It should not be used in patients at risk of cerebral or myocardial ischaemia.

Pharmacological methods
Antifibrinolytics such as tranexamic acid given as an initial loading dose of 10–20 mg kg^{-1} then as an infusion of 1–5 mg kg^{-1} hr^{-1} have been used.

Recombinant factor VIIa may be considered if there is major, ongoing haemorrhage despite adequate replacement of clotting factors and platelets.

There is a theoretical risk of cerebral venous thrombosis with procoagulants and this must be balanced against the risk of ongoing haemorrhage.

Other factors influencing blood loss
Normothermia should be maintained wherever possible. Platelets and coagulation factors lose efficacy <35.5°C. Rapidly degradable hydoxyethyl starch (HES)/gelatine-based solutions and crystalloids have minimal effect on coagulation.

Intra-operative cell salvage
Indications
- Anticipated blood loss >1000 ml or 20% of blood volume
- Low haemoglobin or increased risk of haemorrhage
- Multiple antibodies or rare blood types
- Objections to receiving allogeneic blood, e.g. Jehovah's Witness (but check that the individual is happy for use of cell-salvage techniques).

The use of cell saved blood becomes cost neutral after re-infusion of 1–1.5 units. A dedicated member of staff is required to operate the machine and all staff involved should be adequately trained in the use of cell-saved blood. In addition, patients should be given information about the use of autologous blood and documentation should be accurately completed to ensure its safe administration and allow audit of cell salvage use. Adverse events should be reported (Serious Hazards of Transfusion, SHOT).

Procedure
Blood is collected by suction from the surgical field and from washing surgical swabs in saline. (These may contain up to 50% of the blood lost.) It is drawn into a reservoir and anticoagulated at the point of collection with heparin or citrate solutions. Red blood cell separation is achieved by differential centrifugation and saline washing and the resulting cells are resuspended in saline with a haematocrit of 50–85%. The bag should be clearly labelled with the patient's details and the time collected and can be kept for up to 6 h from the start of collection. Up to 80% of the blood lost can be returned if blood is collected efficiently.

Advantages
- Active 2,3-DPG
- Warm
- High haematocrit
- Lower K$^+$ than bank blood
- Physiological pH
- Greater RBC survival.

CHAPTER 4 General principles of neuroanaesthesia

Cautions and contraindications
Care should be taken not to aspirate harmful substances from the surgical field such as antibiotics not licensed for intravenous use and iodine or topical clotting agents. Attempts should be made to minimize the degree of haemolysis as blood is collected via the suction by setting the vacuum to the least necessary to adequately clear the surgical field. Platelets may still be required as they may be activated during salvage. High concentrations of D-dimers may also be present from clotting and lysis taking place in the wound and this does not reflect disseminated intravascular coagulation. Inflammatory mediators are largely removed by the washing process. Collected blood should infused within 6 h to minimize the risk of bacterial growth.

Malignancy
A risk–benefit analysis needs to be carried out before each case. There is a theoretical risk of re-infusion of malignant cells aspirated from the surgical field causing metastasis, although transfusion of allogeneic blood may itself increase infection and recurrence rates. There is little evidence to support the risk of metastasis associated with cell salvage and NICE guidelines now allow the use of intra-operative cell salvage in urological malignancies. Care should be taken to avoid direct aspiration of tumour cells and salvaged blood should be returned to the patient via a leucodepletion filter.

Acute normovolaemic haemodilution (ANH)

Indications
Anticipated blood loss greater than 20% of the circulating blood volume.

This technique is only recommended in particular cases rather than as a routine. Suitable situations would be consenting Jehovah's Witness patients if the blood can remain in continuity with the patient or in patients who are polycythaemic and who would benefit from venesection to decrease blood viscosity.

Contra-indications
- Anaemia
- Significant cardiovascular disease
- Severe respiratory disease
- Sickle cell disease or trait
- Congenital and acquired RBC abnormalities.

Advantages
- No risk of immunological reaction
- Fresh and functioning clotting components
- Administration error unlikely.

Technique
- The volume of blood to be withdrawn is calculated (= estimated blood volume × (initial haematocrit-final haematocrit)/average haematocrit).
- Blood is collected into citrated collection bags, labelled and stored at room temperature to maintain platelet function.
- Crystalloid or colloid solutions are simultaneously infused to maintain normovolamia.

- Collected blood is then infused during surgery, ideally giving the first unit drawn last when haemostasis has been achieved as this is richest in platelets and clotting factors.

Tips and pitfalls
- Take time to ensure good positioning and adequate venous drainage.
- Pay attention to temperature control.
- Early use of coagulation factors and liaison with the haematology service during major haemorrhage will help to prevent coagulopathy and ensure appropriate blood products are made available.
- Use full asepsis when collecting blood for ANH to minimize septic complications.
- Avoid excessive hypotension as a means of minimizing blood loss.
- Ensure all documentation is filled in when using ANH or cell salvage.
- Infusing autologous blood through a leucocyte-depleting filter is very time-consuming and may not be appropriate when there is major ongoing haemorrhage.

Glycaemic control

Glycaemic control is an important part of neuroanaesthesia, particularly in patients with severe head injury. It is established that intensive insulin therapy to maintain blood glucose 4.5–8 mmol l^{-1} reduces morbidity and mortality in critically ill patients in the surgical intensive care unit. The evidence for *tight* glycaemic control of neurosurgical patients is not so clear, and it must be borne in mind that hypoglycaemia is also harmful.

- Hyperglycaemia is common following head injury and is associated both with severity of injury and with outcome.
  - Hyperglycaemia or a relative insulin deficiency at the time of a severe head injury results in an increase in cerebral metabolism.
  - This occurs at the same time as cerebral blood flow decreases secondary to trauma resulting in anaerobic metabolism since the brain is an obligate glucose user.
- Patients presenting for elective surgery may experience hyperglycaemia because of pre-existing diabetes or due to the effects of corticosteroid therapy (dexamethasone).
- An intra-operative single dose dexamethasone is unlikely to cause prolonged or severe hyperglycaemia in non-diabetic individuals. The peak blood sugar occurs several hours after administration so may not be seen intra-operatively.
- Patients who are at risk of significant hyperglycaemia should have their blood glucose controlled with a continuous intravenous infusion of soluble insulin. The rate is adjusted according to the blood glucose, which should be monitored hourly until the blood glucose level is stable.
- Dextrose-containing solutions should be avoided because of their potential to cause hyponatraemia and to raise blood glucose levels further.

Tips and pitfalls
- Diabetic patients should have their blood glucose managed following the same local guidelines as non-neurosurgical patients.
- The dose of insulin required for diabetic patients taking dexamethasone may be greater than normal.
- Addisonian crisis due to glucocorticoid deficiency may cause hypoglycaemia. A common precipitant in the neurosurgical population is the withdrawal of long-term steroid therapy and following pituitary surgery.

Thromboprophylaxis

The incidence of deep venous thrombosis (DVT) and subsequent pulmonary embolism (PE) in patients undergoing a neurosurgical procedure may be as high as 25%. The term venous thrombo-embolism (VTE) is used here to refer to both PE and DVT.

A variety of factors in the neurosurgical population place them at an increased risk of developing VTE. These include: intracranial surgery; malignancy; duration of surgery; decreased mobilization pre- and post-operatively; postoperative (leg) paralysis; and advanced age. High-dose steroid therapy may also affect the coagulation status of these patients.

The highest risk has been found in those patients with malignant and benign brain tumours (28–43%), followed by those undergoing craniotomy for other pathologies (25%) and those with an acute head injury (20%). The risk of developing a PE appears to be in the region of 5% in the general neurosurgical population, with mortality ranging from 9–50%.

Thromboprophylaxis

The timing and methods of VTE prophylaxis are controversial with the benefit versus the risk of bleeding unclear.

Pharmacological options

Unfractionated heparin

Unfractionated heparin has a short half-life in plasma (1.5 h) and has variable and extensive binding to plasma proteins and cells.

Low molecular weight heparin (LMWH)

Low molecular weight heparin has a more predictable anticoagulant response than unfractionated heparin, and a lower risk of heparin-induced thrombocytopenia. Compared with the unfractionated form, low molecular weight heparin has greater bioavailability, and longer duration of action, allowing for once-daily doses for prophylaxis.

Small amounts of bleeding after intracranial or intradural surgery can be catastrophic. Trial data have shown an increased rate of postoperative intracranial haematoma with pre-operative administration of heparin.

The vast majority of postoperative haematomas occur in the first 48 h. Some units start heparin in high-risk patients after this period. Other units do not use heparin at all. UK and US guidance is that patients at high risk of VTE should receive combined pharmacological and mechanical prophylaxis. Meta-analysis of three trials of LMWH given for 7–10 days starting 18–24 h after intracranial and major spinal surgery found that:

- heparin treatment was effective at reducing thrombotic events:
  - the number needed to treat for VTE overall was around 8
  - for proximal DVT the number needed to treat was around 16.
- heparin increases bleeding complications, but:
  - the number needed to harm for any bleeding complication was around 38
  - the number needed to harm for major bleeding complications was around 115
  - none of the trial patients required re-intervention for bleeding.

Of note, these trials all excluded patients with excessive bleeding risk.

Mechanical options

Graduated compression stockings (GCS)
Compression stockings reduce the risk of DVT by affecting the three aetiological factors: venous stasis; vessel injury; and coagulation. External compression reduces the cross-sectional area of the limb and increases the velocity of blood flow in both superficial and deep veins. This increased velocity of blood reduces venous stasis and decreases the risk of thrombus formation by reducing venous wall distension, local contact time, and the concentration of coagulation reactants. External compression also improves venous valve function, reducing stasis of blood in the cusps. There is some evidence that thigh-length GCS are more effective than knee length.

Complications
- Reduction in cutaneous blood flow leading to impaired subcutaneous tissue oxygenation. Those particularly at risk include patients with peripheral vascular disease or diabetes. Care should be taken with patients with flexed knees for a prolonged period of time.
- Other rare problems include arterial occlusion, gangrene, and thrombosis.

Pneumatic compression devices
Intermittent pneumatic compression (IPC) devices induce specific increases in both venous flow and fibrinolytic function. Their antithrombotic activity is likely to be related to both these mechanisms. There is some evidence that IPC are more effective than graduated compression stockings alone.

The optimal antithrombotic efficacy of these devices is achieved when they are worn continuously in the postoperative period.

Complications
- Nerve compression leading to neuropathy
- Compartment syndrome
- Rare incidence of allergies to the component materials.

There is limited evidence suggesting that IPC confer slightly more benefit than GCS when worn intra-operatively. Overall, intermittent pneumatic compression boots with or without graduated compression stockings provide a safe and partially effective prophylactic regimen for neurosurgical patients postoperatively.

Guidelines for thromboprophylaxis
Local policies should be in place to ensure optimal management of all patients. NICE (UK), SFAR (France) and the American College of Physicians have all produced guidelines which include neurosurgical patients as a specific sub-group. The guidance is similar; the NICE guidance is reproduced here.
- Patients having neurosurgery should be offered mechanical prophylaxis (IPC or GCS).

- Patients having neurosurgery with one or more risk factors for VTE (see Box 4.1) should be offered mechanical prophylaxis and LMWH.
- Patients with ruptured cranial or spinal vascular malformations (for example, brain aneurysms) should not be offered pharmacological prophylaxis until the lesion has been secured.

Box 4.1 Risk factors for VTE in neurosurgical patients

- Active cancer or cancer treatment
- Active heart or respiratory failure
- Acute medical illness
- Age >60 yr
- Anti-phospholipid syndrome
- Behçet's disease
- Central venous catheter *in situ*
- Continuous travel of more than 3 h approximately 4 weeks or less before or after surgery
- Immobility (for example, paralysis or limb in plaster)
- Inflammatory bowel disease (for example, Crohn's disease or ulcerative colitis)
- Myeloproliferative diseases
- Nephrotic syndrome
- Obesity (body mass index ≥30 kg m^{-2})
- Paraproteinaemia
- Paroxysmal nocturnal haemoglobinuria
- Personal or family history of VTE
- Pregnancy or puerperium
- Recent myocardial infarction or stroke
- Severe infection
- Use of oral contraceptives or hormonal replacement therapy
- Varicose veins with associated phlebitis
- Inherited thrombophilias, for example:
  - High levels of coagulation factors (such as Factor VIII)
  - Hyperhomocysteinaemia
  - Low activated protein C resistance (for example, Factor V Leiden)
  - Protein C, S and anti-thrombin deficiencies
  - Prothrombin 2021A gene mutation

Pregnancy

A need for neurosurgical intervention in pregnant women can be precipitated by indications specific to pregnancy, or incidental pathology. In the last two triennial UK Confidential Enquiries into Maternal Deaths intracerebral and subarachnoid haemorrhage were responsible for 6 and 13 deaths, respectively, each year (mean values). (Each triennium covers approximately 2 million maternities.) It is unknown how many women sustain significant morbidity as a result of intracranial haemorrhage, and unclear whether or not pregnancy predisposes to cerebral aneurysmal rupture.

The incidence of meningioma in pregnant women appears to be comparable with that in non-pregnant women of the same age group. However, symptoms can be exacerbated during pregnancy on account of water retention, vessel engorgement, and enhanced tumour growth facilitated by sex hormone receptors on tumour cells.

Timing of neurosurgical intervention

At fetal gestational age before extra-uterine viability (<24 weeks) surgical delivery will not be considered. Women can be treated as if they were not pregnant, with due attention to the salient physiological concerns listed below. In the third trimester, fetal compromise or deteriorating maternal condition might signal the need for Caesarean section. Multidisciplinary communication is essential involving neurosurgeon, neuroradiologist, obstetrician, neonatologist, and anaesthetist. Beyond 32 weeks gestation, fetal lung maturity is likely to be assured.

Physiological concerns

Respiratory
- From the end of the first trimester onwards, there is a decrease in $PaCO_2$ to a mean (with narrow standard deviation) of 4.0 kPa. Arterial blood should be analysed to allow correction of any disparity between arterial and end-tidal PCO_2.
- The reduction in maternal functional residual capacity (FRC) and metabolic demands of the feto-placental unit mean that apnoea leads to extremely rapid arterial haemoglobin desaturation. Pre-oxygenation must be optimized (guided by measurement of end-tidal oxygen concentration).

Cardiovascular
- The risk of aorto-caval compression by the gravid uterus assumes increasing importance as pregnancy progresses beyond mid-second trimester. 15° left-lateral tilt, although difficult to implement, will largely prevent impairment of cardiac output.

Gastrointestinal
- Gastric emptying is normal in the absence of pain and opioid medication, although gastro-oesophageal reflux is extremely common.
- Women awaiting surgery should receive clear fluids until 2 h pre-anaesthesia. Isotonic, non-carbonated drinks prevent both ketosis and dehydration.

Haematological
- Pregnancy predisposes to hypercoagulability. Thromboembolism is the leading cause of death in the UK Confidential Enquiries.
- Graduated compression stockings to reduce risk of VTE should be used as a minimum prophylactic measure, and low molecular weight heparin should be considered.

Pre-eclampsia

Pre-eclampsia is a multisystem disorder of endothelial dysfunction. The diagnosis can be suspected in the absence of hypertension and proteinuria (e.g. by headache and visual disturbance alone). The leading cause of death is intracranial haemorrhage, which can present as a convulsion. Since intracranial haemorrhage (of any cause) is followed commonly by hypertension, and often a convulsion, it can be difficult to exclude severe pre-eclampsia/eclampsia. Hyperuricaemia, decreasing platelet count, abnormal liver enzymes and signs of placental insufficiency on ultrasound will substantiate the diagnosis.

Specific concerns
- The pressor response to laryngoscopy and intubation is markedly exaggerated.
- There is a significant risk of postoperative laryngeal oedema and stridor.
- The duration of action of all non-depolarizing neuromuscular blocking agents is significantly prolonged by therapeutic serum concentrations of magnesium (used as an anticonvulsant).

Caesarean section preceding craniotomy

- Two pre-operative doses of oral ranitidine 150 mg should be given, separated by 6 h.
- The woman should be positioned head-up, with 15° left-lateral tilt to avoid aorto-caval compression.
- Apart from the need to eliminate a period of mask ventilation before tracheal intubation, the anaesthetic induction regimen need not differ from that used for non-pregnant neurosurgical patients.
- Direct arterial pressure monitoring should be established before induction of anaesthesia. Prevention of a hypertensive response to intubation is paramount, particularly if an aneurysm is to be clipped or coiled. If the induction results in hypotension, direct arterial pressure monitoring will allow swift correction with small (50 μg) increments of phenylephrine (the vasopressor of choice in obstetrics).
- Although propofol has largely superseded thiopental in neuroanaesthesia, thiopental remains the time-honoured induction agent of choice for Caesarean section. A generous dose should be supplemented by opioid (remifentanil 0.5–2 μg kg^{-1} or alfentanil 10 μg kg^{-1}), and the attending neonatal paediatrician informed that the baby might require naloxone and ventilatory support.
- Succinylcholine is the most commonly used muscle relaxant for intubation. Some anaesthetists consider rocuronium 1 mg kg^{-1} allows avoidance of succinylcholine whilst retaining a rapid onset of neuromuscular blockade.

Craniotomy with fetus *in utero*
- Two pre-operative doses of oral ranitidine 150 mg are given, separated by 6 h.
- Neither neurosurgery nor anaesthesia should predispose to fetal compromise or precipitate premature labour.
- 15° left-lateral tilt must be maintained at all times.
- Continuous monitoring of the cardiotocogram (CTG) is of dubious value—the trace will be predictably abnormal (reflecting fetal anaesthesia and narcosis) and fetal compromise might be inferred erroneously. Pre-operative discussion amongst the mother, neurosurgeon and anaesthetist should establish a clear strategy—that obstetric intervention will not be considered unless there is risk to the mother's life (e.g. from life-threatening, uncontrollable haemorrhage complicating the neurosurgical procedure). Such a strategy should be clearly documented in the case notes.
- Anaesthesia should be maintained with opioid and volatile agent in air and oxygen. A large cumulative dose of propofol risks propofol infusion syndrome in the fetus.

Spinal surgery
Lumbar disc surgery can be undertaken safely and effectively in a full left lateral position. Aorto-caval compression by the gravid uterus is eliminated.

Postpartum conditions
Conditions requiring neurosurgical or neuroradiological intervention in the postpartum period include:
- Cranial subdural haematoma secondary to accidental (lumbar) dural puncture and consequent intracranial CSF depletion and tearing of a dural vein.
- Epidural abscess or haematoma complicating epidural catheterization in labour.
- Cranial venous sinus thrombosis, possibly amenable to radiologically targeted thrombolysis.

Regional analgesia/anaesthesia in the presence of intracranial lesions
- There is no direct evidence upon which to base recommendations regarding regional analgesia/anaesthesia in the presence of small intracranial neoplasms that do not require neurosurgical intervention.
- The same considerations apply to pregnant women as non-pregnant patients regarding lumbar puncture in the presence of potentially raised intracranial pressure.

Tips and pitfalls
- Intra-operative CTG monitoring is not recommended. Anaesthesia masks the indices of fetal well-being.
- Normal end-tidal CO_2 is reduced from the end of the first trimester onwards (with a compensatory metabolic acidosis). Placement of an arterial line pre-induction will allow measurement of $PaCO_2$ to guide ventilation during a neurosurgical procedure with fetus *in utero*. It is unclear how long it takes for postpartum normalization of $PaCO_2$.
- Left-lateral tilt is imperative, from induction to recovery. Consideration should be given to induction in theatre on an electronically adjustable table. Clearly, the need for left-lateral tilt is removed immediately following delivery of the fetus.
- Many factors influence risk of aspiration; it is reasonable to prescribe ranitidine for women up to 48 h postpartum.

Chapter 5

Positioning and surgical approaches

Positioning *162*
Surgical approaches *171*

CHAPTER 5 Positioning and surgical approaches

Positioning

Patient positioning in neurosurgery requires good communication between the anaesthetist and surgeon regarding surgical and anaesthetic needs and patient physiology. Although a variety of positions are employed, the same general principles apply to all:
- Optimum surgical access to make the procedure as straightforward as possible.
- Good venous drainage to minimize blood loss.
- Avoidance of peripheral nerve injury and protection of pressure areas.
- Planning of where to site intravenous and arterial cannulae to maintain accessibility throughout the procedure.
- Avoidance of unnecessary morbidity by simple measures such as ensuring that ECG leads, vascular lines etc. are not pulled tight across the body.

Occasionally patients' body habitus or physiology makes positioning difficult and compromise may be needed. The surgeon should be present when positioning the patient and there should be sufficient team members to allow it to be done safely. Specific points such as an unstable cervical spine should be communicated to the whole team so that appropriate management is carried out.

Supine

The supine position is used for the majority of intracranial procedures and for anterior cervical discectomy. It provides good surgical access for procedures on the frontal lobe. Turning the head to the side and tilting the patient with a sandbag under the shoulder also gives access to the temporal and parietal lobes and is used for shunt procedures and some 'trauma' craniotomies (Figure 5.1).

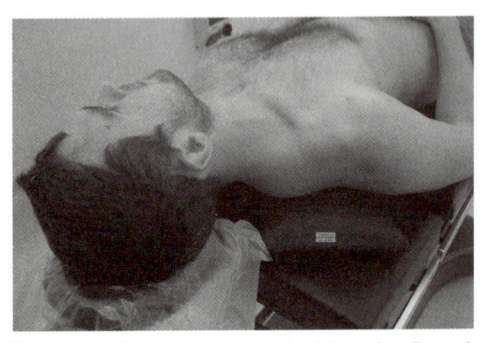

Fig. 5.1 The patient supine, head on horseshoe head ring and sandbag under right shoulder to facilitate access to temporal or parietal lobes.

- Neurosurgical patients are often in the same position for prolonged periods and good pressure area care is essential.
- The eyes should be well covered to protect against trauma from the drapes.
  - Active measures should be taken to prevent any surgical antiseptic skin 'prep' solution from entering or pooling around the eyes.
- The head is usually held on a horseshoe headrest or in Mayfield pins (for a craniotomy), or rests directly on the table for anterior cervical discectomy. Application of the pins is extremely stimulating and there must be good communication with surgical colleagues before and during their application.
- Care must be taken to avoid excessive flexion or extension of the neck with the head in pins which risks inward (flexion) or outward (extension) movement of the tracheal tube and may impede venous drainage.
- The ulnar nerve at the elbow is at risk of compression if not protected.
- The heels should be protected with gel pads.
- A pillow is often placed behind the knees to prevent hyperextension.
- A degree of head-up tilt is often requested; the amount must be balanced against the risk of air embolism and the patient's cardiovascular status.

Prone

This position is used for operations on the spine, occipital lobe or posterior fossa. It may be achieved in various ways depending on local preference and the area to be operated on. The head may rest on a gel headrest or be held in pins depending on the nature of surgery.

The key issues for prone positioning are:
- difficult access to the airway in the event of problems;
- potentially increased airway pressure with positive pressure ventilation:
  - this may also increase epidural venous pressure and hence increase surgical blood loss.
- increased abdominal pressure:
  - this may reduce systemic venous return and hence cardiac output
  - this may also increase epidural venous pressure and hence increase surgical blood loss.
- different pressure points (compared with the supine position) are at risk:
  - eyes
  - axillae
  - breasts
  - genitals
  - liver
  - inguinal region.
- significantly more risk to patient, vascular lines, drains, and staff during patient turning (both into and out of the prone position).

At-risk areas

Airway
The airway must be secure when the patient is positioned prone. Although a minority of anaesthetists use a laryngeal mask airway for straightforward procedures such as lumbar discectomy, standard practice is to use a tracheal tube. The type of tube used, the placement of throat packs and the method used to secure the tube are based more on local custom and practice than evidence of superiority.

Whatever techniques are used care must be taken to ensure:
- the tube will not move in or out significantly during surgical positioning
- the tube will not become kinked
- the circuit will not become disconnected from the breathing system, or if it does it can be reconnected easily.

Breathing
Increased airway pressure with controlled ventilation is not uncommon. This leads to increased intrathoracic pressure which, in turn, may increase epidural or central venous pressure and may result in increased bleeding at the operative site.

Circulation
The physiological changes associated with turning prone are incompletely understood and vary between individuals. A small number of patients do not tolerate being turned prone. Severe hypotension is well described. Changes that may occur include:
- Acute reduction in venous return, particularly if intrathoracic or intra-abdominal pressures are high.
- Increase in systemic vascular resistance (due to compression of resistance vessels)
- Decreased cardiac output and systemic vascular resistance secondary to anaesthesia.

Cardiac output is not usually monitored and routine monitoring of pulse rate and blood pressure may not reveal the underlying physiological changes.

There is no panacea to prevent hypotension on turning prone. Strategies that are commonly used include:
- Not turning patients who are hypotensive already
- Preloading with intravenous fluid
- Administration of vasoactive drugs prior to or soon after turning.

Most patients will tolerate turning prone eventually.

Abdomen
All of the prone positioning techniques described below endeavour to keep the abdomen free and prevent raised intra-abdominal and intrathoracic pressures. This is something of an art form, and may require more than one adjustment of patient position.

Eyes
There are three separate risks to the eyes. Direct trauma, resulting in corneal abrasion, chemical injury from surgical skin 'prep' solution and the spectrum of postoperative visual loss associated with retinal damage.
- A closed eyelid will prevent corneal drying and trauma.

- Different units have different approaches to how this is achieved:
  - some centres advocate padding which distributes any applied pressure more evenly
  - other centres use simple taping to retain the protective contours of the orbit
  - eyeshields and numerous different forms of head support are available.
- Whichever technique is used the anaesthetist must be confident that the eyelids are closed and that direct pressure to the eyes is avoided.

Undiluted surgical skin 'prep' solution may cause corneal damage, so steps must be taken to ensure that it does not get into or remain in the eyes.
- Local practice varies, but some centres aim for a waterproof seal around the eyes with taping.
- Others promote care during surgical preparation and wipe the eyes clear before starting.
- Neither method can guarantee eye safety without due vigilance from the anaesthetist and surgeon.

Postoperative visual loss is a rare but well recognized event after prone spinal surgery with an estimated rate of around 1 in 1000. Identified risk factors include:
- scoliosis surgery and posterior lumbar fusion
- age <18 or >85 years
- prolonged surgery (>6 h)
- peripheral vascular disease
- intra-operative blood loss >1000 ml and anaemia.

Various aetiologies have been described and it is likely that there is no single cause. Ischaemic optic neuropathy is the commonest.

Nerves

Injuries to the brachial plexus, ulnar nerve around the elbow and lateral cutaneous nerve of the thigh have all been reported associated with prone positioning.
- Although there is little direct evidence, best practice is to position the limbs in neutral, relaxed positions avoiding excessive extension, flexion, rotation, traction or compression.
  - For the shoulder a rule of thumb is to aim for <90° in all planes.
  - This is only a guide and the anaesthetist should use clinical judgement.
- Moving limb position periodically is thought to reduce the risk of nerve injury.

Breasts and genitals

- There is no consensus on the best position for breasts when positioned prone.
  - There have been reports of breast tissue necrosis after prone surgery.
- The male genitals should be free of compression. Urinary catheters must be positioned free of tension.

Monitoring and lines
It is possible, but cumbersome, to turn patients with all monitoring attached. In practice, most anaesthetists remove or disconnect the monitoring prior to positioning.

The airway should always be disconnected from the breathing system during turning.

Numerous equipment manufacturers produce positioning aids for prone positioning. There is little evidence to support one approach over another. Regardless of the aids and position used, the anaesthetist must assure him or herself that the patient is positioned as safely as possible.

Variations of the prone position

Knee-chest
Operations on the lumbar spine are often carried out with the patient in the knee-chest position. The knees are flexed under the hips and the chest rests on a bolster. The arms are brought forward to rest at the side of the head and the head rests on a gel cushion. While providing excellent access to the lumbar spine by abolishing the lordosis, it requires several staff to achieve this position safely. For this reason it is less commonly used than previously.

- Care should be taken to avoid excessive shoulder abduction and traction injury to the brachial plexus.
- The axillae should not be under tension and the elbows should be padded to protect the ulnar nerve.
- The eyes must be closed and the forehead should rest on a gel headrest to avoid pressure on the eyes and minimize the risk of visual loss from central retinal artery occlusion.
- The neck should be in a neutral position avoiding hyperextension.

Wilson frame (and similar alternatives)
This is an alternative to the knee-chest position that requires fewer staff and is less labour intensive to achieve. The patient is turned prone onto the frame, which has two support cushions running lengthways (Figure 5.2).

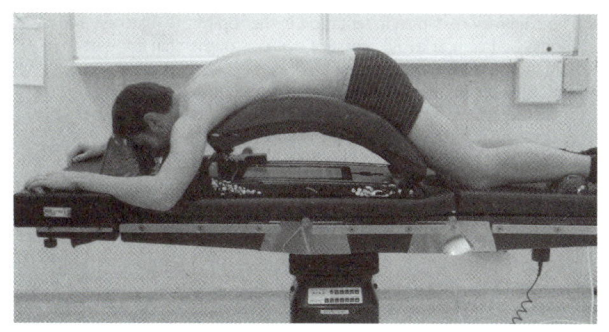

Fig. 5.2 A patient placed prone on a Wilson frame.

- The supports should be adjusted medially or laterally so that they are in line with the patient's nipples.
- The curvature of these supports is then increased to the required amount by turning a handle.
  - The patient's head will move during this manoeuvre; care must be taken to avoid injury.
- The arms are brought to rest at the side of the head and the head rests on a gel cushion.
- The same pressure area precautions as for the knee-chest position apply.
- There is a risk of excessive or prolonged pressure on the axillae from the end of the lateral supports.

Montreal mattress

This is a custom-made mattress with a hole in the centre to allow free abdominal movement during ventilation. It is often used for procedures on the thoracic and cervical spine and posterior fossa (Figure 5.3).

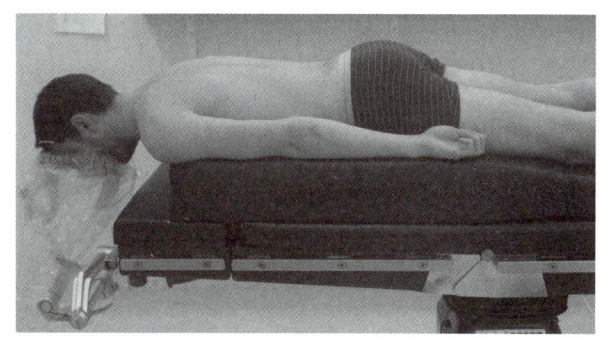

Fig. 5.3 A patient placed prone on a Montreal mattress.

- The chin may rest in an indentation in the top of the mattress and care should be taken to avoid pressure necrosis of the chin if the head is held in excessive flexion.
- The arms rest by the sides and the legs may be supported on a pillow or flexed against a padded board to allow greater stability if head up positioning is to be used and to minimize venous pooling.
- Different sizes are available.

Bolsters

Bolsters positioned under the chest and pelvis may be used for operations on the spine or posterior fossa (Figure 5.4).

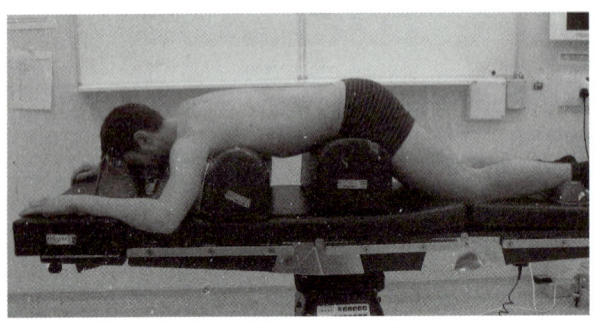

Fig. 5.4 A patient placed prone on bolsters under the chest and pelvis.

- They should be supportive but not too firm and should be positioned so as not to impair venous drainage and cardiac output.
- Care must be taken with the chest bolster to ensure it is not mistakenly positioned under the upper abdomen which may risk hepatic ischaemia. In extreme cases this has been associated with fulminant hepatic failure.

Park bench or lateral recumbent position

Lateral positions are used for operations on the parietal or occipital lobes or the posterior fossa, particularly for acoustic neuroma.

- The patient is turned to the lateral position and the head usually held in pins.
- The upper part of the dependent arm must be protected from prolonged pressure if the patient lies on it. Either place a soft bag of fluid in the axilla (to lift the upper chest off the arm), or support the arm below the table on a frame (Figure 5.5).

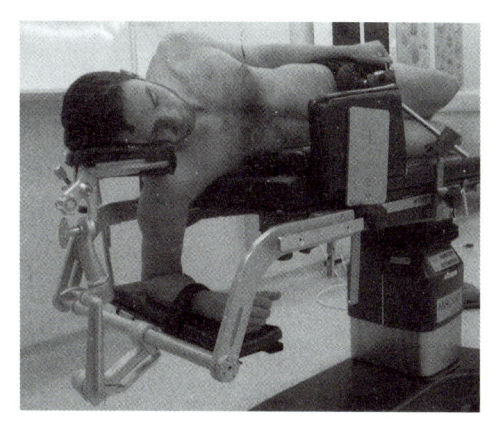

Fig. 5.5 A patient placed laterally. With this particular frame the dependent arm is supported.

- The upper arm rests along the upper side of the torso.
- The lower leg is slightly bent at the knee while the upper is flexed at the hip and a pillow or other padding is placed between the knees.
- Care must be taken that the shoulders and lower arm are comfortably positioned and that all pressure areas are well padded as surgery in this area often takes a very long time.
- The location of intravenous and arterial lines needs to be carefully considered. They should all be sited in the upper arm if possible to allow good access during the procedure and minimize compression.
- The neck should be held in a position to allow good venous drainage and the patient should be secured on the table with straps or surgical supports as the table is often tilted to optimize surgical access.

Sitting

This position is now only used in a few centres. It has the advantages of providing excellent access to the posterior fossa and superior venous drainage, but there is a high risk of air embolism and hypotension. Centres that use the sitting position routinely report a low incidence of serious complications.

- It is achieved by resting the patient at 45° on the operating table and flexing the head forwards onto a headrest.
- Traditionally patients breathed spontaneously during surgery to allow variations in respiratory pattern to be observed as a marker of brainstem ischaemia.
  - This has now been abandoned in favour of controlled ventilation.
- The position is contraindicated in patients with cardiac septal defects, those with cardiovascular instability and patients who are dehydrated.

- Close monitoring for air embolism (see Air embolism, p.142) is mandatory and includes:
  - End-tidal capnography
  - Precordial Doppler.

Tips and pitfalls
- Do not be rushed into accepting an unacceptable position. Some patients require more than one attempt at positioning.
- Always hold on to the head during changes in position. Never assume that someone else will do this for you.
- Be clear about what monitoring you want left on during positioning and what you are happy to disconnect.
- Disconnect the airway and breathing system during major changes in position.
- Ensure adequate paralysis before moving the patient. Sudden movement of the tube is likely to result in coughing otherwise.
- If venous and arterial lines are to remain connected, allocate a named individual to take care of these during positioning. You can not do this at the same time as taking care of the head.
- Be clear about what monitors you want reattached after turning prone and in what order.
- The anaesthetist must assure him or herself of adequate cardiac output very soon after turning the patient prone. If there is any doubt, and it does not respond promptly to simple intervention, the patient should be turned back again.
- Always check the eyes after final positioning.
- Take a walk around the patient after positioning to assure yourself of good positioning.
- Document clearly what position and additional protection was used.

Surgical approaches

The ideal approach for a neurosurgical procedure will be influenced by consideration of:

- patient cosmesis and comfort
- avoidance or protection of critical structures (such as the middle ear, facial nerve branches, venous sinuses) during the approach
- adequate access to the lesion
- satisfactory visualization of any critical structures around the lesion
- the experience and preference of the surgeon.

As a rule, flaps and approaches have become smaller in scale over the last 20 years as a result of technical developments in localization such as image guidance, and a move to more minimally invasive surgery with increased use of the microscope and neuroendoscopy.

Hair

While it may get in the way, particularly during closure, there is no evidence that leaving hair intact increases wound infections or other complications (and indeed there is some evidence to the contrary that shaving increases infection rate). It is increasingly common for the hair simply to be parted for the incision or for a very limited shave to be performed.

Infiltration

Local anaesthetic infiltration can help define tissue planes, reduce bleeding (when combined with adrenaline) and provide some postoperative analgesia.

Burr hole

This will provide adequate access and be the usual approach for:
- evacuation of chronic subdural haematoma
- brain biopsy either by stereotactic means or with image guidance
- aspiration of abscesses or cysts
- siting of ventricular drains for hydrocephalus.

A burr hole appropriate for the underlying pathology can be sited almost anywhere on the cranial vault, as long as the anticipated position of the venous sinuses and expansions or 'venous lakes' from these are avoided.

Surgical steps

- Infiltration and scalp incision.
- Pericranium stripped back, self-retaining retractor inserted.
- Bone drilled with a hand brace or power drill.
- Cruciate-shaped dural opening with dural edges diathermied.
- The whole process, including haemostasis around the edges, should take only 5–10 min.

Craniotomy for trauma

This will provide adequate access and be the usual approach for:
- evacuation of acute subdural haematomas and contusions
- evacuation of extradural haematoma.

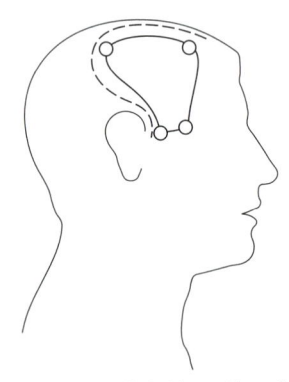

Fig. 5.6 Classical trauma craniotomy skin incision and bone flap.

Steps
- Patient positioned supine, sandbag under the shoulder, and head turned to side.
- Head held in pins or on a horseshoe headring.
- Infiltration and long 'question mark' scalp incision commencing at the pinna and extended to cover the area of anticipated interest, plastic 'Raney' clips to scalp edge (to minimize blood loss).
- Burr holes as shown (Figure 5.6), connected with a craniotome (high speed drill and saw with dural gurad) and bone flap either lifted free or reflected (turned) inferiorly with the temporalis muscle.
- Extradural haematoma evacuated, bleeding points identified and haemostased (usually the middle meningeal artery branches inferiorly).
- Dura opened and subdural haematoma and contused brain evacuated.
- Once haemostasis and satisfactory brain conditions are ensured the dura is closed.
- The bone flap may be held in place with sutures through small drill holes, with metal screws and plates or with fixation clamps.
- Drains may be left subdurally, extradurally or under the scalp.
- An intracranial pressure monitoring wire may be led out alongside drains if ITU care is anticipated.
- Uncomplicated cases will take 60–90 min.

Tips and pitfalls
- Rapid blood loss extra- or intradurally (especially with injuries near to venous sinuses).
- Overwhelming brain swelling (necessitating lobectomy or leaving the bone flap out during closure).

Bicoronal flap craniotomy
This will provide access and be the usual approach for:
- anteriorly situated haematomas and tumours
- the forehead and frontal sinuses in a combined craniofacial repair.

SURGICAL APPROACHES   173

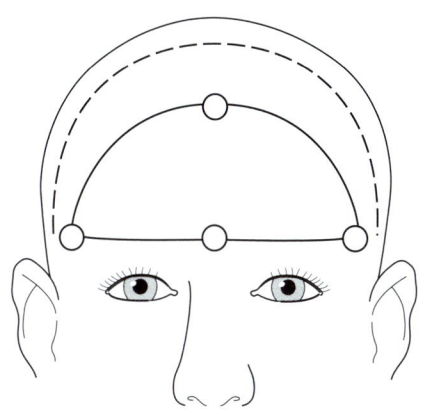

Fig. 5.7 Bicoronal skin incision and frontal bone flap.

Steps
- Patient positioned supine, head neutral held in pins or on a horseshoe headring.
- Infiltration and long bicoronal incision reflecting scalp forwards.
- Burr holes as shown (Figure 5.7) connected with the craniotome and usually a free bone flap lifted avoiding the frontal air sinuses.

Small craniotomies—pterional and straight
These provide limited access to a well-defined area such as:
- the pterional and Sylvian region for approaches to aneurysms
- tumours which can been accurately localized either from their position or with image guidance.

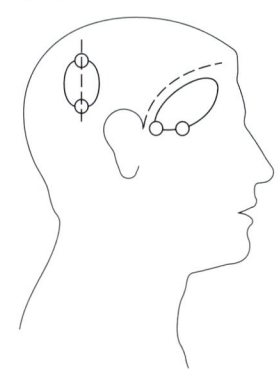

Fig. 5.8 Small parietal skin incision and bone flap. Classial pterional skin incision and bone flap.

Posterior fossa—retrosigmoid craniectomy

This is most commonly used for approaches to the lateral cerebellum and cerebellopontine angle for surgery for:
- acoustic neuromas
- other tumours such as meningiomas and epidermoids in this region.

Steps
- Usually done in either a lateral 'park bench' position, or prone with the head turned to the side and held in pins.
- Either a linear incision or a flap of scalp are turned over the mastoid process and the bone immediately posterior to this (Figure 5.9).
- Bone in this area is drilled inferomedial to the sigmoid sinus—at least some degree of venous bleeding will be encountered from the mastoid emissary vein and other veins.
- Adequate dural exposure avoiding damage to the sinuses may be time-consuming and modifications to this approach such as translabyrinthine surgery can involve several hours of meticulous bone work to expose the cerebellopontine angle while protecting the facial nerve.
- Further venous bleeding (and a risk of air embolism) may occur as the dura is opened and when the superior petrosal vein is encountered.
- The bone dust and in some cases a graft of fat are put back into the defect at closure.

Posterior fossa—midline craniectomy

This is most commonly used for approaches to the medial cerebellum, fourth ventricle and craniocervical junction for:
- the majority of posterior fossa tumours, especially in children
- decompression of the cranio-cervical junction for a Chiari I malformation.

Steps
- Patient usually positioned prone, 'head up', head held in pins with the neck flexed.
- A midline, or occasionally paramedian, linear incision is made (Figure 5.9).
- Posterior fossa bone may either be removed using a drill and rongeurs to create a craniectomy, or a craniotomy may be cut and replaced at the end.
- Depending on the indication for surgery, the posterior arch of C1 is often removed.
- The posterior fossa dura has sinuses of variable size and at least some degree of venous bleeding is usually encountered, though usually short-lived.

Tips and pitfalls
- Rarely the vertebral artery may be injured at the lateral aspect of the arch of C1.

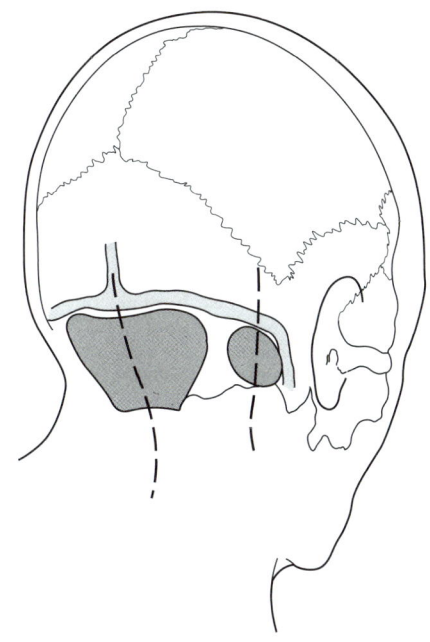

Fig. 5.9 Skin incisions and areas of midline posterior fossa craniectomy and retrosigmoid craniectomy.

Anterior cervical approach
This is used for approaches to the cervical vertebral bodies and discs for:
- anterior cervical discectomy, corporectomy and grafting procedures
- safe access to any other pathology anterior to the cervical spinal cord.

Steps
- Patient positioned supine, head usually in a neutral to slightly extended position.
- A right-sided skin crease incision is made (to avoid the left recurrent laryngeal nerve and the thoracic duct) (Figure 5.10).
- The platysma is divided; the fascia between the strap muscles and larynx and oesophagus medially and the carotid and jugular neurovascular sheath laterally is dissected. Fixed retraction of these structures allows midline access to the spine in between the paired longus colli muscles.
- There is significant and persisting retraction of the trachea to the left —potentially compressing the tracheal tube.
- The spinal level is confirmed with a lateral X-ray and a marker needle in the disc space.

176 CHAPTER 5 **Positioning and surgical approaches**

- The vertebrae are distracted.
- Discectomy and removal of osteophytes is carried out until dural decompression is confirmed.
- The disc space may be left empty (anticipating fusion) or an appropriately sized bone graft or a disc spacer or articulating disc replacements inserted.

Tips and pitfalls
- Venous bleeding during approach or from epidural veins during intraspinal decompression.
- Rarely (but potentially seriously) early postoperative haematoma will necessitate emergency wound re-opening because of airway compromise.

Laminectomy (cervical, thoracic, lumbar)
This is the standard posterior approach to the spinal canal for:
- decompression of a degenerative, stenotic canal
- extradural haematomas, abscesses, and tumours
- the majority of intradural spinal procedures.

Steps
- Patient positioned prone on rolls, mattress or specific positioning frame.
- Midline incision, in some cases with reference to a pre-operative marker X-ray or by using a marker spinal needle placed to confirm the level on an 'on table' X-ray.
- Fat and fascia split, muscles dissected off the spinous processes and laminae.
- The bone of the spinous processes and laminae removed at appropriate levels as far laterally as the facet joints.
- Ligamentum flavum removed to decompress the dura.

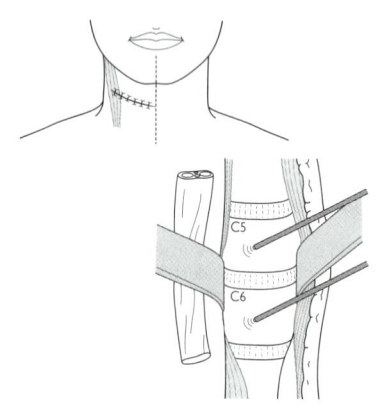

Fig. 5.10 Anterior cervical discectomy: skin crease incision from sternomastoid to midline and then operative view with neurovascular bundle retracted laterally and trachea and oesophagus retracted to the left exposing anterior cervical spine. Distractor posts have been screwed in to C5 and C6 bodies so that discectomy can begin.

Tips and pitfalls
- Occasionally heavy bleeding from paraspinal muscles and bony venous channels.
- Bleeding from epidural veins particularly in lateral gutters towards completion of laminectomy.
- Risk of dural tear causing CSF leak which can be time-consuming to close
- Surgeon may request a Valsalva manouevre to test the integrity of a CSF leak repair.
- 'Re-do' procedures can be prolonged and difficult due to scar tissue and distorted anatomy.

Lumbar microdiscectomy
The daily 'bread and butter' of spinal neurosurgery, but variable in apparent difficulty and duration.

Steps
- Patient positioned prone on rolls, mattress or specific positioning frame.
- Short midline incision usually using a spinal needle to confirm the level on an 'on table' X-ray.
- Fat and fascia split, muscles dissected off the spinous processes and lamina.
- Retractors and microscope introduced.
- Ligamentum flavum opened to identify the exiting nerve root and dura.
- Exposure increased taking care not to further injure the already compressed nerve root.
- Root and dura retracted medially with any free disc fragments anterior to this withdrawn.
- Disc space entered via an incision in annulus with any further loose material withdrawn (surgical enthusiasm for amount of material to be removed varies).
- Limited bony decompression along the nerve root exit canal.

Tips and pitfalls
- Wrong level surgery (and having to start again at the adjacent level when this is realized).
- Occasional CSF leaks.
- 'Re-do' procedures can be difficult and prolonged.

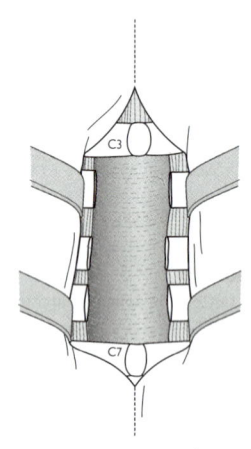

Fig. 5.11 Cervical laminectomy: operative view with retractors holding back overlying muscle and spinous processes, laminae and ligamentum removed, decompressing in this case C4, C5 and C6.

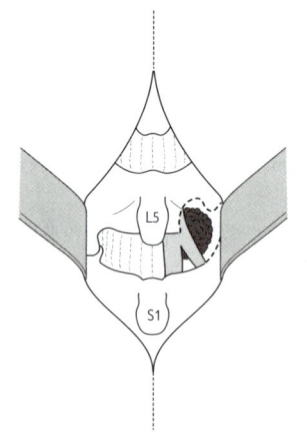

Fig. 5.12 Lumbar microdiscectomy; diagrammatic operative view (exposure exaggerated for clarity) to show fenestration through the ligamentum flavum and parts of laminae of L5 and S1 allowing access to the right S1 nerve root and disc fragment or bulge anterior to this.

Chapter 6

Intracranial surgery (non-vascular)

Tumours in adults (meningioma, glioma, lymphoma, metastasis) *180*
Tumours (children) *191*
Acoustic neuroma *196*
Pituitary tumours *200*
Posterior fossa surgery *206*
Shunts and ventricular drains *214*
Neuroendoscopic surgery *220*
Colloid cysts *222*
Midline surgery *224*
Seizure surgery *228*
Functional neurosurgery *234*
Cranial neuralgias *238*
Awake craniotomy *242*
Stereotactic surgery *246*
Cerebral abscesses *250*
Decompressive craniectomy *254*

Tumours in adults (meningioma, glioma, lymphoma, metastasis)

Tumour surgery forms a large part of neurosurgical practice. In many patients surgery can be electively planned for the next available elective surgical list, although some patients require more urgent temporizing measures or even resection.

Epidemiology

- Approximately 2% of all adult cancers are primary CNS tumours. Statistics vary as the incidence of tumour subgroups seen in neurosurgery is different from those seen in radiotherapy, palliative care or at autopsy.
- Around half of all primary CNS cancers are gliomas.
- Meningioma represents about 15% of CNS tumours.
- Cerebral lymphoma represents around 3% of intracranial tumours.
- Metastases from primaries outside the CNS represent up to 40% of lesions; however, only a small proportion of these patients present for neurosurgery.
- In addition to the more common tumours discussed here, a huge variety of subtypes exists, including tumours with overlapping or mixed histological features. A full discussion is beyond the scope of this text.

Pathology

The concept of benign or malignant differs from that used for tumours outside the CNS. A benign meningioma can show invasive spread into adjacent bone, while metastases from brain primaries, even from malignant gliomas, are unknown. The grading of brain tumours takes into account their histological characteristics.

Meningioma

These develop from arachnoid cells and are defined by site, size and WHO grading (I–III). More than 90% of meningiomas are benign, and they can grow for a long time and reach considerable size before becoming symptomatic, or even be incidental findings at autopsy.

Typical sites for meningiomas are parasagittal, falcine, convexity, sphenoid ridge, suprasellar, olfactory groove, and optic nerve sheath. Their shape is dependent on the site and the space available; convexity meningiomas are often spherical, while optic nerve meningiomas are fusiform. Meningiomas can invade dura and bone; the bone often responds with hyperostosis. While invasion of bone can be seen in grade I meningiomas, invasion of brain is a sign of more malignant growth typical of grade III lesions. Multiple meningiomas occur in less than 10% of cases. Meningiomas occur at increased frequency following radiotherapy.

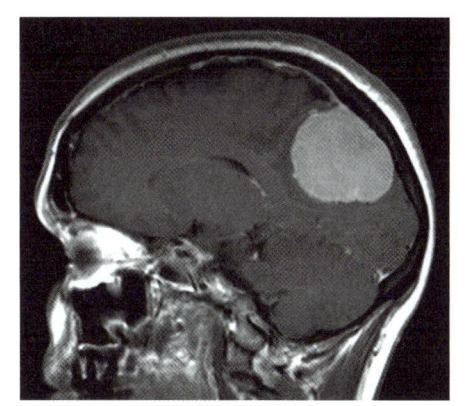

Fig. 6.1 Meningioma. Post-contrast sagittal T1-weighted MRI scan showing a parietal meningioma.

Gliomas

Gliomas or neuroepithelial tumours originate from glial cells, most commonly astrocytes and oligodendrocytes. The WHO classification is the most commonly used system for gliomas, but other classifications exist.

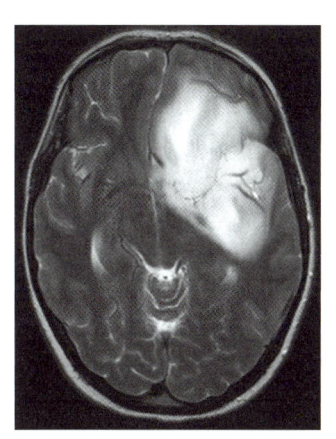

Fig. 6.2 Glioma. Axial T2-weighted MRI. Large left fronto-temporal low-grade glioma which encases the branches of the left middle cerebral artery. Note the presence of midline shift to the right.

CHAPTER 6 Intracranial surgery (non-vascular)

Astrocytoma
A characteristic feature of astrocymomas is their ability to transform from a low-grade or diffuse astrocytoma (WHO Grade II) to an anaplastic astrocytoma (WHO Grade III) and ultimately to a high-grade tumour—glioblastoma (WHO Grade IV). This transformation can take over 10 years, and acquired genetic changes are implicated. Different histological grades can exist in the same tumour simultaneously. High-grade gliomas can also arise *de novo*. These represent around 90% of high-grade lesions. Unfortunately, high-grade tumours (gliobastomas) account for about half of the gliomas seen in neurosurgery with about 4 new cases per 100,000 population per year in northern Europe. Low-grade gliomas account for approximately 20%. Pilocytic astrocytomas (WHO Grade I) characteristically present in childhood (see p. 191), and do not usually transform to a more malignant tumour.

Astrocytomas grow diffusely, are poorly demarcated from surrounding tissue, may distort normal anatomy and can produce oedema, raised intracranial pressure and brain shift. Low-grade gliomas are often located in the subcortical or white matter, commonly in the fronto-temporal area, and are relatively avascular, in contrast to high-grade lesions. Cysts containing yellow fluid can be seen. Tumour areas highlighted by contrast enhancement on a CT scan are a feature of anaplastic transformation, while necrosis and haemorrhage are typical for high-grade lesions. Aggressive growth patterns of glioblastoma can result in spreading of tumour to distant parts of the brain, leading to appearance of lesions at multiple sites.

Oligodendroglioma
Oligodendrogliomas represent about 10% of primary CNS tumours and can be subdivided into slow growing (WHO Grade II) and anaplastic (WHO Grade III) lesions. Anaplastic transformations from grade II to grade III are known, as are *de novo* grade III lesions. They are often located in the cortex or subcortical areas of the frontal lobe. Mucoid cysts, necrosis, and calcifications are typical for these lesions.

Lymphoma

Primary CNS lymphomas represent up to 3% of intracranial tumours; they are non Hodgkin's lymphomas, mostly large diffuse B-cell lymphomas. Their typical location is in the cerebrum. Secondary lymphomas, mainly spreading to the subarachnoid space and meninges, are seen in 5–10% of patients with primary sites outside the CNS, and are commoner than primary lymphomas. CNS lymphomas can be multifocal. Peritumour oedema is common, although not as extensive as in gliomas. The last two decades have seen a significant increase in the incidence of primary CNS lymphomas, due to the increase in organ transplants and immunosuppressive therapy and an increase in patients with HIV/AIDS. The incidence is also rising in immunocompetent patients.

Metastasis

Metastases account for up to 15% of CNS tumours in neurosurgical patients and approximately 40% of CNS tumours seen at autopsy. Half of these tumours are caused by lung cancer; other common primaries are breast cancer, malignant melanoma, renal, and gastrointestinal tumours. About a quarter of all cancer patients have intracranial metastases. Many CNS metastases are solitary, and 15% present before the primary lesion becomes symptomatic. Frontal and parietal lobes are the commonest locations, proportional to the blood supply, as seeding is via the bloodstream. Metastases tend to form a spherical mass with surrounding oedema. Haemorrhage within the lesion is often seen in malignant melanoma and metastasis from renal carcinoma. Malignant melanoma cells can also show typical pigmentation.

Associated conditions

While most CNS primaries are of unknown aetiology, genetic factors, such as neurofibromatosis, are associated with up to 5% of CNS primaries. Ionizing radiation is associated with late development of menigioma and the meningiomas induced by radiation tend to have a higher histological grade. There is an association between meningiomas and both breast and endometrial cancer.

Numerous environmental and occupational factors have been linked to the development of brain tumours such as formaldehyde, vinyl chloride, herbicides, fungicides, viruses (e.g. SV 40 virus), industrial products (metal and rubber industries). There is, however, no convincing evidence of a causal link described in the literature.

Presentation

As space-occupying lesions within the cranial vault, tumours present either with local effects (neurological deficits, seizures) or general symptoms and signs of raised ICP.
- Low-grade gliomas typically present with epilepsy, which may precede the diagnosis for several years.
- In patients with a known low-grade glioma, new neurological deficits or symptoms can be a sign of anaplastic transformation of the tumour.
- Anaplastic lesions are characterized by faster growth leading to oedema and midline shift, while high-grade gliomas typically have a short history of less than 3 months, presenting with neurological deficits or signs of raised intracranial pressure.
- Symptoms vary with location and size of the tumour, frontal lobe lesions can affect the patient's personality, while even small tumours in eloquent areas of the brain can give rise to significant neurological deficits, such as limb weakness or dysphasia.
- The level of consciousness can be altered—a sign of markedly increased ICP.
- In contrast to lesions outside the CNS, weight loss is not a typical feature.
- CNS lymphomas can manifest themselves through raised intracranial pressure, focal neurological symptoms or epilepsy. Lymphomas originating from outside the CNS also affect the CNS indirectly, e.g. mediastinal lymphomas leading to cord compression, or plasmocytomas leading to vertebral collapse.
- Metastases typically present with headache, neurological deficits or behavioural changes.

Patient population

Menigioma
Meningiomas affect women more often than men at a ratio of approximately 2:1. The incidence increases with age, with a peak incidence between 60 and 70 years. Meningiomas can remain asymptomatic during life and be an incidental finding at autopsy in as many as 3% of people aged over 60. Abnormalities on chromosome 22 are common in patients with meningioma. Development of multiple meningiomas is associated with genetic syndromes, such as neurofibromatosis. In these patients they present at an earlier age.

Glioma
Glioma is commoner in men than women. The mean age of patients with astrocytomas ranges from 35 years for low-grade tumours to ~55 years for high-grade lesions. Oligodendrogliomas commonly present in patients aged 30–50 years, showing a similar incidence in males and females. Patients with high-grade gliomas which have developed from low-grade lesions are typically younger than patients with *de novo* high-grade tumours. Caucasians are more often affected than those of other racial backgrounds.

Lymphoma
Primary CNS lymphomas are more common in males than in females (3:2). Affected immunocompetent patients are usually in their sixties, while immunocompromised patients are commonly in their forties.

Metastases
CNS metastases are typically seen in patients in their sixties and seventies.

Pre-operative assessment

In addition to the normal pre-operative assessment the anaesthetist should be vigilant for common associated conditions and investigations.

GCS/ICP
A low GCS due to high ICP is a sign of a severely impaired cerebral perfusion. Raised ICP can also lead to classical signs of hypertension, bradycardia and low GCS. Vomiting can also be a feature. Patients can be dehydrated, and have electrolyte/metabolic imbalances. This needs to be addressed prior to surgery. Hydrocephalus can develop if tumour obstructs the CSF flow, causes excessive CSF production of interferes with CSF absorption.

Neurologial deficits
The clinical picture depends on size and site of the lesion, and can include limb weakness or paresis, dysphasia, vision disturbance or visual field defects, bulbar symptoms and can, on occasions, mimic a stroke.

Epilepsy
Patients with newly diagnosed seizures will have been commenced on anti-epileptic medication. This, as well as existing epilepsy drugs, should be continued prior to surgery.

Imaging
A review of available scans can provide information about the size and location of the tumour, the amount of oedema and midline shift, compression of ventricles, and the risk of herniation of the brain. It also gives information about the vascularity of the tumour and involvement of significant feeding vessels or proximity to a sinus. Midline shift of more than 10 mm is a sign of a severely compromised brain.

Medication
Use of antiplatelet agents such as clopidogrel and aspirin is common in the ageing population. These need to be stopped before planned neurosurgery (unless significant contraindications exist) to minimize risk of postoperative haemorrhage and to ease peroperative haemostasis.

Dexamethasone will impair glucose homeostasis, particularly in patients with diabetes. An insulin sliding scale may be necessary.

Blood cross-match
Blood should be cross-matched according to local protocol. A group and save should be performed as a minimum.

Plan for postoperative care
A significant compromise of conscious state, impairment of cough or swallowing, tumour location in a sensitive area or massive oedema indicate a need for a higher level of postoperative care; some patients require postoperative ventilation.

Urgency
Most operations will be carried out semi-electively, and a few days of dexamethasone therapy will often show a marked improvement in raised ICP or neurological dysfunction in patients with tumour-related oedema. Occasionally urgent craniotomy or insertion of an external ventricular drain is required to prevent herniation of the brain.

Surgical approach
Tumours, especially meningiomas, can have large feeding vessels. Patients will sometimes be scheduled for embolization of these vessels, especially if they are not accessible at an early stage of the operation. A shunt can be inserted as a palliative procedure in patients with tumour-related obstructive hydrocephalus.

Meningioma
Meningiomas can be managed conservatively in patients with asymptomatic lesions or lesions in an inaccessible location. Surgical removal of tumour is the treatment of choice for most patients, and complete resection in benign tumours can offer a complete cure. Location and involvement of vital structures can make complete removal impossible, and a reduction in tumour mass can be undertaken prior to radiotherapy. Stereotactic radiotherapy or radiosurgery can be used as a sole treatment or following subtotal resection.

Glioma

For low-grade gliomas conservative management with anticonvulsants can be a treatment option, as surgery is not without risks and complications. The location of the tumour, whether superficial, close to eloquent areas of the brain, or deep within the basal ganglia is relevant as this determines accessibility and the risks of the surgical procedure. Some patients with low-grade glioma can be cured by complete resection, if necessary aided by advanced intra-operative monitoring and by performing an awake craniotomy (see p. 242). Debulking can be the preferred option as attempting complete resection comes with the risk of serious postoperative neurological deficits. A biopsy alone, rather than resection, can serve to confirm the histological diagnosis and aid the discussion about further treatment options. Biopsies can be obtained via a burr hole or as an open biopsy via mini-craniotomy. In a high-grade glioma the surgical option will usually be a biopsy or debulking.

Lymphoma

Steroid therapy has a dramatic though temporary effect by shrinking the tumour and possibly depleting the lesion of B-cells. If the diagnosis is suspected in the pre-operative period, patients are not started on steroids before a sample of tissue for histology is obtained. Stereotactic or image guided biopsy is commonly performed if a lymphoma is suspected.

Metastasis

Surgical resection of a solitary CNS metastasis offers a good prognosis. Small metastases respond well to stereostactic radiosurgery. Sometimes it is necessary to perform a biopsy to find a histological diagnosis if the primary is uncertain. A pragmatic view should be taken in patients with metastasis and advanced systemic metastic disease.

Positioning

- Most operations are carried out with the patient positioned supine; a sandbag under one shoulder can often facilitate surgical access.
- Other positions can be required as well, depending on the site of the lesion.
- Occipital and posterior fossa lesions often require prone positioning.
- Care should be taken not to obstruct venous return of the neck veins.

Intra-operative issues

Craniotomy for tumour is the 'typical' intracranial procedure. General considerations as discussed in General principles of neuroanaesthesia, pp. 110–119 will apply. The aim of anaesthesia is to provide optimal cerebral perfusion and good surgical access and operating conditions.

- Induction of anaesthesia is usually intravenous. Inhalational induction may be appropriate if intravenous induction is likely to cause excessive anxiety.
- Large bore intravenous access should be obtained, as significant bleeding can occur unannounced.
- The degree of stimulation varies considerably during the procedure. Insertion of pins is painful as are skin incision, reflection of the galea and closure. Local anaesthetic or systemic analgesia needs to be administered in time to prevent hypertension and increases in cerebral volume.

TUMOURS IN ADULTS

- Scalp blocks following induction may improve cardiovascular stability.
- Local anaesthetic infiltration of the scalp by the surgeon is widely used.
- Remifentanil infusion provides easily titratable analgesia.
- Once the dura is opened, direct inspection of the brain is possible.
  - A slack brain will demonstrate pulsations synchronous with heartbeat and respiration. A tight brain will show attenuated pulsations, or none at all, or might be bulging outwards, only restricted by the dura.
  - If indicated, administration of mannitol or furosemide, temporary hyperventilation and head-up tilt have all been used to reduce the bulk of the brain and minimize the risk of herniation upon opening of the dura (see p. 140). A bolus of dexamethasone is often requested by surgeon at the start of the operation.
- Intra-operative air embolism (see p. 142) can occur when the craniotomy is carried out over major sinuses such as the sagittal sinus.
- Intra-operative bleeding can be sudden and massive, with sometimes no immediate way to stop it. The extensive use of intra-operative wash and blood pooling under drapes can make estimation of blood loss difficult. It is important to communicate clearly with the surgeon if bleeding is a concern. Bleeding may come from a variety of sources and can occur at any time.
  - Skin flap—the scalp is vascular and unnoticed failure of initial haemostasis may result in a steady blood loss throughout the operation.
  - Bone flap—hyperostosis or tumour invasion by menigioma may result in significant bleeding from the bone.
  - Sinuses and venous lakes. Craniotomies which cross or are close to the midline may result in planned access through, or accidental injury to the major sinuses or the feeding large veins. Deliberate transection is much easier for the surgeon to control.
  - Tumours with increased vascularity can cause troublesome bleeding and can prolong surgery. Sometimes the feeding vessels are at the bottom of the tumour cavity and cannot be controlled until an access is made.
- Post-resection haemostasis should be meticulous. Hypotension should be avoided. Some anaesthetists and surgeons deliberately raise the blood pressure at this point.
- Hypertension at emergence and in the early postoperative period should be avoided.
  - Appropriate analgesia should be provided.
  - Numerous pharmacological techniques to prevent or control post-operative hypertension are available.

Monitoring

- Invasive arterial blood pressure measurement is used as routine for these patients.
  - Individual practice varies but direct arterial pressure monitoring is usually commenced prior to induction in patients with a tight brain, to allow for close monitoring during this part of the procedure.

- Temperature monitoring is routine.
- Urinary catheterization is normally performed both to allow monitoring of urine production and also to avoid bladder distension during long procedures.
- Some anaesthetists routinely place long-lines/central venous catheters for known vascular tumours.
- Some units are starting to use intra-operative MRI to help determine resection margins. This needs to be taken into account when choosing monitoring equipment.
- Other monitoring such as transcranial Doppler (TCD), jugular bulb oximetry, brain tissue oxygen probes have their advocates, but are not used as a matter of routine in most units in the UK.

Postoperative care
- Most craniotomy patients should be woken up extubated at the end of the procedure.
- Some units send all tumour craniotomies to a high dependency unit (HDU).
- Patients are usually nursed with a 15–30° head-up tilt.
- Adequate analgesia is important; a significant number of patients will have moderate to severe pain after craniotomy unless this is treated appropriately.
  - Morphine is a useful and safe analgesic, which can be given as PCA or orally according to local practice.
- PONV is common after neurosurgery and should be aggressively prevented and treated (see Anti-emetics and PONV, p.62).
- Most bleeding occurs in the first few hours following surgery. Reduction in conscious level, or failure to achieve full recovery to pre-operative neurological status should prompt urgent CT. This will usually require general anaesthesia.
- New neurological deficits can manifest themselves in the recovery room. Some of these deficits can be predicted by the surgeon, and recovery staff can be advised accordingly. Otherwise, new deficits should trigger urgent action.
- Seizures need to be recognized and treated promptly (see p.374). Recognition in the immediate postoperative period can be difficult, so a high index of suspicion is required.
- Postoperative ventilation can be required in patients with pre-existing significant neurological deficits, especially when airway reflexes or breathing can be affected, or when significant cerebral oedema is present.
- ICP monitoring might be indicated in ventilated patients postoperatively.
- Dexamethasone will usually be reduced over a few days following the operation.

Some tumours or tumour locations are associated with particular problems postoperatively.
- Prolonged retraction of the frontal lobes for resection of an olfactory groove meningioma can lead to postoperative oedema. Postoperative

sedation and ventilation may be considered though there is little evidence that this affects incidence or outcome of the complication.
- Following temporal lobe resection patients can be lethargic for a few days.
- Gliomas with tumour-related oedema occasionally respond to resection with the development of massive and fatal brain swelling within the early postoperative period. Postoperative sedation and ventilation will be required if this occurs.
- Patients with posterior fossa tumours may develop significant bulbar palsy following surgery, and may not be able to protect their own airway postoperatively (see Posterior fossa surgery, p. 206).

Prognosis

Prognosis is dependent upon tumour type, grade and location.

Meningioma

- Complete resection of a meningioma is often curative.
- Tumour location and possible involvement of local structures are the most important prognostic factors as they determine surgical accessibility.
- Histological features are relevant, as a higher-grade tumour is more likely to show malignant growth with invasion of surrounding structures.
- About 15% of apparently completely resected meningiomas recur.

Glioma

- A small percentage of low-grade gliomas can be cured by complete surgical resection.
- Low-grade astrocytomas can take 10 or more years to transform to a more malignant tumour.
- Anaplastic astrocytomas usually have a survival of 2–3 years from presentation.
- Glioblastomas have a median survival of 6 months if untreated.
  - The survival benefits of surgical debulking, chemotherapy and radiotherapy are additive. With 'triple' therapy 25% are alive at 2 years; with just radiotherapy 10% are alive at 2 years.
  - Selected patients with good functional status and recurrent tumour may be offered further debulking and insertion of chemotherapy wafers (carmustine).
- Some oligodendrogliomas are more chemosensitive than other gliomas; a particular chromosome abnormality is thought to be related to a better response. Younger age and lower WHO grade are related to a better prognosis.

Lymphoma

- Overall survival is around 40% at 5 years with combined radiotherapy and chemotherapy.

Metastasis

Patients with CNS metastases survive less than two months if untreated.
- Dexamethasone can prolong survival by about 2 months.
- Radiotherapy can prolong survival.

- Cerebral metastases appear to have a similar response to radiotherapy, independent of the primary tumour.
- Surgery for single CNS metastasis with a slow progressive primary lesion can extend survival by about a year; stereotactic radiosurgery produces similar results if the lesion is <3cm.
- Chemotherapy is currently indicated in metastases from breast cancer, small cell lung cancer and choriocarcinoma.

Tips and pitfalls
- Dexamethasone is usually withheld by surgeons prior to a biopsy if a lymphoma is suspected.
- Meningioma and metastases from malignant melanoma and renal cell carcinoma have the potential to bleed significantly during surgery.
- Patients undergoing resection of epidermoid cysts can develop chemical meningitis from the cyst content.
- The prognosis for patients with high-grade glioma is poor. The aim of surgery is to buy a limited amount of high-quality survival. The anaesthetist should endeavour to minimize morbidity as much as possible.

Tumours (children)

Intracranial tumours are the most common solid childhood tumours and the second most common paediatric malignancy after leukaemia. The incidence is increasing and varies across the globe from 15–31 per million. There is a greater incidence in boys.

Pathology
- In contrast to adult tumours, the majority (> 60%) of childhood tumours are infratentorial in the posterior fossa
- Presentation peaks at 1–8 years of age
- Histology varies with age; around 30% are gliomas, 30% medulloblastomas, 30% astrocytomas, 7% ependymomas and 3% other tumours, including acoustic neuromas and meningiomas
- If age <3, ependymomas account for ~30%.

A debulking procedure may allow symptom relief, slow disease progression, and depending on tumour histology may be curative if complete resection is achieved. Adjunctive radiotherapy may follow surgical excision, but is usually avoided in children <3 years due to adverse effects on brain development. Chemotherapy is used for some tumours.

Associated conditions
- The majority of brain tumours occur in previously healthy children
- Some tumours are more common in children with the inheritable neurocutaneous syndromes—neurofibromatosis and tuberous sclerosis
- Some astrocytomas show autosomal dominant inheritance
- Intracerebral lymphomas may be associated with immunodeficiency syndromes, e.g. Wiskott–Aldrich syndrome.

Presentation
Presentation of childhood tumours varies according to the age of child, the tumour site and the speed of growth of the intracranial lesion.
- In the very young, symptoms and signs are often non-specific. Infants and neonates can present with feeding difficulties, irritability or lethargy and loss of developmental milestones. Hydrocephalus (bulging fontanelle, increased head circumference, sunset eyes) may be seen.
- Older children often complain of headaches and/or vomiting, with visual disturbance, which develops over days or weeks.
- There may be signs of raised ICP or focal neurology according to the site of the tumour.
- New onset seizures or altered level of consciousness.
- Endocrine dysfunction may indicate a midline lesion.
- Cranial nerve palsies—especially with posterior fossa and midbrain tumours.

Pre-operative assessment
In addition to the normal pre-operative assessment the anaesthetist should be vigilant for common associated conditions and the effects of the lesion on the patient. History and examination are directed at detecting raised ICP and neurological deficits.

Parents
The presumed diagnosis of a brain tumour will be catastrophic news for the parents and the child. A compassionate approach to questions they may have, however trivial they may seem, is paramount.

Neurological deficits
The extent of cerebellar and cranial nerve dysfunction should be documented. Significant impairment of the lower cranial nerves increases the risk of pre- or postoperative gastric aspiration.

Hydration and nutrition
Children with a longer history may present with significant malnutrition due to a combination of vomiting, reduced conscious level and sometimes difficulty with swallowing. It will not be possible to correct all of these prior to surgery, but the anaesthetist should make an assessment of hydration and check the serum electrolytes.

Imaging
A review of available scans can provide information about the size and location of the tumour, associated oedema, the proximity of the fourth ventricle and the degree of hydrocephalus. The vascularity of the tumour, presence of feeding vessels or proximity to venous sinuses can all be assessed.

Blood cross-match
Blood should be cross-matched according to local protocol. Posterior fossa surgery has a higher risk of significant bleeding than other sites.

Plan for postoperative care
Children should be nursed postoperatively on specialist neurosurgical wards or in critical care areas. Elective ventilation is not usually necessary.

Urgency
Children presenting with posterior fossa tumours are usually operated on as soon as practical.
- If there are concerns about a risk of decompensation secondary to hydrocephalus, an external ventricular drain (EVD) may be inserted as a temporizing measure before formal debulking.
- ICP should be controlled before proceeding to definitive surgery, e.g. steroid treatment to reduce peritumour oedema, or drainage of hydrocephalus.
- Endocrine abnormalities, diabetes insipidus, SIADH and seizures should be treated or optimized pre-operatively, if possible.

Surgical approach
- The craniotomy site depends on the site of the tumour.
- Stereotactic surgery is used to locate deep-seated lesions to reduce the risk of neurological trauma.
- Frameless techniques now obviate the need to transfer patients to and from the CT suite.

Positioning
- A 10° head-up tilt improves cerebral venous return.

- In the supine position the head is turned to the side to expose the surgical site.
  - Rotation of the torso, along with the head and neck, is necessary to avoid venous obstruction.
  - A sand bag under the shoulder is helpful.
- Posterior fossa surgery is usually conducted with the patient prone, supported on bolsters or a specialized frame to allow free abdominal movement and facilitate IPPV.
  - The head may be supported on a horseshoe rest, or held in pins.
  - In children <3 years the use of pins may cause bony injury, intracranial haemorrhage or a dural tear.
- In some centres the sitting position is preferred for posterior fossa surgery to improve surgical access, reduce blood loss, lower intracranial pressure, reduce the likelihood of cranial nerve injury, and improve postoperative recovery.
- The benefits of using good surgical access need to be balanced against the risks of hypotension and VAE.
  - Centres using the sitting position regularly have reported low incidence of complications from VAE.
  - However, most units prefer the prone position on the basis of a lower risk of hypotension and VAE.

Intra-operative management

The general principles of paediatric neuroanaesthesia apply (see Paediatric neuroanaesthesia, p.120). The aim of anaesthesia is to provide optimal cerebral perfusion and good surgical access and operating conditions.

- Sedative premedication is usually avoided because of the risk of respiratory depression, hypercapnia, and potential adverse effects on ICP and airway integrity.
- If ICP is raised an intravenous induction is preferred, followed by tracheal intubation and ventilation to low-normal $PaCO_2$.
- Rapid sequence induction and cricoid pressure may be used where there are concerns about gastric emptying and the risk of aspiration. However, practicalities often override theoretical concerns and an inhalational induction is superior to fraught attempts at cannulation.
- A reinforced oral tracheal tube is placed if the patient is to be positioned prone, and may be stabilized using a throat pack, which will also soak up secretions. For the supine patient a 'south facing' RAE tube is an alternative. A nasal tube may be preferred in very young children, or if postoperative IPPV is planned.
- The child should be kept warm during this period and during positioning, usually using a forced air blower.
- Large bore intravenous access should be obtained, as significant bleeding can occur unannounced.
- A nasogastric tube is usually inserted at induction for posterior fossa tumours in case of new or continuing problems with swallowing following surgery.
- The degree of stimulation varies considerably during the procedure. Insertion of pins is painful as are skin incision, reflection of the galea and closure. Local anaesthetic or systemic analgesia needs to be administered in time to prevent hypertension and increases in cerebral volume.

CHAPTER 6 **Intracranial surgery (non-vascular)**

- Scalp blocks following induction may improve cardiovascular stability.
- Local anaesthetic infiltration of the scalp by the surgeon is widely used, though in practice the period between infiltration and incision is often short.
- Remifentanil infusion provides easily titratable analgesia in children.
- Most tumour surgery proceeds with minimal blood loss. However, rapid unexpected loss can occur and large bore intravenous access is mandatory.
  - Cross-matched blood should be available in the operating theatre suite
  - Losses are hard to measure and may be mixed with large volumes of wash or concealed in the drapes
  - Excessive amounts of crystalloid should be avoided as this may exacerbate oedema formation
  - Fluid management can be problematic if osmotic diuretics have been used to treat raised ICP
  - Dehydration increases the likelihood of hypovolaemia and hypotension and colloid boluses may be required.
- Surgery or decompression near or involving the brainstem and fourth ventricle may provoke considerable cardiovascular disturbance:
  - Bradycardia
  - Hypertension and hypotension
  - Dysrhythmia.
  - There is little that can be done to prevent these from occurring. Good communication with the surgeon is vital, both to warn of likely disturbance and to request a temporary halt to dissection if possible.
  - If cardiovascular disturbance persists after surgical dissection has stopped this suggests significant neural compromise. Postoperative admission to a critical care unit may be indicated.
- Most children are extubated at the end of surgery. This allows prompt neurological assessment.
- The aim is a smooth rapid emergence.
  - Prior to emergence analgesics and anti-emetics are administered and neuromuscular blockade is reversed.
- The choice of analgesia depends on the age of child, pre-operative morbidity and extent of surgery.
  - Intravenous paracetamol and a short-acting opioid can be used to cover the emergence period.
  - Opioid analgesia is required after craniotomy or posterior fossa craniectomy. If remifentanil has been used intra-operatively, morphine (0.1 mg kg^{-1}) should be given at least 40 min before the end of surgery. Further boluses can be titrated during emergence and recovery.
  - Opioid analgesia can be continued postoperatively as patient-controlled analgesia (PCA), nurse-controlled analgesia (NCA) or orally, depending on local protocols and processes for monitoring analgesia.
  - It is usually possible to discontinue opioid analgesia at 12–36 h postoperatively and replace with simple oral analgesia. Analgesic requirements are however variable.

Monitoring

In addition to routine monitoring:
- An arterial line is placed to allow invasive blood pressure monitoring and peri-operative blood sampling.

- Temperature monitoring is routine.
- Urinary catheterization is normally performed both to allow monitoring of urine production and also to avoid bladder distension during long procedures or when mannitol or furosemide are to be used.
- Oesophageal stethoscopes may be used in small children, particularly if there is a significant risk of VAE. Most anaesthetists consider that other monitoring techniques have superseded these.
- Central venous pressure monitoring is not routine, but should be considered if the risk of VAE is high, if significant blood loss or CVS instability is anticipated.
- Frequent assessment of haemoglobin and coagulation status should be performed if significant bleeding is encountered.

Postoperative care
- Postoperative care is usually in a HDU environment. Invasive monitoring may be continued if there are concerns about cardiovascular instability.
- The child's neurological status is monitored as a change may indicate intracranial haemorrhage or seizure and needs urgent assessment, investigation and treatment.
- Postoperative IPPV is considered if the child is hypothermic, has severe neurological injury, or seizure control or airway protection are inadequate.
- Posterior fossa surgery may cause brainstem oedema, with disruption to cardiovascular and respiratory centres or damage to cranial nerves innervating the vocal cords, leading to stridor or respiratory obstruction.

Prognosis
Overall, mortality from childhood brain tumours has declined to less than 0.9 per 100,000 per year.

Tips and pitfalls
- Large blood loss may be swift and unexpected, or insidious and concealed. Have cross-matched blood available in the theatre suite.
- Posterior fossa surgery may cause intra-operative CVS instability. Ask the surgeon to stop manipulation or to relax retraction.
- Delayed emergence, hiccoughs, hypoventilation or inadequate airway protection may indicate brainstem dysfunction secondary to surgical trauma.
- Stridor in the immediate postoperative period indicates vocal cord paralysis. Fibre-optic transnasal laryngoscopy can help assessment of vocal cord function.
- The parents will need a compassionate, unhurried explanation of what anaesthesia and postoperative care will involve. Do not be afraid to ask the neurosurgical team to come back to answer their questions if they fall outside your expertise.
- Correctly titrated opioid analgesia does *not* impair postoperative neurological assessment. A child in pain may become hypertensive or develop raised intracranial pressure, both of which should be avoided.

Acoustic neuroma

The majority (~80%) of cerebello-pontine (CP) angle tumours are acoustic neuromas. The term 'acoustic neuroma' is a misnomer as they usually occur on the vestibular portion of the nerve and the term vestibular schwannomas is more accurate. They are benign tumours, but can recur.

The cerebello-pontine angle is bordered by the petrous temporal bone laterally and the lower pons and medulla (antero-medially) and the cerebellum (postero-medially).

The principles presented in this chapter also apply to other types of CP angle surgery.

Presentation

Acoustic neuromas usually present in adults (most commonly in the fifth and sixth decades). They may be associated with neurofibromatosis type II.

- Hearing loss—usually unilateral, but may be bilateral particularly when associated with neurofibromatosis type II
- Tinnitus
- Balance disturbance
- Other cranial nerve dysfunction due to local compression, e.g. Vth cranial nerve with facial numbness, or trigeminal neuralgia.
- Hydrocephalus—secondary to large tumours preventing normal circulation of CSF.

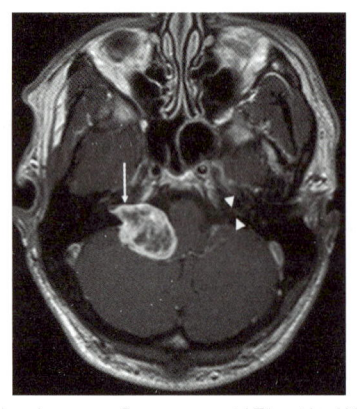

Fig. 6.3 Vestibular schwannoma. Post-contrast axial T1-weighted MRI. Right-sided vestibular schwannoma impressing into the cerebellum. The intracanalicular portion of the tumour (white arrow) expands the internal auditory canal. (White arrowheads—normal-appearing left internal auditory canal.)

ACOUSTIC NEUROMA

Management
- Initial management depends on size and symptoms; 40–60% may not grow after discovery.
- If <2.5 cm and with no symptoms other than hearing loss or tinnitus, interval scanning is performed until growth is proven.
- Tumours that are growing and <3 cm can be treated by surgery or stereotactic radiosurgery. (This can be delivered by a dedicated machine for the CNS—called a 'gamma knife', or using a linear accelerator. Both employ the stereotactic frame used for biopsy.)
- Larger tumours require surgical excision.

Surgical approaches
- The cerebello-pontine angle may be reached through the inner ear (translabyrinthine), behind the ear (retrosigmoid), through the middle fossa or suboccipitally (using the sitting position). The first two are used most commonly.
- The VIIIth cranial nerve is nearly always permanently damaged by surgery (its function is usually already affected by the tumour), and the translabyrinthine approach (used for larger tumours) sacrifices the inner ear.
- The function of the VIIth cranial nerve is monitored by EMG during the procedure. Brainstem auditory evoked responses have also been used.
- These procedures can be last up to 8 h.

Positioning
- The patient is positioned supine for a translabyrinthine approach and in the park bench or lateral position for a retrosigmoid approach.
- In both the operating table is rolled frequently during surgery to bring different aspects of the craniotomy into the view of the surgeon. It is necessary to prevent the patient slipping or falling off the table by placing supports at the level of the pelvis and the upper torso.

Pre-operative assessment
In addition to the normal pre-operative assessment the anaesthetist should be vigilant for commonly associated conditions such as other manifestations of type II neurofibromatosis such as meningiomas and spinal cord tumours.

Intra-operative issues
The main anaesthetic considerations relate to prolonged surgery, the requirement for facial nerve monitoring and stimulation of cardiovascular responses during surgery.
- Careful positioning must be utilized, and then checked due to the length of the cases:
  - pad pressure areas;
  - place a urinary catheter;
  - keep the patient warm;
  - move the pulse oximeter probe to a new digit at least every 4 h;
  - if placed lateral, place a roll under the axilla (to reduce pressure on the arm and shoulder) and a pillow under the lower leg.

- Use a technique without nitrous oxide; use TIVA or volatile–based anaesthesia.
- Neuromuscular blockades (NMBs) should be avoided during maintenance as they interfere with facial nerve EMG monitoring.
- NMBs can be used to facilitate tracheal intubation, transfer to the operating table and positioning.
- Spontaneous respiration can be suppressed with high-dose opioid infusion—remifentanil infusions are used.
- CVS instability including marked bradycardia, hypo- and hypertension can occur with either direct stimulation of brainstem structures or of other cranial nerves.
  - Most anaesthetists do not give prophylactic vagolytic drugs.
- These operations can be painful—use simple analgesics and moderate doses of long-acting opioids such as morphine 0.05–0.1 mg kg^{-1} before stopping remifentanil and emergence.

Postoperative care
- Usually provided on a neurosurgical ward or HDU.
- Because of the length of the procedure there is a risk of hypothermia, fluids shifts and oedema of dependent areas.
- Pain and nausea and vomiting may be problematic.

Postoperative complications
- VIIth nerve palsy—temporary or permanent
- CSF leak
- Meningitis
- Haematoma formation
- Facial numbness (Vth)
- Swallowing difficulties (IXth, Xth).

Tips and pitfalls
- Low dose NMBs have been used with EMG monitoring, but as they are not necessary it is best to avoid them.
- Maintain close communication with the surgeon if CVS instability occurs. Simply stopping the surgery for a minute or so usually results in complete resolution.
- Use prophylactic anti-emetics. PONV is very common in these patients.
- Craniotomy through the relatively thick temporal or skull base bones can be painful, use carefully titrated doses of long-acting opioids in the recovery room.

Pituitary tumours

Pituitary tumours present either as functional tumours causing endocrine syndromes or with visual disturbance due to local compression of the optic chiasm.

These tumours start in the pituitary fossa (sella turcica) and may extend superiorly above the fossa. Most tumours are non-secreting, although they may cause endocrine effects by pressing on the hypothalamic–pituitary axis, resulting in hypopituitarism. Secreting tumours can cause a variety of syndromes.

Craniopharyngioma is covered elsewhere (p. 224).

Pathology
Pituitary tumours are benign adenomas of the anterior pituitary gland. They are relatively common, with an estimated population prevalence of around 15%, though most are asymptomatic. Around 10% of intracranial neoplasms are pituitary tumours.

Patient population
Women are more likely to be diagnosed with pituitary tumours. Most patients are middle aged. Pre-pubertal diagnosis is rare.

Hypersecreting tumour syndromes

Growth hormone—acromegaly
Prior to puberty and fusion of the epiphyses growth hormone excess results in gigantism. After puberty, excess growth hormone results in acromegaly (an increase in size of the extremities):
- Increased shoe and ring size
- Frontal bossing
- Enlargement of mandible
- Soft tissue and connective tissue abnormalities:
  - Airway swelling
  - Nasal and pharyngeal tissue hypertrophy
  - Glottic narrowing
  - High incidence of obstructive sleep apnoea
- Hypertension
- Glucose intolerance
- Cardiomyopathy, cardiomegaly, and congestive heart failure (CCF)
- Osteoarthritis
- Sweating.

ACTH–Cushing's syndrome
- Centripetal obesity (and buffalo hump)
- Hirsutism
- Skin striae, acne
- Infection and poor wound healing
- Amenorrhoea
- Increased blood pressure
- Hyperkalaemia
- Glucose intolerance
- Muscle weakness (proximal myopathy).

TSH
- Thyrotoxicosis.

Sex hormones
- Various abnormalities (usually clinically silent).

Prolactin
Moderate increases in prolactin may be due to compression of the hypothalamic–pituitary structures by a non-secreting tumour. High levels of prolactin are due to prolactin-secreting tumours (prolactinomas).
- In women:
  - Galactorrhoea
  - Infertility
  - Amenorrhoea.
- In men:
  - The mass effect usually seen first (optic nerve compression)
  - Decreased libido, impotence
  - Oligospermia.

Pituitary apoplexy

A rare acute presentation due to haemorrhage or infarction of a pituitary adenoma leading to meningeal irritation, effects of a space-occupying lesion (SOL) and sudden visual impairment along with sudden onset of hypopituitarism.

Pituitary apoplexy may be seen during pregnancy (Sheehan's syndrome). This is associated with hypotension after a postpartum haemorrhage.

Visual disturbance

Mass effect from pituitary tumours may cause compression of the optic chiasm, nerves or tracts.
- The optic chiasm is most commonly affected. This causes varying degrees of bitemporal hemianopia.
- Eccentric or extensive tumour growth may affect other parts of the visual pathway causing less classical symptoms.

Treatment options

Observation
Asymptomatic or incidental tumours may be managed purely expectantly, with serial scanning. This option may be most appropriate for patients with serious medical comorbidity.

Drug treatment
Prolactinomas may be managed solely with dopamine agonists (bromocriptime or cabergoline). Endocrine symptom control may be required for secreting tumours (e.g. insulin, metapyrone) but medical management alone is usually insufficient.

Radiotherapy
Stereotactic radiosurgery has been used either as a primary therapy or as a postoperative adjunct.

Surgery

Surgical treatment is aimed at debulking the tumour. It is the treatment of choice for patients presenting with visual loss and for secreting tumours which cannot be controlled medically.

Pre-operative assessment

In addition to the normal pre-operative assessment, the anaesthetist should be vigilant for the commonly associated conditions. Elective patients will have had a formal endocrine assessment prior to surgery. Emergency patients (presenting with acute visual loss) are unlikely to have had this performed.

- Diabetes mellitus.
- Hypertension.
- Obstructive sleep apnoea.
  - A large proportion of patients with acromegaly are reported to have a degree of obstructive sleep apnoea and a subset may also have central sleep apnoea.
  - Many of these may be undiagnosed. Aside from careful history taking, formal sleep studies or overnight pulse oximetry may be useful investigations.
  - Pre-operative continuous positive airways pressure (CPAP) may be beneficial for some patients.
- Cushing's patients are likely to be receiving metyrapone to reduce corticosteroid production.
- Prolactinoma patients may be receiving cabergoline to reduce symptoms and to shrink the tumour.

Surgical approaches

Trans-sphenoidal

The standard approach.
- Midline access to pituitary fossa through the sphenoid sinus.
- Reached via the nasal passages (or sometimes sublabially) either with X-ray control or naso-endoscopically guided.
- Patient placed supine, with neck a little extended (more so for X-ray-guided approach). Some surgeons use a semi-sitting position and stand in front of the patient.
- If a CSF leak is detected the surgeon may wish to pack the nose with fat harvested from the abdominal wall.

Supratentorial

- Approached by a frontal craniotomy
- Usually used for large tumours that have extended (upwards) out of the pituitary fossa.

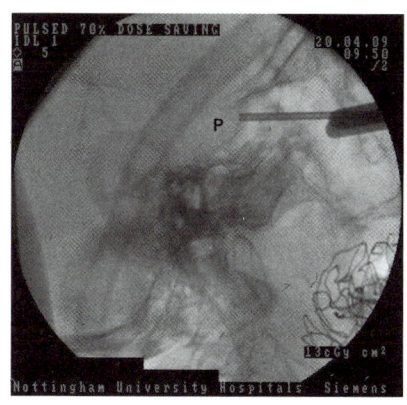

Fig. 6.4 Lateral intra-operative radiograph demonstrating the radio-opaque probe pointing towards the pituitary fossa (P).

Anaesthetic considerations

Trans-sphenoidal surgery is neurosurgery via an ENT approach. The anaesthetic considerations are similar, however.
- The nasal mucosa is prepared by the surgeon before commencing surgery with a topical vasoconstrictor. Drugs commonly used include adrenaline (on swabs) or cocaine paste, solution (on swabs) or spray.
- The approach through the nasal passages is stimulating, even with local anaesthesia of the mucosa. Watch for sudden increases in blood pressure.
- Large tumours which cause pressure symptoms should be managed like any other space-occupying lesion.
- Balanced anaesthesia with either volatile agents or TIVA is appropriate.
- If short-acting opioids (in particular remifentanil) are used, give a long-acting opioid before emergence.
- Bleeding may be sudden and brisk. A throat pack is placed to reduce laryngeal soiling.
- To force remaining tumour into the surgical field or to see if there is a CSF leak the surgeon may request a Valsalva manoeuvre.

Postoperative management
- In uncomplicated cases the immediate care is like that for any other nasal (airway) operation.
- Ensure the airway is likely to be well-maintained before extubation (have the patient as awake as possible).
- Remove the throat pack and suck out the oral cavity and nasophayrnx (behind the soft palate).

- If nasal packs are used the patient will not be able to breathe normally through the nose (although most packs do have a small passage inside them to allow some air though).
- Hormone replacement should be given according to local policies.
- Patient with known or at high risk of obstructive sleep apnoea (OSA) (e.g. acromegalics) should be nursed in HDU for at least 24 h.

Complications

Immediate
- Airway obstruction.
- Bleeding—nasal mucosa, veins around the pituitary, carotid artery.
- VAE if head-up tilt is excessive.
- Carotid-cavernous fistula.

Later
- Infection.
- CSF leak:
  - May require return to theatre for repacking.
- Diabetes insipidus (DI):
  - This may start very soon after surgery. In most patients it is temporary although it may last for up to 10 days. It may be permanent in a few patients.
  - Regular (at least daily) measurements of urea and electrolytes, plasma and urinary osmolarity.
  - Replace fluids on a 'like-for-like' basis in addition to normal fluid requirements.
  - Use hypotonic solutions as the fluid lost is mainly water (low sodium content).
  - Desmopressin is used for more severe or prolonged DI.
- Endocrine disturbance:
  - Most units have associated endocrine medicine departments who manage the more difficult postoperative endocrine disturbances.

Prognosis
- Complete resection of small tumours is expected.
- For larger tumours, the surgeon may accept debulking rather than excision.
- Some degree of endocrine disturbance is usual. This may change with time.
- Visual disturbance improves to an extent in ~80% or patients.
- Tumours may recur.

Tips and pitfalls
- **❶ Do not** use adrenaline and cocaine together. Cocaine sensitizes the heart to catecholamines and there is a risk of ventricular arrhythmias.

- A throat pack is essential to reduce laryngeal and tracheal contamination with blood from the nose and nasopharynx.
- Trans-sphenoidal resection is a relatively short operation by neurosurgical standards.
- Trans-sphenoidal resection is an operation where significant bleeding can occur very soon after the start of the operation. Ensure that adequate venous access is in place.
- Meticulous attention should be paid to ensuring that any nasopharyngeal clot is removed prior to extubation.

Posterior fossa surgery

Posterior fossa surgery is carried out for a variety of pathology. Tumours and haemorrhage are the most common. Although the general principles of anaesthesia for tumour and haemorrhage surgery apply to the posterior fossa, there are some aspects which are more specific. The location of the pathology has a significant impact on the presentation, surgical access and outcome. Lesions may be extra-axial, midline or lateral. Hydrocephalus may be present and require management in its own right (EVD or endoscopic third ventriculostomy).

Pathology
- Posterior fossa tumours account for ~60% of childhood brain tumours, compared with ~20% of adult brain tumours.
- Astrocytoma, ependymoma, primitive neuroectodermal tumours and other mixed glial tumours account for most of the paediatric posterior fossa tumours.
- Metastasis is the commonest posterior fossa tumour in adults, followed by haemangioblastoma and brainstem glioma.

Astrocytoma
Around 1/3 of childhood posterior fossa tumours are cystic cerebellar astrocytoma. These usually present in later childhood.

Primitive neuroectodermal tumours (PNET)
Primitive neuroectodermal tumour in the posterior fossa is usually referred to as medulloblastoma. It is more common in younger children, though may present at any age. It originates in the fourth ventricle and often presents with a gradually progressive history of listlessness, headache, and localizing symptoms and signs such as nystagmus and cranial nerve palsies. Complete resection may be impossible for tumours which have brainstem involvement or which are metastatic at presentation.

Ependymoma
Ependymomas typically occur within the fourth ventricle. With the potential to extend to and through the foramina of Lushka and Magendie, these tumours can be surgically challenging. The extent of resection is vital for prognosis so surgery may be prolonged, or undertaken as a staged approach with repeat operations for residual tumour.

Haemangioblastoma
As the name suggests these are tumours of vascular origin. They occur more frequently in middle age and are usually lateral. They present with progressive history of headaches, diplopia, nystagmus, and ataxia. They are often associated with polycythaemia. Some are predominantly cystic with a small mural nodule. Others are larger, solid tumours which can bleed significantly during resection.

Associated conditions
- Most posterior fossa tumours are isolated entities.
- Haemangioblastoma may be part of the von Hippel–Lindau syndrome (haemangioblastoma in cerebellum, spinal cord and retina, café au lait spots, phaeochromocytoma, renal tumours etc.).
- Intracerebral haemorrhage (ICH) in the posterior fossa has the same associations as for ICH elsewhere, including smoking and hypertension.

Presentation
As space-occupying lesions within the posterior fossa vault, tumours present either with local effects (cerebellar or lower cranial nerves) or general symptoms and signs of raised ICP. Typically diagnosis is delayed as more common explanations are ruled out.
- Cerebellar symptoms and signs may include:
  - Ataxia
  - Past pointing
  - Horizontal nystagmus
  - Dysarthria.
- Lower cranial nerve palsies may result in:
  - Dysphagia and swallowing problems, which in turn may lead to nocturnal cough, recurrent chest infections
  - Dysarthria
  - Diplopia.
- The symptoms and signs off raised ICP vary with speed of onset and age of the patient:
  - Listlessness/failure to thrive
  - Confusion
  - Reduction in conscious level
  - Headaches (classically in the morning)
  - Vomiting
  - Diplopia and squint.

Posterior fossa haematoma usually presents with an abrupt reduction in conscious level.

Pre-operative assessment
In addition to the normal pre-operative assessment the anaesthetist should be vigilant for commonly associated conditions.

Neurological deficits
The extent of cerebellar and cranial nerve dysfunction should be documented. Significant impairment of the lower cranial nerves increases the risk of pre- or postoperative gastric aspiration.

Hydration and nutrition
Patients with a longer history may present with significant malnutrition due to a combination of vomiting, reduced conscious level and difficulty with swallowing. It will not be possible to correct all of these prior to surgery, but the anaesthetist should make an assessment of hydration and check the serum electrolytes.

Imaging

A review of available scans can provide information about the size and location of the tumour, the proximity of the fourth ventricle and the degree of hydrocephalus. It also gives information about the vascularity of the tumour and involvement of significant feeding vessels or proximity to a sinus.

A history of recurrent chest infection may occasionally warrant a chest X-ray, though this is unlikely to alter management in the short-term.

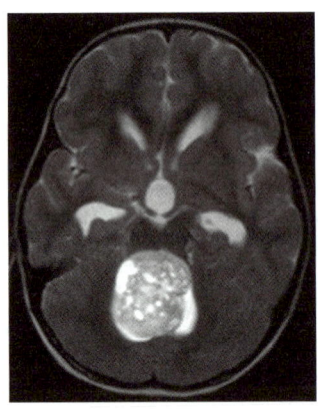

Fig. 6.5 Posterior fossa tumour. Axial T2-weighted MRI scan of an 8-year-old child with a posterior fossa pilocytic astrocytoma centred on the 4th ventricle. Note the third and lateral ventricles are dilated, consistent with supratentorial hydrocephalus.

Blood cross-match

Blood should be cross-matched according to local protocol. Posterior fossa surgery has a greater risk of significant bleeding than other sites. This is particularly the case for patients with solid haemangioblastoma and some metastases (notably renal).

Postoperative care

A significant compromise of conscious state, impairment of cough or swallowing, or tumour location in a sensitive area indicate a need for a higher level of postoperative care; some patients require postoperative ventilation.

Urgency

Posterior fossa haemorrhage is a true emergency, and as with other operations for bleeding, there may only be limited time available for assessment.

Children presenting with posterior fossa tumours are usually operated on as soon as practical. Symptomatic supratentorial hydrocephalus may be treated by insertion of an EVD prior to formal debulking.

Positioning

The commonest position in adults and children is with the patient prone.
- Lateral positions may be used for lateral access.
- The sitting position is used relatively rarely, and only by centres that undertake it regularly.
- The advantages of the sitting position of better access to midline structures are felt by many to be outweighed by the potential risks, particularly hypotension and venous air embolism.
- Care should be taken not to obstruct venous return of the neck veins particularly as the neck is usually flexed.

Surgical approach

The approach is usually through a craniectomy (not a craniotomy). The cranium overlying the posterior fossa is not suited to removal of a bone flap, and the neck muscles provide good protection postoperatively.
- The craniectomy is either midline, or biased towards the side of the lesion.
- Multiple burr holes are performed above the foramen magnum and the craniectomy completed with rongeurs and punches.
- Dural venous sinuses vary widely in their size and layout and brief periods of heavy blood loss may occur during craniectomy and dural opening.
- Midline or deep tumours will be close to or within the fourth ventricle.
- An EVD may be inserted before the craniectomy either to reduce ICP, or to allow intra-operative drainage of CSF. This may improve surgical access by allowing the cerebellum to fall back into the posterior fossa, away from the edges of the craniectomy.
- Dural opening inferiorly to the cisterna magna may also be used to release CSF and relieve pressure.

Intra-operative issues

Patients with posterior fossa pathology should be assumed to have raised intracranial pressure, and the anaesthesia technique should reflect this.

Smooth induction is the ideal, though may not always be possible in children.
- Large-bore intravenous access should be obtained, as significant bleeding can occur unannounced.
- A nasogastric tube is sometimes inserted at induction in case of new or continuing problems with swallowing following surgery.
- The degree of stimulation varies considerably during the procedure. Insertion of pins is painful. Posterior fossa craniectomy requires a considerable degree of muscle dissection and bony work and therefore tends to be more stimulating than supratentorial surgery.
- Local anaesthesia for posterior fossa craniectomy is more difficult to achieve reliably than for supratentorial craniotomy.
- Systemic analgesia needs to be administered in time to prevent hypertension and increases in cerebral volume. Remifentanil infusion provides easily titratable analgesia

CHAPTER 6 **Intracranial surgery (non-vascular)**

- Once the dura is opened, direct inspection of the contents of the posterior fossa is possible.
  - A slack brain will demonstrate pulsations synchronous with heartbeat and respiration. A tight brain will show attenuated pulsations, or none at all, or might be bulging outwards, only restricted by the dura or craniectomy.
- Intra-operative air embolism (see p. 142) can occur at any point during surgery.
  - Open large veins may be encountered during muscle reflection, craniectomy, and intracranial dissection.
- Intra-operative bleeding can be sudden and massive, and there may be no immediate way to stop it. The extensive use of intra-operative wash, and blood pooling under drapes can make estimation of blood loss difficult. It is important to communicate clearly with the surgeon if bleeding is a concern. Bleeding may come from a variety of sources and can occur at any time.
  - Soft tissues. Even in the most experienced hands bleeding from the neck muscles can be troublesome at times.
  - Sinuses and venous lakes. The site of the craniectomy is usually planned to avoid the major sinuses but inevitably accidental or deliberate injury to the major sinuses or the feeding large veins may occur. Deliberate transection is much easier for the surgeon to control. Tearing of the side wall of a sinus may cause prolonged and relatively uncontrolled bleeding.
  - Tumour excision. Vascular tumours will bleed. This is particularly true for haemangioblastoma. Sometimes the feeding vessels are at the bottom of the tumour cavity, so cannot be controlled directly until near the end of surgery.
- Surgery or decompression near or involving the brain stem and fourth ventricle may provoke considerable cardiovascular disturbance:
  - bradycardia
  - hypertension and hypotension
  - dysrhythmia.
- There is little that can be done to prevent these from occurring. Good communication with the surgeon is vital both to warn of likely disturbance and to request a temporary halt to dissection if possible.
  - Some anaesthetists routinely give vagolytic drugs, others only give them if bradycardia is persistent and associated with adverse effects on cardiac output.
- Post-resection haemostasis should be meticulous. Hypotension should be avoided. Some anaesthetists and surgeons deliberately raise the blood pressure at this point; others do not.
- Hypertension at emergence and in the early postoperative period is common and may be associated with postoperative haemorrhage.
  - Appropriate analgesia should be provided.
  - Numerous pharmacological techniques to prevent or control postoperative hypertension are available (see Vasoactive drugs, p.44).

Monitoring
- Invasive arterial blood pressure measurement is used as routine for these patients.
  - Individual practice varies but direct arterial pressure monitoring is usually commenced prior to induction in patients with a 'tight' brain, to allow for close monitoring during this part of the procedure.
- Temperature monitoring is routine.
- Urinary catheterization is normally performed both to allow monitoring of urine production and also to avoid bladder distension during long procedures.
- Some anaesthetists routinely place long lines or central venous catheters for known vascular tumours.
- Frequent assessment of haemoglobin and coagulation status should be performed if significant bleeding is encountered.

Postoperative care
- Most posterior fossa surgery patients should be woken up and extubated at the end of the procedure.
- Patients with intracranial haemorrhage or extensive brainstem involvement may require a period of postoperative sedation and ventilation.
- Patients with posterior fossa tumours may develop significant bulbar palsy following surgery and may not be able to protect their own airway postoperatively. The anaesthetist should have a high index of suspicion for these problems and not be afraid to re-intubate if airway protection is not satisfactory.
- Some centres perform MRI imaging of children with tumours in the immediate postoperative phase. Local logistics may determine whether this is performed as the final phase of surgery, or as a separate event. Intra-operative MRI is also beginning to be used in some centres for some of these cases.
- Patients are usually nursed with a head-up tilt.
- Adequate analgesia is important; most patients will have moderate to severe pain after craniectomy unless this is treated appropriately.
  - Morphine is a useful and safe analgesic, which can be given as PCA, NCA or orally according to local practice.
- PONV is common after posterior fossa surgery and should be aggressively prevented and treated (see Anti-emetics and PONV, p.62).
- The EVD, if inserted, is usually left in place postoperatively. This can be opened to allow acute reduction in ICP if necessary.
- Most bleeding occurs in the first few hours following surgery. Reduction in conscious level, or failure to achieve full recovery to pre-operative neurological status, should prompt urgent CT. This will usually require sedation, intubation, and controlled ventilation.
- Injured neural tissue or pathways (from haemorrhage, tumour, surgery or instruments) tends to recover slowly from the effects of anaesthesia, so slow return of neurological deficits is relatively common.

Complications

Intra-operative
- Bleeding.
- Venous air embolism.
- Cardiovascular disturbance.

Postoperative
- Raised ICP.
- Cranial nerve palsies.
- Injury to respiratory centre.
- Cerebellar mutism:
  - A condition of unknown aetiology in children following posterior fossa surgery. Despite apparently normal cognition children show apathy and do not speak for anything from a few days to several months following posterior fossa surgery. Risk factors include medulloblastoma histology and vermis/paravermian damage. It resolves spontaneously.

Late
- CSF leakage through the wound.
- Infection.
- Pseudomeningoocoele.
- Obstructive hydrocephalus, which may require VP shunting.
- Tumour recurrence.

Prognosis
Prognosis is dependent upon the lesion.

Posterior fossa haemorrhage
- Lateral cerebellar haemorrhages may do relatively well.
- Midline bleeds have a poor prognosis.

Pilocytic astrocytoma
- Resection is often complete resulting in a cure from surgery alone.

Medulloblastoma/ependymoma
- With combined chemo- and radiotherapy, 60–70% have progression-free survival at 5 years.

Haemangioblastoma
- Surgery is usually curative.

Metastasis
Patients with CNS metastases survive less than 2 months if untreated.
- Dexamethasone can prolong survival by about 2 months.
- Radiotherapy can prolong survival.
  - Cerebral metastases appear to have a similar response to radiotherapy, independent of the primary tumour.
- Surgery for single CNS metastasis with a slow progressive primary lesion can extend survival by about a year; stereotactic radiosurgery produces similar results if the lesion is <3cm.
- Chemotherapy is currently only indicated in metastases from breast cancer, small cell lung cancer, and choriocarcinoma.

Tips and pitfalls
- Beware of malnutrition and dehydration in patients with a prolonged history.
- Venous air embolism is not solely a complication of the sitting position.
- Be prepared for significant bleeding.
- Patients with haemangioblastoma may start off with relatively high haemoglobin; significant bleeding may have occurred before anaemia becomes evident.
- Be prepared for significant cardiovascular disturbance, particularly with:
  - Evacuation of haematoma
  - Resection of brain stem and 4th ventricle tumours
  - These disturbances usually, but not always resolve intra-operatively. Some patients continue to have problems in the postoperative phase.
- Do not be afraid to ask the surgeon for a surgical pause if you feel you are in need of time to achieve fluid or coagulation homeostasis.
- If necessary resections can be completed at a second operation.
- Hypothermia will worsen bleeding.

Shunts and ventricular drains

Shunt and drain insertions are some of the commonest neurosurgical procedures, and are performed both electively and as emergencies. The fundamental purpose of a shunt or drain is to divert CSF, either internally or externally, and thereby reduce or control intracranial pressure.

Shunt insertion is a common procedure in premature or newborn infants. One in 500 live births develops hydrocephalus. Shunt revision surgery is also common. Two-thirds of shunt procedures are revisions of previously placed shunts—usually due to a problem with the distal catheter. Up to 50% of shunts fail within the first two years.

Shunt is the commonest surgical procedure for treatment of hydrocephalus. An alternative is neuroendoscopic third ventriculostomy (p. 220).

Pathology

The physiology and pathology of intracranial pressure and cerebrospinal fluid are described more fully in p. 22. Raised intracranial pressure requiring shunts or drains is due to:
- Space-occupying lesions/haematoma/contusion.
- Obstruction of CSF flow—the commonest cause. The obstruction is within either the ventricular system or subarachnoid space, e.g. blockage of cerebral aqueduct or interventricular foramina secondary to tumours, blood, infection or congenital malformations.
- Increased production of CSF, e.g. choroid plexus papilloma.
- Decreased re-absorption. This may be secondary to obstruction of major dural venous sinus, e.g. tumour or thrombosis, or idiopathic (normal pressure hydrocephalus).

Based on the cause, hydrocephalus can be classified into communicating and non-communicating. Either of these may be congenital or acquired.

Communicating hydrocephalus
Also known as non-obstructive hydrocephalus. There is no obvious obstruction to CSF flow from the ventricles to the subarachnoid space, but the CSF is not reabsorbed from there. This may be secondary to subarachnoid haemorrhage, meningitis, congenital abnormality of the arachnoid villi, or be associated with a Chiari malformation.

Normal pressure hydrocephalus
A type of communicating hydrocephalus. The ventricles are enlarged but the CSF pressure may be normal if isolated measurements are taken. The pressure may only be raised intermittently. Diagnosis is made on the basis of history, CSF pressure at lumbar puncture (LP) and the response to removal of lumbar CSF either at LP or via a lumbar drain. Sometimes pressure infusion tests are performed. The clinical signs of acutely raised ICP may not be seen (such as headache, nausea, and vomiting) but the triad of disturbed gait, mental decline, and urinary incontinence mimicking dementia are seen.

Benign intracranial hypertension
A chronic increase in ICP that is not associated with any other acquired or congenital abnormality. It is a diagnosis of exclusion. Usually diagnosed

in overweight women aged between 20 to 40 years. Headaches and visual loss secondary to papilloedema are the cardinal features. Nausea and vomiting, tinnitus, cranial nerve palsies (in particular those controlling the external ocular muscles) may also occur. Treatment includes weight loss, medical therapy with carbonic anhydrase inhibitors such as acetazolamide. Lumbar puncture and shunts are used primarily for headache. Optic nerve sheath fenestration is used for visual loss.

Non-communicating hydrocephalus
This is an obstructive hydrocephalus due to a blockage of CSF flow. Bleeding, tumour, colloid cysts, and congenital abnormalities are the commonest causes.

Presentation
- Acutely raised ICP causes headache, nausea, and vomiting, papilloedema, abnormalities of upward gaze, and altered consciousness.
- In normal pressure hydrocephalus there is another common triad of symptoms: gait disturbance, mental decline, and urinary incontinence.
- Chronic hydrocephalus in children with unfused cranial bones causes the skull to enlarge.
- The nature of presentation is dependent upon the pathology. Slow increases in ICP seen in association with tumours and failing shunts may have relatively subtle presentations.
- Acute increases in ICP, often associated with trauma and subarachnoid haemorrhage, may result in rapid deterioration in conscious level.

Surgical considerations
The commonest diversion procedure involves insertion of a catheter into one of the lateral ventricles.

External drains
In acute or infected cases, the ventricular catheter is externalized (EVD). This allows controlled drainage of CSF, direct measurement of ICP, microbiological sampling and intraventricular administration of drugs (antibiotics).

EVDs may also be used intra-operatively for posterior fossa surgery as controlled drainage of CSF may improve surgical access.

Lumbar drains may also be placed pre-operatively for patients undergoing craniotomy or pituitary surgery, particularly if surgical access is expected to be difficult. This is relatively unusual in the UK.

Ventricular shunts
For long-term control of ICP the ventricular catheter is connected to a one-way valve, which in turn drains into an internal catheter. The ultimate destination of the CSF is most commonly peritoneal (ventriculo-peritoneal (VP/shunt), or pleural (more common in children) or rarely atrial, (ventriculo-atrial (VA)/shunt).

Access to the ventricle is through a burr hole placed either frontally or parieto-occipitally. The valve is placed subcutaneously at or just below the burr hole.

216 CHAPTER 6 **Intracranial surgery (non-vascular)**

The distal catheter is passed under the skin of the neck, chest and upper abdomen to the site of an abdominal incision where the catheter is fed into the peritoneum through a small laparotomy. A metal tunnelling 'shunt passer' is used to pass the distal catheter under the skin.

The one-way valves come in a variety of forms, mainly related to the pressure required to open the valve (e.g. high/medium/low pressure valves). Programmable valves are also used, which allow alteration of the opening pressure externally via an electromagnet once the shunt has been inserted.

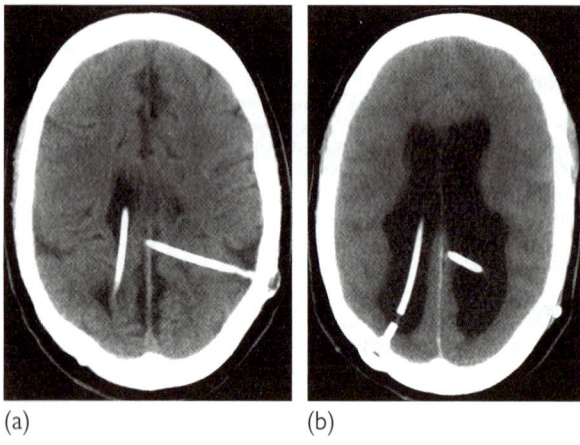

(a)　　　　　　　　　　　　(b)

Fig. 6.6 Blocked ventriculoperitoneal (VP) shunt. Unenhanced CT scans of a child with bilateral VP shunts, taken 6 months apart. The initial scan (a) shows that ventricles adequately drained, but the subsequent scan (b) shows new bilateral lateral ventricular dilatation indicating dysfunction of both shunts.

Lumboperitoneal shunts

Lumboperitoneal (LP) shunts are used for patients where VP shunts have failed or are anatomically difficult to place, and for selected younger patients who wish to avoid the driving implications of intracranial surgery.

A limited spinal dissection is performed and the catheter inserted into the lumbar sac through a Tuohy needle. The distal portion of the catheter is tunnelled to the abdomen and placed intraperitoneally as for a VP shunt.

Pre-operative assessment

Regardless of presentation, all patients requiring shunt surgery should be considered as having raised ICP. Some will be obtunded, whereas some may appear to be normal.

- Pre-operative neurological status should be carefully assessed, for example using GCS, presence of lateralizing signs, and pupillary responses.
- Many patients will be returning for shunt revisions. The anaesthetist should be aware that the patient may not be in the same medical state as previously.
- Patients requiring emergency drainage procedures are true emergencies and should not be delayed for unnecessary investigations.

Intra-operative issues

- Adequate analgesia for the burr hole and, in particular, the passage of the shunt passer under the skin is essential.
- A remifentanil infusion is not usually used, unless as part of a TIVA technique.
- Boluses of short-acting agents such as fentanyl are adequate.
- TIVA or volatile-based anaesthesia are both acceptable.
- Use local anaesthesia at the site of the abdominal incision (if a VP/LP shunt) to reduce the requirements for postoperative opioids.
- The surgical procedure itself is relatively short. Uncomplicated cases in experienced hands should take less than 30 minutes.

In small children:

- The anaesthetic issues are as much about anaesthesia in small children as they are about the neurosurgical condition.
- When the shunt passer is in place under the skin it may press against the thorax of small children and normal thoracic movements may be inhibited. This time should be kept as short as possible.

Monitoring

- The procedure is relatively non-invasive, so there is usually no need for invasive monitoring for the procedure *per se*.
- Some of these patients have significant comorbidity (e.g. subarachnoid haemorrhage, trauma) which may necessitate more invasive monitoring. Even in these cases, the anaesthetist should consider the risks of delaying treatment of intracranial hypertension against the benefit of invasive monitoring.

Postoperative care
- Complications of shunt insertion are unusual and these patients can usually return to the neurosurgical ward.
- Failure to recover suggests the presence of another cause for neurological deterioration (e.g. bleeding or seizure) or a misplaced shunt and should be investigated.
- Simple analgesia is normally all that is required, though some patients experience significant pain postoperatively, most commonly from the tunnelling. This may require strong opioids.
- EVDs may either be capped off, or more commonly connected to a combined manometer and drainage set. The zero line on this should be set level with the patient's external auditory meatus. The drainage pressure is usually set between 5 and 15 cm H_2O.

Tips and pitfalls
- Make sure the patient recovers to at least their pre-operative status in the immediate postoperative period.
- Insertion of the shunt passer is very stimulating—pre-empt with a bolus of short-acting opioid analgesia.
- Assume the ICP is raised in all patients—even those who are apparently well.
- In small children a large part of the body may be exposed during surgery and other areas should be covered and forced warm air warming used.
- The shunt passer has been reported to have damaged most neighbouring structures: liver, pleura and lungs, neck vessels and nerves, posterior fossa. In children it is prudent to have a chest drain available.
- Ensure that the staff caring for the patient postoperatively know how to manage an EVD and the desired pressure.
- Occasional catastrophic drug errors have occurred with EVDs. Make absolutely certain that drugs are not inadvertently administered into an EVD.
- Patients with VP shunts not infrequently present with intra-abdominal issues such as pregnancy, appendicitis. Ideally such patients should be managed in a centre with neurosurgeons on site for review and advice. Sometimes the distal end of the VP shunt will be exteriorized.

Neuroendoscopic surgery

Neuroendoscopy involves the use of rigid, semirigid or flexible endoscopes introduced through a cranial burr hole and then through brain parenchyma into the ventricular system. Surgery can then be performed on areas accessible from the ventricular system.

Neuroendoscopic third ventriculostomy (NTV)
- Indicated for the management of obstructive hydrocephalus.
- Maybe performed immediately prior to exploration of the posterior fossa.
- The endoscope is introduced into the lateral ventricle and then navigated into the third ventricle. Diathermy is used to make a venticulostomy in the base of the third ventricle establishing a direct communication with the subarachnoid space and arachnoid villi and bypassing any obstruction to CSF flow at the level of the aqueduct of Sylvius or foramina of Magendie or Lushka.
- NTV has ~70% success rate (compared with 80% failure rate for shunts over 15 years).
- Morbidity associated with NTV is ~4 % (compared with 5–10% for shunts—mostly infection and shunt failure).

Other neuroendoscopic procedures
- Biopsy of intraventricular and periventricular tumours
- Craniopharyngioma cyst marsupialization
- Arachnoid cyst marsupialization
- Pellucidotomy.

Pre-operative assessment
The usual principles of assessment of the child presenting for neurosurgery apply.
- A review of imaging is useful for procedures involving marsupialization of cysts.
- As with other surgery for longer term raised intracranial pressure, there may be poor nutrition or dehydration.
- Symptoms of raised intracranial pressure or radiographic evidence of mass effect from cysts should increase intra-operative alertness for cardiovascular instability secondary to sudden changes in pressure between intracranial compartments.

Intra-operative management
The general principles of neuroanaesthesia apply.
- If NTV is to precede formal exploration of the posterior fossa then the anaesthetic technique should be tailored to this.
- Intra-operative cardiovascular instability, particularly bradycardia, is usually surgical in origin and is most commonly related to:
  - Aggressive irrigation or blocked irrigation efflux
  - Diathermy near sensitive areas.
- Intra-operative analgesia can be provided with fentanyl.
- Postoperatively, simple oral analgesia is sufficient.

Monitoring

Direct arterial blood pressure monitoring may be reassuring during NTV but is not essential. For more involved neuroendoscopic procedures such as cyst marsupialization, such monitoring is useful.

Complications

Cushing's response
- Hypertension and bradycardia secondary to raised intracranial pressure.
- Most commonly caused by the outflow for surgical irrigation becoming blocked.

Cardiovascular instability or dysrhythmia
Can arise secondary to direct surgical trauma or as a result of aggressive irrigation to control hemorrhage.

Haemorrhage
May result in abandoning surgery. An EVD will usually be left in place.

Ipsilateral pupillary dilation
The optic nerve and chiasm are closely related to the third ventricle and may be injured during diathermy for NTV resulting in a transient ipsilateral dilated pupil in the early postoperative period. No active management is required but the presence of a dilated pupil should be clearly documented to avoid later confusion.

Diabetes insipidus (DI)
Seen particularly after surgery for craniopharyngioma cysts. These patients should be specifically monitored for the possibility of DI in the postoperative period.

Tips and pitfalls
- If there is CVS instability tell the surgeons, e.g. 'stop irrigating'!
- Watch the anaesthetic monitors, not the interesting endoscopic pictures.
- The procedure itself is not stimulating, it is usually the irrigation that causes problems.
- In infants and neonates do not continue to try and insert an arterial cannula if you can't get one in easily. The benefits of invasive monitoring are limited in such small children.

Colloid cysts

Pathology
Colloid cysts are benign, relatively unusual, congenital epithelium-lined cysts. They almost always arise in the anterior third ventricle and comprise ~1% of all intracranial tumours. They consist of an epithelial-lined cyst, which contains serous or viscous fluid of varying composition. They are generally very slow growing. They cause symptoms either if they become sufficiently large to cause mass effect or more commonly if they cause obstruction of the foramen of Monro.

Presentation
Most colloid cysts are found incidentally during investigation for other pathology. The classic presentation is of 'drop attacks' where the colloid cyst moves to obstruct the foramen of Monro, causing an abrupt rise in ICP. With movement the cyst may then move away, and intracranial hypertension resolves. Colloid cysts are also one of the causes of sudden death in otherwise healthy individuals. Other patients may present with a longer history of headache, often positional, which presumably reflects incomplete and remitting obstruction to CSF flow through the foramen of Monro.

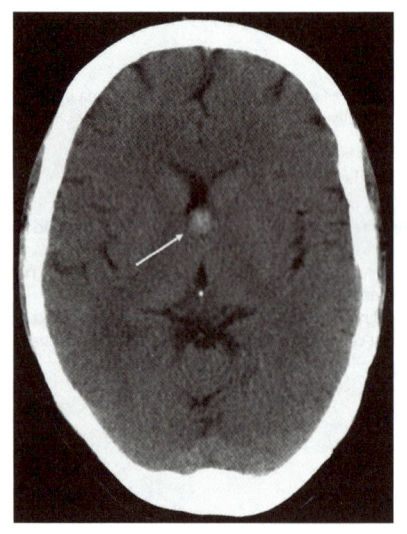

Fig. 6.7 Colloid cyst. Unenhanced CT showing a rounded hyperdensity (white arrow) located in the anterior third ventricle, adjacent to the foramen of Monro. The absence of hydrocephalus indicates that this is currently a non-obstructing colloid cyst.

Pre-operative assessment
If the cyst is an incidental finding, or if it is causing drop attacks, the patient is usually fit and well.

Surgical approach
The cysts may either be removed through a neuroendoscopic approach or via a formal craniotomy and corticotomy.

Positioning
Supine.

Intra-operative management
The anaesthetic issues are the same as for other endoscopic procedures or craniotomy.
- Intra-operative blockage of the foramen of Monro may cause an abrupt rise in ICP if there is no other route of efflux for CSF.

Postoperative management
Full and prompt recovery should be expected. If this does not occur then causes of deterioration should be sought and treated, for example haemorrhage and seizure.

Tips and pitfalls
- As with other endoscopic procedures, if there is CVS instability tell the surgeons, e.g. 'stop irrigating'!
- Unlike tumour resection, the interval between cyst resection and skin closure may be quite short.

Midline surgery

Craniopharyngioma
Embryologically craniopharyngiomas arise from a remnant of Rathke's pouch. Craniopharyngioma is the most common perisellar tumour in childhood and accounts for ~1% of all intracranial tumours.

Pathophysiology
- Two pathological forms of craniopharyngioma are described—adamantinous and papillary.
- The adamantinous type is typical in childhood tumours and is characterized by the presence of cholesterol crystals and fibrous thickening of the tumour wall.
  - The tumours are often cystic.
  - 15% arise in ectopic sites such as the optic chiasm.
- Papillary tumours are predominantly a finding in adults and often arise in the third ventricle.

Presentation
- Craniopharyngioma may present acutely with signs of raised intracranial pressure.
- Other findings include visual field defects and disorders of endocrine function secondary to impairment of the hypothalamo–pituitary axis.
- Hypothyroidism, diabetes insipidus, and failure to thrive secondary to impairment of growth hormone, may also be present or develop.
- Impairment of the ACTH-cortisol axis and the potential for Addisonian crisis exists and requires pre-operative investigation and treatment.

Pre-operative assessment
- Endocrine investigations should include TFT, cortisol, prolactin and growth hormone (GH). Many patients present for repeat anaesthesia and a careful note should be taken of the current management of their endocrine function. This must be maintained throughout the peri-operative period.
- In new patients a full evaluation of the hypothalamo–pituitary axis may not be available and it is prudent to provide steroid cover for the peri-operative period.
- Diabetes insipidus is unusual in the pre-operative period. It is unlikely to present intra-operatively unless surgery is prolonged but is likely to present postoperatively.

Surgical procedures
- Patients may present for various procedures including EVD insertion, insertion of Ommaya reservoir (into the craniopharyngioma cyst) and neuroendoscopic marsupialization of the craniopharyngioma cyst.
- Surgical resection of the tumour is uncommon because of the difficult surgical approach and subsequent complete disruption of the hypothalamic–pituitary axis.
- Older children may be referred for treatment with radiotherapy.

Ommaya reservoir

A reservoir usually implanted at the site of a cranial burr hole. It has a single catheter which extends intracranially. The tip of the catheter can be placed either in an intracranial fluid-containing space such as the ventricular system or in a pathological cyst such as a craniopharyngioma cyst or arachnoid cyst.

It can be accessed percutaneously to allow fluid to be aspirated to control pressure symptoms and can also be used as a conduit to deliver intrathecal chemotherapy.

Anaesthetic technique

The anaesthetic technique will be dictated by the proposed surgical procedure. Surgery for craniopharyngioma requires the anaesthetist to be attentive to monitoring for, and managing the complications associated with, this type of surgery—in particular diabetes insipidus (DI).

Diabetes insipidus

Usually develops postoperatively because the posterior pituitary has stores of antidiuretic hormone (ADH) which may last for several hours after complete disruption of the hypothalmo–pituitary axis. DI presents as a high output of low osmolality urine with progressive hypernatraemia secondary to loss of free water.

Management
- Monitor hourly urine output, serum and urinary electrolytes and osmolality.
- Replace excess urine output (urine output >1–2 ml kg^{-1} hr^{-1}) with 5% dextrose and monitor electrolytes. If the patient is conscious, replace excess urine output with water given orally.
- Desmopressin is indicated if high urine output is maintained. This may be given nasally or intravenously. Nasal administration is preferred outside ICU.
- Native ADH production may resume some days after surgery. Failure to stop desmopressin in this situation may result in cerebral oedema.

Tumours of the pineal gland

Approximately 50% of pineal region tumours are germ cell tumours; the remainder originate from cell lines native to the pineal region. Management is dependent on accurate tissue diagnosis.

Surgery is high risk, and relief of hydrocephalus, followed by radio- and chemotherapy is sometimes used as the first line, with surgery reserved for non-responding or progressive cases.

Presentation

Tumours tend to present during the early teenage years and early adult life. Pineal region tumours account for 0.4–1% of adult and 3–8 % of childhood intracranial tumours. The presenting signs and symptoms of pineal tumours are related to the effects of compression or direct invasion into surrounding structures.

Raised intracranial pressure
This may arise directly as an effect of tumour mass or because pineal tumours arise from the diencephalon and may extend into the third ventricle across the foramen of Monro causing obstructive hydrocephalus. Typical signs of raised ICP include headache, nausea, vomiting and depressed conscious level.

Pressure effect on the superior colliculus
May result in Perinaud's syndrome characterized by IIIrd cranial nerve palsy and resulting in loss of upward gaze, loss of convergance, impaired light reflexes and nystagmus.

Pressure on the peri-aqueductal grey matter
May give a similar range of symptoms to that seen in Perinaud's syndrome but also with cerebellar signs due to effects on the superior cerebellar peduncle.

Endocrine symptoms
Most usually seen as an effect of tumours with suprasellar extension. Includes DI, growth retardation, precocious puberty, secondary amenorrhea and panhypopituitarism.

Visual field defects
Caused by direct pressure effects on the optic nerves. Requires assessment by an ophthalmologist.

Pre-operative considerations
- Careful assessment of endocrine function is required. However, in the presence of life-threatening hydrocephalus these investigations should not delay stabilizing surgery.
- A plan must be established for the management of peri-operative DI. Corticosteroid cover is likely to be required for surgery.
- Visual field defects should be documented pre-operatively.

Anaesthetic technique
This is largely dictated by the operative procedure. Tissue diagnosis will most commonly be achieved by stereotactic or neuroendoscopic biopsy. Once a tissue diagnosis is achieved subsequent management is most commonly with chemotherapy or radiotherapy.

Tumour resection carrries significant risk. It may be approached by the supra- or infratentorial routes. The patient may need to be positioned sitting, prone or semi-prone depending on the particular surgical approach.

Stereotactic biopsy
Anaesthesia will be required during transfer from the CT scan room to the operating room. This is most commonly achieved with a propofol infusion. Simple oral analgesia is sufficient for management of postoperative pain.

Neuroendoscopy
📖 See p. 220.
Consideration should be given to direct monitoring of arterial blood pressure if neuroendoscopic biopsy is undertaken.

Open surgery
Requires a major craniotomy.

Postoperative complications
- Seizures.
- Haemorrhage into the tumour bed.
- DI.
- Abnormal movement of the extra-ocular muscles.
- Ataxia.

Immediate postoperative care following craniotomy should be in a critical care environment.

Prognosis

Craniopharyngioma
Overall, ~90% of patients with treated craniopharyngioma are alive at 10 years. Functional outcome is related to the degree of pre-operative damage and the endocrine effects of resection.

Pinealoma
The prognosis is dependant on the histological diagnosis. Approximately 60% of tumours arising from germ cell lines are germinomas and carry a good prognosis. The remaining 40% include carcinomas, teratomas, and yolk sac tumours which tend to be less responsive to treatment.

Tips and pitfalls
- Be sure that you are aware of the results of the endocrine work-up.
- Check what you need to do for corticosteroid replacement intraoperatively.
- Ensure there is a clear plan for management of postoperative DI.
- DI is one occasion in neuroanaesthetic practice when it is acceptable to use hypotonic crystalloid solutions such as dextrose saline (0.18% saline and 4% dextrose). Isotonic solutions may result in hypernatraemia.

Seizure surgery

Epilepsy is a relatively common condition; around 1 in 200 people in the UK are receiving treatment for epilepsy. For some patients, medical management is inadequate. The aim of epilepsy surgery is to achieve a better seizure control so as to improve patient's quality of life without causing any functional loss. Some patients can become seizure-free after epilepsy surgery.

Pathology

Seizures are the result of excessive excitation, or failure of termination of abnormal excitation resulting in synchronized discharge of large groups of neurons and temporary loss of coordinated neuronal activity.

A single seizure, or a small number of isolated fits, will be experienced by ~5% of people during their lifetime. The diagnosis of epilepsy is reserved for those suffering from repeated episodes of seizures of a certain type. These may be accompanied by characteristic EEG changes.

Associated conditions

Seizures can be:
- idiopathic with no identifiable cause
- part of an ongoing disorder:
  - metabolic e.g. electrolyte abnormalities, abnormal glucose levels
  - substance withdrawal e.g. benzodiazepines, alcohol
  - substance toxicity e.g. tricyclics, amphetamines, cocaine, alcohol
  - CNS or systemic infection e.g. meningitis, encephalitis
  - space-occupying lesion, primary or metastatic tumour, hydrocephalus
  - eclampsia
  - vascular injury e.g. thrombosis, haemorrhage
  - head injury
  - hypoxia
  - brain malformation, cerebral palsy, atrophy, progressive neurological disorder
  - fever e.g. febrile convulsions, especially in young children
- a symptom of a previous injury to the brain following:
  - infections, intoxications, head trauma, vascular injury or following brain surgery.

While any brain tumour can cause epilepsy, it is usually low-grade gliomas which present with seizures.
- A history of recurrent fits can precede the diagnosis by many years.
- Gangliogliomas are the commonest cause of temporal lobe epilepsy and account for ~40% of these
- Dysembrioplastic tumours and pilocytic astrocytomas are about half as common.

Presentation

There are numerous classifications of seizures based upon location of onset, impairment of consciousness, effect of the seizure (e.g. tonic, tonic-clonic, myoclonic, automatacity), EEG patterns, and associated syndromes.
- Generalized seizures with loss of consciousness can be tonic or tonic-clonic.
  - May be preceded by headaches, dizziness, nausea, sweating, unrest, or mood disturbance.
  - About 10% of patients with generalized seizures experience an optical or acoustic aura.
  - A post ictal period and amnesia are typical.
  - Injuries may occur in association with generalized seizures, e.g. tongue biting, falls with fractures, head injuries, burns or aspiration of stomach contents.
- Focal seizures affect a part of the body (at onset). The manifestation of seizure activity is dependent upon the anatomical location e.g. motor, sensory, absence, psychomotor.
- Some seizure patterns are typically seen in children
  - Febrile convulsions are most often seen in patients under the age of 5.
- Status epilepticus is a prolonged single seizure, or several seizures with the patient remaining unconscious between these episodes (see Status epilepticus, p.374).

Patient population

The diagnosis of epilepsy is associated with many undesirable effects:
- Social stigma
- Dependence on medication
- Compromised independence if epilepsy is intractable
- Restrictions on employment choice and decreased productivity
- Increased requirement for social/financial support
- The mortality rate amongst newly diagnosed epileptics is 2–4 times higher over 10 years than normal population
- Death is related to seizure, injury, suicide and sudden unexpected death in epilepsy (SUDEP).

Pre-operative assessment

The general approach to assessment is the same as for other patients undergoing intracranial surgery. In addition:
- A history of the aura and the type and frequency of the patient's seizures should be taken.
- If intra-operative patient assessment or an awake procedure is planned, premedication producing sedation and interference with neurophysiological monitoring, or affecting the patient's ability to co-operate during awake procedures, should be avoided.
- Anti-epileptic medication should be discussed with the surgical team. These medications may need to be stopped prior to intra-operative neurophysiological monitoring procedures, but should be continued for resection of lesions without such monitoring.

Surgical approach

There are several different types of procedure undertaken in the surgical management of epilepsy.

To aid diagnosis—invasive neurophysiology

These procedures aim to localize an epileptogenic area in the brain. Resective or disconnective epilepsy surgery requires precise understanding and localization of an epiletogenic area, before such area can be neutralized. Conventional neurophysiological investigations like scalp EEG, video-telemetry or structural imaging (MRI) remain the mainstay of investigation of patients for epilepsy surgery.

Depth electrodes
- These are very fine electrodes, placed with stereotactic guidance, within the brain parenchyma.
- Usually more than one electrode is placed and often they are placed bilaterally.
- The surgical procedure is similar to any stereotactic procedure with multiple targeting (see p. 246).
- Bilateral temporal depth electrode placement is commonly performed to lateralize and localize temporal onset epilepsy.
- Once placed the electrodes are connected to a receiver and are examined similar to videotelemetry over a period of time in the neurophysiology suite.
- The patient does not need a general anaesthetic for removal of these electrodes; they can usually be removed safely with the patient awake.

Cortical grids
- These need guided (image guidance) placement.
- The grids contain an array of electrodes which are placed through a craniotomy over a suspected epileptogenic area and the surrounding normal brain.
- The electrodes are then connected to an amplifier and the electrocorticogram is analysed over a period of time in the ward.
- Removal of these grids requires a general anaesthetic.
- As most of the assessment will happen in the postoperative period, no specific precautions are needed during anaesthesia regarding interference with seizure activity.

Epilepsy-modifying surgery

Disconnective:
- Corpus callosotomy
- Functional hemispherectomy
- Multiple subpial transections.

The white fibre tracts that are involved in propagation of epileptogenic discharge from an epileptic focus are selectively severed (disconnected). The aim is to restrict the epileptiform activity to a confined area, thus preventing a generalized seizure or drop attack.

These procedures require craniotomy and general anaesthesia.

Resective
- Lesionectomies
- Temporal lobectomy
- Anatomical hemispherectomy.

Epileptogenic lesions are removed for symptomatic control of epilepsy. This surgery may accompany intra-operative cortical mapping to delineate eloquent areas or areas of cortex involved in seizure activity to plan resection. Surgery may be done with the patient awake in appropriate cases.

Vagal nerve stimulators
This procedure involves the peripheral stimulation of the left vagus nerve in the neck.
- The mechanism of action is speculative.
- It is indicated in intractable partial epilepsy not amenable to resective or disconnective surgery.
- The operation involves dissection in the neck and implantation of an internal pulse generator over the left infraclavicular area.
- No intra-operative monitoring is required regarding the epilepsy.
- The patient may feel irritation in the throat after an episode of vagal nerve stimulation.

Positioning

Patients are usually positioned supine, but other positions may be required depending on the location of the lesion. If the patient is to be woken up, a compromise may have to be found between an ideally positioned patient from a surgical point of view and patient comfort.

Intra-operative issues

The same general principles apply as for patients undergoing other intracranial surgery or awake/functional surgery.
- Hypothermia should be avoided, as this affects the EEG.
- For general anaesthesia a propofol/remifentanil-based regime is often described, but other drugs or combinations have been used successfully.
- Propofol should be discontinued for about 15 min prior to neurophysiological monitoring.
- Intra-operative seizures should be treated with small doses of propofol if occurring before corticography, as longer-acting substances like anti-epileptics or diazepam can interfere with the recording. A cold saline wash of the operative field is also effective. Once recording is completed, conventional medications can be used to terminate seizures.
- Cardiac arrhythmias and bradycardias have been described intra-operatively following implantation of a vagal nerve stimulator. Cardiological advice may be required in patients with pre-existing conduction abnormalities prior to implantation of a vagal nerve stimulator (VNS).
- Airway obstruction in patients with laryngeal masks has been described in association with VNS placement.

Monitoring

Standard anaesthetic monitoring is used, as described elsewhere. Although awake patients may only require minimal anaesthetic intervention, close attention to detail and constant careful supervision is essential. Complications can be sudden and may require immediate intervention.

Postoperative care

The postoperative care of these patients follows general neuroanaesthetic principles. Implantation of a vagal nerve stimulator has implications for future operations and investigations:
- Ultrasound-based investigations or procedures, shock wave lithotripsy, radiofrequency ablation can all cause damage to the device.
- MRI can cause damage to the device and can cause injury to the patient.
- Interference can occur between these devices and cardiac pacemakers as well as implanted cardioconverters and defibrillators.
- The neurosurgical team or device manufacturer should be contacted if these procedures are planned.
- Monopolar diathermy should not be used.
- External defibrillation or cardioversion can cause damage to the device.
  - In an emergency the paddles should be placed as far away from the device as possible, and the minimum amount of energy used.
- ECG recordings may show artefacts.

Prognosis

The aim of epilepsy surgery is to achieve better seizure control. Some patients may become seizure free following surgery. In a carefully selected group of patients undergoing temporal lobectomy with amygdalo hippocampectomy for medial temporal sclerosis, a seizure-free status of 70% was achieved.

Tips and pitfalls
- A cold saline wash of the operative field is effective at terminating seizures.
- Bolus doses of alfentanil can be used to provoke seizures selectively during electrocortigraphy. This may be of benefit in distinguishing non-epileptogenic from epileptogenic brain tissue during resection surgery.
- Chronic use of anticonvulsants can result in enhanced or prolonged effects of neuromuscular blocking agents.

Functional neurosurgery

Functional neurosurgery aims to modify the function of the nervous system through a variety of procedures.

Pathology
The range of conditions being treated in this way is increasing.

Deep brain stimulation
- Parkinson's disease
- Essential tremor
- Dystonia
- Neuropathic pain
- Epilepsy (see Seizure surgery, p. 228)
- Depression.

Procedures for chronic pain
- Spinal cord stimulation
- Deep brain stimulation
- Motor cortex stimulation
- Programmable (Implantable) intrathecal drug delivery.

Procedures for chronic neuralgic pain
Covered separately (see Cranial neuralgias, p. 238).

Surgery for epilepsy
Covered separately (see Seizure surgery, p. 228).

Surgery for spasticity
Intrathecal baclofen (see p. 314).

Patient population and associated conditions:
Patients usually present with a complex medical history and can be extremely disabled by their disease process. Other organ systems may be affected. Common conditions include:
- Gastric reflux in cerebral palsy
- Epilepsy following trauma
- Swallowing problems in multiple sclerosis (MS).

The underlying aetiology is varied:
- Degenerative (Parkinson's disease)
- Inflammatory (MS)
- Traumatic (traumatic brain and spinal cord injury)
- Congenital/hereditary/neonatal (cerebral palsy)
- Vascular (stroke)
- Neoplasms.

Pre-operative assessment
Assessment of patients for awake deep brain stimulation (DBS) should include patient, procedural and anaesthetic factors.

Assessment for procedures under GA
- If procedures are carried out with the patient anaesthetized, long-acting anti-movement medication, that can interfere with electrophysiological monitoring, should be changed to shorter-acting drugs.

Assessment for awake procedures
- Comprehensive explanation about every step of the procedure is essential to alleviate anxiety, and to allow the patient to cooperate as much as possible.
- Assessment of the patient's GCS and the degree of any physical disability including restlessness/involuntary movements, or degree of stiffness with Parkinson's disease should be made.
- Sedative premedication should be avoided to allow optimal intra-operative monitoring of brain function.
- Many patients scheduled for intrathecal drug delivery devices or spinal cord stimulation have a limited ability to cooperate or suffer from spasticity or deformities, which makes positioning more difficult.

Special considerations for DBS patients
- Continuation/discontinuation of pre-admission medication should be discussed with the multidisciplinary team and the patient. The team will usually wish to stop the medication for Parkinson's disease to allow accurate assessment of the stimulation procedure without the masking effect of the medication.
  - The morning dose of anti-Parkinson's medication is usually omitted. Drugs for essential tremor are usually omitted for longer.

Surgical approach

Deep brain stimulation
- The target for deep brain stimulation is diagnosis-specific.
- Generally patients with essential tremor, Parkinson's disease, and chronic pain will have placements of electrodes whilst awake, whilst implantation of the battery is carried out under general anaesthesia.
- In some cases accurate scanning under general anaesthesia is required, and the patient is subsequently woken up for the placement of the electrodes.
- Clinical feedback helps in accurate placement of the electrodes.
- Neurophysiological monitoring is continued during the procedure.
- With improvements in imaging and targeting many centres are positioning DBS implants under general anaesthesia.

Intrathecal drug delivery
- An epidural catheter is placed in to the CSF through a Tuohy needle, usually under local anaesthesia. Sedation or general anaesthesia may be required for some patients.
- A trial injection is performed and the effect of the intrathecal drug assessed.
- If the trial is deemed successful a catheter is subsequently placed via a surgical approach under direct vision, tunnelled and connected

to a pump, which is implanted in the anterior abdominal wall. This procedure is usually performed under general anaesthesia.

Spinal cord stimulation
- A stimulator probe is placed epidurally through a Tuohy needle. This is carried out with the patient awake as the patient will be required to confirm that the stimulation is in the area affected by pain.
- The wires are connected to an external stimulator for the trial, and if successful, permanent wires are placed and connected to a subcutaneous stimulator box placed under local or general anaesthesia.

Positioning
- Patients will usually be positioned supine for DBS procedures and lateral for intrathecal catheter placements and catheter/pump implants.
- A variation on the prone position may be used for insertion of spinal cord stimulator placements, with a sandbag under one hip and the ipsilateral leg flexed at the hip and knee. This allows surgical access to the lateral abdomen for insertion of the battery/controller.

Intra-operative issues
For awake DBS procedures the application of the headframe and the burrholes can be carried out under general anaesthesia, with sedation, or with the patient awake using local anaesthesia only.
- Propofol and remifentanil are commonly used, though other short-acting drugs can be used.
- Neurosurgical/neurophysiological monitoring should be performed without the interference of anaesthetic drugs.
- Insertion of the generator box can again be carried out under general anaesthesia at the end of the procedure, as patient cooperation is not required at this stage.
- Regardless of the anaesthesia/sedation technique used, the anaesthetist needs to be vigilant for intra-operative problems:
    - intra-operative seizures can be life-threatening
    - patient movement while being in the headframe is dangerous
    - hypertension may lead to bleeding and needs to be treated effectively
    - a reduction in consciousness (drug or procedure related) can interfere with a patent airway and breathing.
- Due to the length of the procedures, particular attention should be paid to patient comfort, i.e. soft padding, warming blanket, theatre temperature etc.
- Excessive intravenous fluids should be avoided as this risks bladder distension and discomfort. Sheath catheters are preferable to urethral as they are less irritant.
- Long-acting opioids should be avoided in patients with catheter placements for intrathecal drug application to avoid interaction of drugs and oversedation of the patients.

Monitoring
- Routine non-invasive monitoring is employed for shorter procedures.
- An arterial line avoids the need for repeated non-invasive blood pressure readings in awake DBS patients.

Postoperative care
General principles apply.
- If normal medication has been withheld for intra-operative monitoring it should be restarted as soon as possible in recovery (especially Parkinson's/anti-epileptic medication).
- Patients having intrathecal drugs should only receive their intrathecal medications once the effects of the anaesthetic drugs have worn off.
- DBS devices, spinal cord stimulators, intrathecal drug delivery systems and vagal nerve stimulators can be damaged by or interfere with other procedures, e.g. ultrasound, cardiac pacemakers etc. Monopolar diathermy is contraindicated, MRI scans can cause injury to the patients and also damage the device.

Prognosis
The aim of functional neurosurgery is to improve quality of life or facilitate care without compromising neurological function. In carefully managed patients these procedures bring significant benefit.
- Patients suffering from Parkinson's disease require significantly lower dosage of dopaminergic medication and stay longer in the 'on' stage.
- Spinal cord stimulation is associated with reduction in pain by more than 50% in failed back surgery patients.

Tips and pitfalls
- Intra-operative hypertension has a variety of causes. Each of these should be assiduously sought and treated if hypertension occurs:
  - pain either operative or musculoskeletal from prolonged immobility
  - bladder distension
  - anxiety.
- Venous air embolism is unusual but may occur. Normal monitoring is either impractical or unreliable.
  - Cough is the most common presenting symptom in the awake patient.
- Drugs exacerbating Parkinsonian symptoms should be avoided in these patients, e.g. butyrophenones, phenothiazines, and metoclopramide.

Cranial neuralgias

Cranial neuralgias describe a spectrum of conditions in which there is episodic, often severe pain, in the distribution of one of the cranial nerves. Trigeminal neuralgia is the commonest, but glossopharyngeal neuralgia also occurs. Hemifacial spasm is the motor equivalent with involvement of the facial nerve. Patients may present for surgical intervention if medical treatment has failed or produces intolerable side effects.

Pathology

The underlying cause is often compression of the nerve near its exit from the brain by a blood vessel. The trigeminal nerve may be in contact with the superior cerebellar artery, the facial nerve by the anterior inferior cerebellar artery, and the glossopharyngeal nerve by the posterior inferior cerebellar artery.
- The contact between vessel and nerve is believed to cause damage to the nerve sheath. There are many theories explaining the cause of neuralgia from a vascular contact. One theory suggests that spontaneous excitation of the dorsal root ganglion cells and cross-talk between touch and pain fibres are the cause of the symptoms.
- It is not clear why most patients present in later life since the vessel will have been present since birth. Possibilities include:
  - that the injury is a very slow process
  - that as the vessel ages it lengthens and comes to rest against the nerve.

Patient population

Generally patients are older (>50 years) and women are affected more than men. There may be an inherited predisposition, presumably as a result of inherited anatomical variants.

Associated conditions

Severe neuralgia is associated with depression and (rarely) suicide.
There are other conditions which can cause or mimic the cranial neuralgias:
- Multiple sclerosis
- Tumour
- Epilepsy syndromes
- Paget's disease (causing bony compression of the nerve).

Presentation

Classically, patients present with episodic pain in the distribution of the affected nerve or one of its branches. Atypical presentations raise the suspicion of non-vascular origin or alternate diagnoses.
- The area may be allodynic, and many patients have trigger points which can initiate the pain.
- The type of pain varies. Some patients predominantly have short, shock-like pain, others have more aching or burning symptoms. Classical trigeminal neuralgia is described as bursts of electric shock with no pain in the intervening period. Persistence of some pain or ache in-between the shocks suggests atypical features.

CRANIAL NEURALGIAS

- Episodes of pain often come in waves, which may become more frequent over time.
- Some patients have premonitory symptoms of aching or tingling in the affected area.

Treatment options

Drug treatment
Medical management with oxycarbamazepine, carbamazepine, gabapentin, and pregabalin is the mainstay of treatment for most patients. Other drugs such as lamotrigine, phenytoin and baclofen have also been found effective. These may be complemented by a variety of alternative therapies such as acupuncture and herbal remedies.

Ablative therapies
A variety of procedures can be performed to injure or destroy the affected nerve branches. These generally involve accessing the trigeminal ganglion through the cheek and foramen ovale under X-ray guidance. The relevant branch of the nerve is then ablated using either compression (balloon), heat (radiofrequency) or less commonly glycerol.
- This approach is relatively less invasive, but carries the risk of dysaesthesia and early or late failure of the technique.
- Corneal anaesthesia is a complication and if it occurs requires eye care to avoid corneal ulceration.
- Balloon compression is specially suited for patients with V1 trigeminal pain.
- Balloon compression is done with the patient asleep while radiofrequency ablation will need the patient to be awake to confirm position of the needle during the procedure.

Microvascular decompression
The trigeminal nerve is exposed through a retrosigmoid craniotomy. An inert sponge (Teflon®) is interposed between the nerve and the overlying vessel.

This technique is more invasive, but has the greatest short- and long-term success rates, with a low rate of neural injury. Even in the absence of an overlying vessel, manipulation of the nerve results in symptomatic improvement in around 70%.

Pre-operative assessment
- These patients are often elderly, and may have significant medical comorbidity. Since surgery is not the only option, consideration of the most appropriate technique should be made in those who are medically unfit.
- A careful drug history should be taken, as many of these patients may have tried numerous therapies in an attempt to control their pain.
- Patients for radiofrequency ablation will need to be prepared for a wake-up test during the procedure. They need to be aware that their pain will be stimulated. Patient, surgeon, and anaesthetist need to agree on appropriate terminology.

Intra-operative issues

Ablative procedures
- Local anaesthesia is rarely sufficient for placement of the percutaneous needles. As the foramen ovale is bordered by the pterygoid plates, the needle cannot be 'walked' off the base of the skull and multiple passes may be required. A 'light' GA or deep sedation will be needed for patient comfort.
- Radiofrequency ablation requires identification of the correct branch of the trigeminal nerve. This is most reliably achieved by stimulating the nerve with the needle and asking the patient whether it reproduces their pain. This will necessitate waking the patient. Most of these patients will not have their airway secured during this procedure.
- The ablative procedure itself is short-lived (a few minutes) but intensely painful and the patient will require short-lived general anaesthesia or deep sedation to tolerate this. Various techniques including propofol and remifentanil infusions are used.
- Balloon ablation is normally performed under general anaesthesia. There is no patient communication required.
  - Marked cardiovascular changes, including asystole can occur during compression. Some anaesthetists advocate prophylactic vagolytic drugs; others 'wait and see'.
  - The needle used for balloon ablation is much larger than that for radiofrequency ablation. Consequently any bleeding (usually from an emissary vein in the foramen ovale) will be more severe, and can result in a significant hyperacute subdural haematoma which will require surgical drainage.

Microvascular decompression
This is an intracranial operation, which requires the same principles and practice as any other.

Interposing the Teflon sponge can provoke marked cardiovascular changes, including asystole. The anaesthetist should be alert to the possibility and communicate clearly with the surgeon. These effects should stop if the sponge is removed.

There are some large vessels encountered by the surgeon on the approach to the trigeminal nerve and significant venous bleeding can occur.

Other cranial neuralgias
Surgical treatment of other cranial neuralgias requires exploration of the cerebello-pontine angle through a retrosigmoid posterior fossa craniectomy. The patient is positioned in a lateral 'park bench' position.

Although the surgical approach varies, the anaesthetic issues are largely the same as for trigeminal neuralgias.

Prognosis
The long-term results are better with microvascular decompression than with percutanuous ablation, but the short-term risks are higher. All types of treatment have a risk of recurrence.

Tips and pitfalls
- If a patient presents for microvascular decompression who is medically unfit, other less invasive options can be explored.
- There is no single 'best' way to sedate patients for percutaneous procedures.
- Be prepared for marked cardiovascular changes when manipulating the trigeminal nerve.
- During radiofrequency ablation, ECG interference mimicking dysrhythmia is common.

Awake craniotomy

This technique has become popular recently for excision of lesions close to so-called eloquent areas (e.g. the motor strip and speech centres). While somatosensory evoked potentials and electrical cortical stimulation mapping of the motor cortex can be carried out with the patient anaesthetized, an awake craniotomy allows the surgeon to directly assess the patient's speech, motor and language functions and overall condition during surgery.

Generally awake craniotomy is used for patients with tumours (p. 180). An awake craniotomy will typically be carried out in a patient with a low grade lesion to achieve the best possible resection margin. These low grade lesions tend to present earlier in life than the higher grade lesions. Some functional neurosurgery and epilepsy surgery is also performed with an awake patient (see Seizure surgery, p. 228, and Functional neurosurgery, p. 234).

Patient population

Although awake craniotomy is most commonly performed in adults, with appropriate selection and pre-operative counselling, awake craniotomy has been successfully carried out in adolescents and children.

Pre-operative assessment

The most important component of pre-operative assessment for this group is adequate preparation of the patient.
- Patients need to be informed of what they are going to experience during their procedure.
- They need to be motivated to undergo the procedure.
- Good cooperation and communication between patient, anaesthetist, and surgeon is paramount.
- Patients need to be aware that movement, especially head movement, will be restricted during the procedure, as the head will be held in a frame and most patients experience a tight band around their head. The patient's vision will be restricted by the limitation of head movement and by the surgical drapes.
- The patient needs to be informed that the theatre team is often large as it may include specialist staff to conduct intra-operative monitoring.
- Awake monitoring of cerebral function may not be straightforward, and the patient should understand what questions they will be asked and how they should respond.
- Sites for intravenous access and monitoring should take into account the patient's preference, and be informed by the surgical requirements to monitor the patient. It is helpful to leave a particular limb free of drips and monitoring devices if the patient will be asked to move this regularly during the procedure.
- Patients often appreciate (if they can choose) whether or not to have a bladder catheter.
- Closure of the wound can be carried out with the patient awake, or under general anaesthesia, according to the patient's preference.

Positioning
- Positioning is a compromise between optimal surgical access and patient comfort.
- Patients will usually be positioned supine, often with the head end of the operating table elevated (10–15°), which also helps the patient to look forward and aids communication.
- Soft padding and sufficient warming (theatre temperature and warming blanket) are important for the patient. The single most important factor is to support the neck. This can be achieved with a pillow wedged between the arms of the Mayfield head frame.

Intra-operative issues
These procedures are usually carried out using an asleep–awake–asleep technique, although it can be performed with the patient awake for the whole procedure.

Anaesthesia and analgesia
- Effective local anaesthesia to the pin sites and for skin incision is essential using long-acting local anaesthetics (e.g. a 50:50 mixture of levo-bupivacaine 0.5% and lidocaine 1% with adrenaline 1:200,000). In addition, blocks of the supra-orbital, supratrochlear and auriculo-temporal nerves can be performed.
- To minimize the pain of durotomy diluted local anaesthetic can be applied on to the exposed dura.
- Using an asleep–awake–asleep technique, the patient is woken up once the craniotomy is completed.
- Systemic analgesia with paracetamol is often all that is required in addition to local anaesthesia for pain relief. A carefully titrated remifentanil infusion can also be used.
- General anaesthesia is maintained with either a volatile/remifentanil or propofol/remifentanil (TIVA) technique. The latter has less effect on cortical monitoring.
- Closure of the wound can be carried out under general anaesthesia, however many patients are happy to remain awake for this part of the procedure.
- Oversedation needs to be avoided, as an uncooperative patient can put him/herself at risk of injury with the head fixed in the headframe. Also, a drop in GCS can endanger a patient airway and breathing. Sedative agents can also interfere with neurophysiological monitoring.

Airway management
- During the asleep phase, airway maintenance is usually provided by a supraglottic airway device, as this allows for smooth emergence.
- Emergency reintubation during the awake phase of the procedure can be more challenging due to the frame as well as surgical drapes. The usual techniques for difficult intubation can be applied.
  - Appropriate positioning of the frame is essential to achieve reintubation.
  - Frames with detachable front parts for easy access to the airway are available.
  - Frameless image guided techniques are now being adopted and obliviate this problem.

- Placement of a tracheal tube can be difficult when the frame is in position, particularly if required urgently. Smooth emergence may be more challenging with a tracheal tube in place, but can be achieved. Various techniques for intra-operative tracheal intubation have been described:
  - airway exchange catheters
  - awake fibre-optic intubation. This requires prior local anaesthesia of the airway
  - asleep fibre-optic intubation, sometimes through a laryngeal mask airway (LMA).

Patient comfort
- Care should be taken to avoid striking the headframe with metal objects, as this sound is transmitted through the frame and the pins going into the patient's skull. This applies to dailling of the bone as well.
- Lying still for several hours may be very uncomfortable for the patient.
  - The anaesthetist should be meticulous about padding and support.
  - Bladder distension due to excess intravenous fluid should be avoided.
- Additional sedation should be used judiciously as it can lead to respiratory depression, a rise in CO_2 and the risk of brain swelling.
  - Oversedation may also result in an uncooperative patient with the head fixed in a head frame.
  - Anxiolytics may be necessary, but continuous communication with the anaesthetist is often sufficient.
- Achieving a comfortable head and neck position is key.

Control of brain swelling during the awake phase
The usual cerebral depressant effects of anaesthesia are not present during craniotomy. Brain swelling can be secondary to seizure, airway obstruction or surgery and management is related to the cause. The anaesthetist should be alert to other factors which will potentially increase cerebral volume.
- Securing of the airway and ventilation may become necessary at any time during the procedure.
- Similarly, conversion to a general anaesthetic can become necessary at any time during the procedure and requires appropriate preparation.
- Durotomy is delayed until the patient is fully awake, to prevent brain herniation if the patient strains before being conscious.
- Blood pressure rises are common during awakening and boluses of a hypotensive agent, such as labetalol, should be used as required.
- Hypoventilation due to excess sedation should be avoided.
- Pain and anxiety should pre-empted and managed promptly.

Seizures
- The patient should continue to take all anti-epileptic medications until the morning of surgery.
- Treatment of seizures depends on the stage of the procedure.
  - Small dosages of propofol may be effective.
  - Longer acting anti-epileptics or a benzodiazepine may interfere with corticography (during seizure surgery).
  - A cold saline wash of the operative field is also effective.

Postoperative management
- In uncomplicated cases postoperative management is the same as for any other craniotomy.
- Pain relief with paracetamol is usually sufficient. Some patients will require opioids when the local anaesthesia wears off.

Tips and pitfalls
- The key to successful awake craniotomy surgery is patient selection and planning.
- The whole theatre team needs to be aware that major complications can manifest themselves at any time, and will require immediate action to safeguard the patient on the theatre table in the head frame, to maintain a patent airway, to convert to a general anaesthesia, and support vital functions.
- Local anaesthesia infiltration and nerve blocks minimize the need for supplemental intravenous analgesia.
- Take time to maximize patient comfort with positioning and padding.
- Good communication with the patient reduces the need for sedation.
- Have a 'back-up' plan for rescue general anaesthesia with suitable airway control.

Stereotactic surgery

Accurate localization of lesions and minimization of trauma to surrounding brain tissue are of paramount importance during intracranial surgery. An increasing number of neurosurgical procedures are now being performed using stereotactic guidance. These range from the minimally invasive such as needle biopsy, insertion of deep brain stimulating electrodes and ventricular catheters through to full craniotomy and tumour excision. Image guidance is also used for radiotherapy procedures.

There are several methods of stereotactic guidance but they can be classified as 'framed' or 'frameless'. The basic principles are the same. A high resolution scan of the area of interest is performed and the area is defined by the surgeon or radiologist. The scan is then mapped to some reference points on the patient. Using 3-D trigonometry or real-time 3-D position location, the precise position of a surgical instrument can be defined.

Patients present with a variety of pathologies for stereotactic surgery. Biopsy is the commonest for framed surgery, and tumour debulking or excision for frameless. As confidence with the technology improves it is likely that more procedures will be carried out with stereotactic assistance.

Framed stereotactic techniques

Framed surgery is particularly suited for small lesions and those that are deep seated within brain tissue.

There are two main types of framed system, both of which use the principle of a target centred arc, accurate to around 1mm. In the BRW/CRW systems (Brown–Roberts–Wells/Cosman–Roberts–Wells) a halo-frame is fixed to the patient using pins. A removable fiducial frame is then fixed to this and the patient then has a head CT. The fiducial frame consists of a cylindrical array of carbon-fibre rods between two metal frames. By virtue of the size and relative position of the cross-section of the carbon-fibre fiducial rods, the position of the frame relative to the patient's head can be defined very accurately.

During surgery the fiducial frame is removed and replaced with a sterile stereotactic frame. The relative position of the needle carrier to the halo can be adjusted in three orthogonal dimensions. The needle guide on the carrier can rotate in two planes. The centre of the frame (i.e. the end of the needle) remains a fixed point within the patients head, regardless of the external orientation. (Imagine putting the point of a pencil on your finger. The point can remain in the same spot, even though the other end of the pencil can move.) The position of the needle is defined by the relative position of the stereo frame and the head halo.

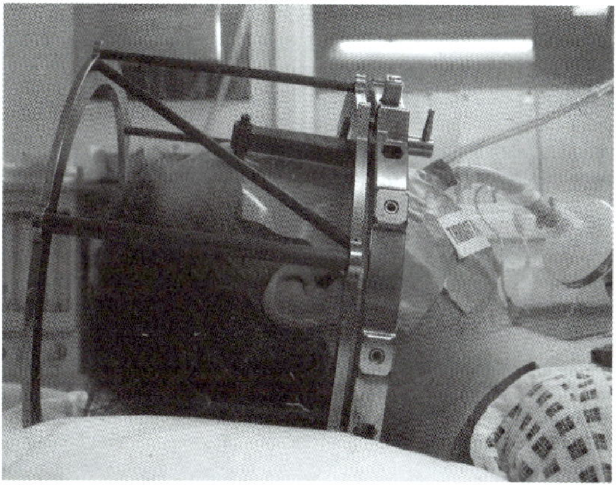

Fig. 6.8 Stereotactic surgery halo frame (lower) applied to patient, with fiducial frame (upper) attached.

In the Leksell system, there are no fiducial rods, but the principles are ostensibly the same.

In some cases the CT may be merged with MRI images to aid in localization of the lesions, or to define safe paths for the needle.

Frameless surgery

A pre-operative MRI is performed and the region of interest defined by surgeon or radiologist. The external contours of the head may be marked using fiducial stickers.

At surgery, the head is pinned and some form of positioning technology is fixed to the pin frame (infra-red) or head (magnetic field). The relative position of the head is then mapped to the stereotactic guidance machine, either using the fiducials as predefined points or using contour mapping.

During surgery a sterile probe, or a modified surgical instruments, can be localized in real time, helping to guide surgical approach and limits of resection.

Stereotactic biopsy

These patients usually present with a presumed tumour which requires tissue diagnosis, but is not causing sufficient mass effect to require debulking. Occasionally, biopsy is carried out for diagnosis of inflammatory or degenerative diseases.

Positioning

As appropriate for the site of the lesion.

Intra-operative issues

- The airway must be secured before frame positioning as airway access may be impossible with the frame in place.

- Placement of the halo frame is painful and in the UK, is usually performed with the patient anaesthetized. In some countries, stereotactic biopsy is performed routinely under local anaesthesia.
- Scalp blocks or local anaesthetic infiltration at the pin sites can be used. Boluses of opioid analgesic are commonly given to attenuate the cardiovascular response to pinning.
- The frame locking key should travel with the patient at all times, in case the frame needs to be removed urgently.
- Depending upon local practice, the patient may be anaesthetized in the theatre complex or in the scanning suite. Either way there will be at least one transfer, from CT to theatre. Preparation for this transfer should be the same as for any other patient. TIVA with muscle relaxation is the usual technique for transfer.

The surgical procedure itself is relatively short.

- The frame is set up with the required coordinates and a small burr-hole created.
- The biopsy is performed using a specially designed suction biopsy needle.
- There is a risk of bleeding from puncture of a vessel by the biopsy needle.
- Most units send the specimens for urgent 'frozen section' histology to ensure that a diagnostic biopsy has been taken.
- More than one target may be used. Biopsies may be sequential, waiting for the results of the 'frozen section' before taking the next.

Monitoring

The procedure is relatively non-invasive and the patients are usually well, with no need for invasive monitoring.

Postoperative care

Complications of stereotactic burr-hole biopsy are rare and these patients can return to the normal ward. Simple analgesia is normally all that is required.

Indications for frameless surgery

This is most commonly used for tumour surgery. It may have a valuable role in placement of anatomically difficult shunts.

- The anaesthetic and surgical considerations are those of the parent procedure.
- MRI and CT scans are carried out with the patient awake. Anaesthesia, controlled ventilation, and surgery itself all cause movement of brain tissue. The result is that *in vivo* lesion margins may not be mapped accurately to the scans.
- Intra-operative ultrasound scanning overcomes this problem by providing real-time assessment of lesion margins. This may necessitate the presence of an experienced radiologist in theatre to interpret the imaging, whilst the surgeon manipulates the probe.
- The operative field needs to be horizontal for this to allow the field to be flooded with saline so that scanning can take place.

Tips and pitfalls
- Positioning of the frame can be difficult. Always check that no part of the frame is digging in to the patient after positioning. If it is, then padding may be sufficient. If padding is insufficient the frame should be repositioned.
- Keep your fingers and thumbs out of the way of the pins when positioning the frame.
- The frame locking key must be with the patient at all times. This is usually achieved by putting it in the anaesthetist's pocket.
- Watch the frame being applied, so that you know how to take it off again in a hurry.
- Some frames make direct laryngoscopy and tracheal intubation extremely difficult. It may be impossible even to hold a face mask. If there is an airway emergency, do not be afraid to remove the frame.
- Do not hold the frame by the fiducial rods. They are relatively delicate and easily bent or broken. When moving the patient hold the patient's head and the pin frame, not the top portion.
- Using the correct coordinates for framed surgery is absolutely imperative. Wrong side stereotactic biopsy has occurred.
- Try to avoid techniques that result in major changes in cerebral physiology during the procedure as the resulting shift of the brain within the cranium can move the lesion away from the set target. A change in ventilation, in particular, should be avoided.
- Setting up frameless surgery can take a relatively long time. Keep the patient warm.
- Local anaesthesia is a perfectly acceptable alternative to GA for framed surgery.

Cerebral abscesses

Pathology
A brain abscess is a focal, intracerebral infection that begins as a localized area of cerebritis and develops into a collection of pus surrounded by a well-vascularized capsule.

Cerebral abscesses are rare (incidence ~2 per 100,000 population per year) due to the impermeable nature of the BBB. The bacterium responsible is determined by the cause and location of the primary lesion. Anaerobic bacteria such as streptococci and enterobacteria are the most common, but in 30–60% of cases multiple organisms are identified. Immunocompromised patients are at greater risk of cerebral abscesses and may have differing causative organisms including nocardia, candida and toxoplasmosis. Patients with HIV and AIDS are more likely to suffer from unusual pathogens such as mycobacterium tuberculosis, toxoplasma and cryptococcus.

De novo cerebral abscesses are unusual. There is usually a primary focus of infection elsewhere which if left untreated may result in a relapse. The site of the abscess may give some pointer to the primary source. Middle ear infection tends to result in middle or posterior fossa abscesses; frontal or ethmoidal sinus infection spreads to subdural collections; right-to-left shunts results in abscesses in the distribution of the middle cerebral artery.

The mainstay of treatment is antibiotics. The role of surgery is to reduce intracranial pressure, reduce the volume of infected tissue and confirm the diagnosis.

Associated conditions
The passage of bacteria through the BBB may occur due to:
- Spread of adjacent infection, e.g. sinusitis, mastoiditis, otitis media (50%).
- Infection disseminated from a distant site, e.g. infective endocarditis (25%).
- Direct introduction either by penetrating trauma or postoperatively (10%).
- No cause is identified in 15–25% of cases.
- Congenital cyanotic heart disease is a leading cause of cerebral abscesses in children.

Presentation
Patients normally present with a short history of symptoms, but in immunocompromised patients the course may be insidious. The primary complaints are headache, fever and focal neurological deficits that are determined by the site of the lesion. These will occur in conjunction with symptoms of any underlying conditions. An altered level of consciousness is common and seizures occur in up to a third of cases.

Patient population
Cerebral abscesses occur most commonly in adults aged between 20–40 years (with a higher incidence in males) and in children between the ages of 4 and 7.

Pre-operative assessment

The diagnosis is usually made by CT or MRI imaging. Cerebral abscesses can result in significant cerebral oedema, hydrocephalus or mass effect, making surgical intervention urgent. Operative delay may result in intraventricular rupture of an abscess, which is associated with a mortality of over 80%.

Patients may show evidence of sepsis or septic shock, and a careful assessment of their haemodynamic and fluid balance status is essential. In these cases, patients should be optimized according to sepsis care protocols.

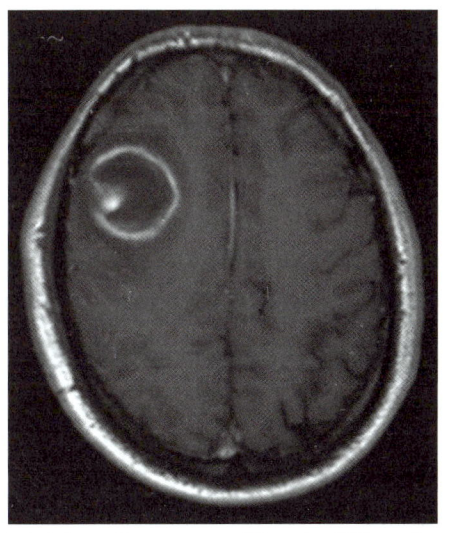

Fig. 6.9 Cerebral abscess. Post-contrast axial T1-weighted MRI scan demonstrating a right frontal ring-enhancing lesion. The patient, with known congenital heart disease, presented with seizures and pyrexia.

Surgical approach

Lesions >2.5 cm in size require surgical intervention. The approach is determined by the site of the lesion. Surgery may involve stereotactic image-guided aspiration, aspiration via a burr hole, or craniotomy and excision.

Intra-operative issues
Aspiration of the lesion may lead to transient cardiovascular instability due to 'septic showers'. If necessary, short-acting vasopressors can be used. Prolonged instability may require infusions of inotropes or vasopressors. The septic patient may be significantly dehydrated, and aggressive replacement of intravascular volume with crystalloid and/or colloid may be necessary.

Monitoring
- Arterial line and central venous pressure monitoring is indicated if there is evidence of cardiovascular compromise due to sepsis.
- Temperature. These patients may be pyrexial, and monitoring is essential to avoid excessive warming.

Postoperative care
- Most patients can be woken at the end of surgery and returned to the neurosurgical ward. Patients with evidence of end-organ dysfunction due to sepsis or with a persistently low GCS may require admission to critical care areas.
- Patients who have had seizures pre-operatively should be given prophylactic anticonvulsants, as there is a high incidence of seizures in the postoperative period.

Prognosis
This has dramatically improved with the increased availability of CT imaging and improved antimicrobial agents.
- Mortality is currently 5–10%.
- Mortality is higher in those patients with a low level of consciousness at the time of presentation and in those who are immunocompromised.
- Mortality for multiple lesions is identical to that of solitary lesions but long-term neurological deficits are more frequent.

Tips and pitfalls
- Avoid intra-operative antibiotic administration until after samples have been obtained for microbiological analysis.
- Make sure that someone talks to the microbiology laboratory directly about any samples that are taken.
- Antimicrobial therapy may be required for 6–8 weeks, so the placement of a long line or central venous catheter may be necessary.
- Corticosteroid use should be reserved for patients with significant cerebral oedema who are at risk of uncal herniation.

Decompressive craniectomy

Pathology
Some patients will develop, or be very likely to develop, refractory intracranial hypertension which is unresponsive to maximal medical therapy or surgical evacuation of space-occupying lesions. There are several precipitating causes, all resulting in cerebral ischaemia and marked oedema. Traumatic brain injury is the commonest cause, but it may also occur following elective tumour resection and following 'malignant' (distal internal carotid or proximal middle cerebral artery) infarction.

The 'RESCUEicp' randomized study of maximal medical therapy versus decompressive craniectomy for refractory intracranial hypertension is expected to finish its two-year follow-up in 2012.

Presentation
- Patients with TBI present with either sudden or gradual deterioration in consciousness, or increases in ICP. ICP may initially be responsive to medical management, but becomes unresponsive.
- Patients with 'malignant CVA' may actually appear quite well, as decompressive craniectomy is a prophylactic operation in this group. The indications for decompressive craniectomy include:
  - Gradual decrease in consciousness to a GCS score of ≤13 for right-sided lesions or an eye and motor score of ≤9 for left-sided lesions.
  - Ischaemic changes on CT that affect two-thirds or more of the territory of the middle cerebral artery and the formation of space-occupying oedema; displacement of midline structures on CT is not required.
  - <48 h since onset of stroke.

Pre-operative assessment
If a decision has been made to perform a decompressive craniectomy then there will be limited time for assessment and investigation. Patients with TBI are likely to be transferred, already intubated and ventilated, from either ICU or CT.

Some patients may be operated on at an earlier stage in their course, providing more time for pre-operative assessment.

Particular attention should be paid to current drug treatments, and which of these can safely be stopped during transfer and anaesthesia.

Surgical approach
The aim of the craniectomy is to convert the cranium from a closed to an open box.
- A sufficiently large craniectomy must be performed to avoid a 'toothpaste' effect where brain tissue is squeezed against the sides of the craniectomy.
- The craniectomy is usually an extensive frontal or fronto-temporo-parietal (hemispheric).

- The dura will be opened, and there is a risk of tearing of venous sinuses or associated dural veins.
- At the end of surgery the skin is closed. The bone flap may be kept either in a bone bank, transplanted to a subcutaneous pocket in the abdominal wall or discarded.

Positioning
Usually supine.

Intra-operative issues
A sudden reduction in ICP may cause cardiovascular instability. The anaesthetist should endeavour to provide adequate stable analgesia and anaesthesia throughout, though this may be difficult.

Monitoring:
Monitoring will be the same as for any other patients with acute brain injury.

Central venous access
TBI patients are likely to have already had central venous access secured for administration of inotropes. There is no need to insert a central venous catheter (CVC) purely for the procedure.

Intracranial pressure
This will be monitored postoperatively in patients with TBI.

Postoperative care
TBI patients should all return to ICU for further management.

Patients with MCA infarction should be woken up and return to HDU or a stroke unit for observation. Reported complications following decompressive craniectomy include:
- expansion of contusions
- haemorrhagic transformation of infarcts
- new extra- and subdural haematoma in the contralateral hemisphere.

Prognosis
The overall benefit of decompressive craniectomy is currently unclear.
- Without decompressive craniectomy many of these patients would be expected to die or have a very poor outcome.
- There is an early improvement in ICP and brain oxygenation in many TBI patients.
- Some patients make a full recovery and return for cranioplasty to restore cosmesis.
- Case series suggest that younger patients have a better outcome.
- There are concerns that decompressive craniectomy may result in very poor quality survival ('extremely dependent' or 'persistent vegetative state') in TBI patients that would otherwise have died.
- Meta-analysis of three trials of decompressive craniectomy following MCA infarction suggests that it converts 60% mortality to 20%,

without increasing poor outcomes, when performed within 48 h of stroke onset.

Tips and pitfalls
- By definition these are very sick patients and the prognosis is often poor.
- There is little merit in taking TBI patients to theatre if they have other injuries which make survival unlikely.
- Patients with malignant infarction may look deceptively well; the operation is essentially prophylactic.

Chapter 7

Cerebrovascular surgery

Extradural haematoma *258*
Subdural haematoma *262*
Intracranial haematoma *268*
Intracranial aneurysms and arterio-venous malformations (AVMs) *272*
EC–IC bypass procedures *276*
Carotid endarterectomy *278*

Extradural haematoma

Pathology
Extradural haematoma (EDH) is a consequence of acute arterial bleeding into the extradural (epidural) space, causing a rapid rise in intracranial pressure and reduction in cerebral perfusion.
- Brain injury is often secondary to compression by the haematoma, but may also be a direct result of trauma.
- The underlying cause of EDH is most commonly trauma, though surgery, infection, and coagulopathy may also precede the event.
- Spontaneous EDH has been described.
- Traumatic EDH is often associated with a fracture of the temporal bone, or 'springing' of the pterion overlying the middle meningeal artery.
- Most EDH occur in relation to the middle meningeal artery, but basal and posterior fossa EDH have also (rarely) been described.

Associated conditions
- EDH is commonly an isolated injury, but other trauma, intracranial, cervical or systemic, must be positively excluded.
- Epilepsy is risk factor for EDH.

Presentation
Classically patients with EDH are described as having sustained a head injury, with or without brief loss of consciousness followed by a lucid interval with normal conscious level. After an interval of a few minutes to hours there is a rapid deterioration in conscious level.

Reduced consciousness may be accompanied by:
- ipsilateral IIIrd cranial nerve palsy (dilated pupil) due to uncal herniation
- bilateral uncal herniation
- ipsilateral IIIrd palsy and hemiplegia (Kernohan's herniation)
- tonsillar herniation (coning).

Patient population
As with other traumatic injuries, EDH occurs most commonly in young males (18–40 years) or children following road traffic accidents, falls or sporting injuries.

Pre-operative assessment:
- EDH with signs of uncal herniation (dilated pupil and lowered GCS) is a true surgical emergency and these patients should go straight to theatre.
- Operation should not be delayed for investigation of non-life threatening issues.
- Blood should be cross-matched when the patient is in the anaesthetic room or operating theatre; bleeding may be significant and hidden particularly in children.
- Pre-operative CT will always have been performed and may demonstrate other intracranial pathology.

- The GCS and pupillary signs immediately before anaesthesia and surgery should be documented (□ p. 98).
- Patients without signs of uncal herniation should be operated on promptly before deterioration occurs. This may allow more time to complete the normal pre-operative assessment.

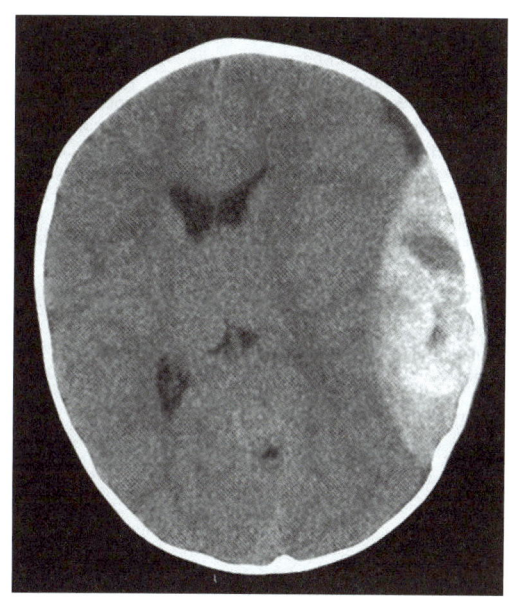

Fig. 7.1 Extradural haemorrhage. Unenhanced CT scan. EDH with marked midline shift to the right. The biconvex haematoma is limited anteriorly by the coronal suture and posteriorly by the lambdoid suture. The low attenuation within the haematoma is consistent with unclotted blood, and is indicative of active bleeding.

Surgical approach
A temporal or pterional craniotomy is used for most lesions. Posterior fossa craniectomy is used for posterior fossa lesions.

Positioning
Supine, with the temporal bone uppermost.
- Beware of concomitant cervical spine injury.
- Appropriate tilting of the theatre table will allow adequate positioning without undue rotation of the neck.

Intra-operative issues
Most patients will be transferred to the operating theatre already intubated and ventilated.

- For those patients requiring induction of anaesthesia, a modified rapid sequence induction should be used.
  - Suxamethonium is associated with a small rise in ICP but provides optimal intubating conditions. High-dose rocuronium is an alternative.
  - The pressor response to laryngoscopy should be suppressed with short-acting opioids.
  - Hypotension and hypoxia should be assiduously avoided.
- Patients with known or suspected other sites of trauma should be managed according to trauma guidelines.
- Surgical haemostasis of the scalp edges may be suboptimal due to the need for urgent decompression. Significant blood loss from scalp or other wounds may already have occurred.
- Decompression of the brain may lead to transient cardiovascular instability with hypotension and dysrhythmias.
  - If necessary, short-acting vasopressors can be used.
  - Prolonged cardiovascular instability should lead to consideration of other causes such as scalp bleeding, chest, abdominal or orthopaedic trauma and spinal cord injury.
- Prolonged cerebral ischaemia or other intracranial injuries may lead to secondary brain injury with oedema.
  - Take a look at the brain when exposed if possible.
  - Target management of cardiorespiratory parameters (PaO_2, $PaCO_2$, MAP etc.) as per TBI guidelines (see Immediate care, p. 340).

Monitoring
- An arterial line is useful but can wait until the patient is being prepared in theatre if uncal herniation is present.
- Temperature should be monitored. These patients are often transferred from peripheral hospitals, and may be significantly hypothermic.
- Near-patient testing of haemoglobin concentration can be used to facilitate the decision to transfuse if necessary.
- Check and correct any coagulation abnormalities.
- If secondary or other primary brain injury is suspected then postoperative ICP monitoring may be used (see Intracranial pressure, p. 68 and General management, p. 350).

Post-operative care
- Some patients can be woken at the end of surgery and return to the neurosurgical ward.
  - These are patients without other major injuries, minimal brain injury, a short duration of reduced consciousness and prompt return of full consciousness.
  - If the patient remains obtunded then consider HDU or ICU as appropriate.
- Sedation and ventilation on ICU is used for patients with brain swelling or other significant injuries.
- Ensure that secondary trauma survey has been completed and documented (see General management, p. 350).

Prognosis
Patients with isolated EDH do well, with over 90% survival and good recovery. Patients with associated intracranial injuries do less well with around 15% mortality and around 35% having a poor functional outcome. Prognostic factors for poor outcome include:
- low GCS prior to surgery
- presence and length of time with uncal herniation
- abnormal motor posturing
- size of haematoma (>30–50 ml)
- presence of other intracranial pathology.

Tips and pitfalls
- Patients with signs of herniation or neurological deterioration are true emergencies and every effort should be made to get them decompressed as quickly as possible. Do not delay the process with unnecessary monitoring, blood tests, changing tracheal tubes etc.
- Be alert to the possibility of other traumatic injuries; hypotension in an adult is rarely a consequence of an EDH alone.
- Children may bleed a significant volume of blood (in comparison with their total blood volume) into an EDH.
- Transferred patients are often hypothermic which will worsen coagulopathy.

Subdural haematoma

Pathology
Subdural haematoma (SDH) is usually a consequence of venous bleeding into the subdural space, causing a relatively slowly expanding haematoma with consequent brain compression and rise in intracranial pressure. The initial injury is generally a rotational or shearing injury which disrupts the bridging veins which cross the subdural space. This may follow minor trauma in at risk populations or high-energy trauma. Brain injury following subdural haematoma is multifactorial.
- Direct trauma to the underlying or distant brain tissue at the time of injury.
- Direct compression by the haematoma.
- Raised intracranial pressure.
- Expansion of chronic haematoma through water osmosis.
- Vasoconstrictive effects of substances within the haematoma.

Subdural haematoma is often divided into acute, subacute, and chronic based on the time since the injury.
- Patients with chronic subdural haematoma have had time to compensate for the haematoma and may present days to weeks after the initial bleed.
- Acute traumatic subdural haematoma is one form of (usually severe) TBI.

Most SDH are supratentorial, though posterior fossa SDH are recognized.

Associated conditions
- Acute SDH is usually associated with high-energy trauma such as road traffic accidents.
- Subacute and chronic subdurals are associated with disturbances of coagulation, particularly warfarin therapy for atrial fibrillation or prosthetic cardiac valves.
- Alcoholics frequently present with SDH due to a combination of cerebral atrophy, falls, and coagulopathy.
- Rarely metastatic malignancy may present with bloody subdural collections, which tend to recur.

Presentation
Acute SDH presents in similar fashion to other traumatic brain injury with a history of trauma, reduction of consciousness, and associated trauma. Chronic subdural haematoma may present in various ways:
- an acute reduction in consciousness, usually due to new bleeding or expansion of the haematoma
- stroke-like symptoms (e.g. hemiparesis, dysphasia) due to local compressive effects
- gradual reduction in cerebral function (e.g. confusion, 'off legs', memory loss, balance or vision disturbance, personality change).

Many patients or their carers will be able to give a history of recent (mild) head trauma, but in 50% of cases no cause is found.

Patient population
- As with other traumatic injuries, acute SDH occurs most commonly in young males (18–40) or children following road traffic accidents.
- Young children may present with SDH following violent shaking (part of the 'shaken baby syndrome') though SDH can occur in a young child for other reasons.
- The elderly and individuals with atrophic brains (dementia, alcohol abuse, previous neurosurgery) are most likely to present with chronic SDH (CSDH).
- The incidence of CSDH is around 60 per 100,000 population per year in those aged >70, but <4 per 100,000 per year in those <65.

Preoperative assessment
Acute traumatic SDH
Acute traumatic SDH is a neurosurgical emergency with a poor prognosis. There may be limited time for pre-operative assessment, and the patient should be assessed in the same way as other patients with TBI.

Warfarin
The patient presenting acutely with SDH due to warfarin should have the effects of warfarin reversed in a timely fashion. Individual units will have their own protocols but a general guide is:
- For non-urgent reversal give vitamin K iv or orally.
- For urgent reversal use prothrombin complex concentrate iv (in consultation with a haematologist). This will normalize the INR within a few minutes. There is little to be gained from waiting for repeated coagulation studies after administration. Intravenous vitamin K should also be given at the same time to provide longer-lasting effects.
- Fresh frozen plasma (FFP) is unpredictable in effect, requires large volumes (15–30 ml kg^{-1}) and the response needs checking. It is not the first choice for reversal of warfarin-induced coagulopathy.
- The absolute risk to the patient from continued bleeding far outweighs the small risks of thrombosis across prosthetic valves or stroke associated with atrial fibrillation.

Chronic SDH
Patients with chronic subdural haematoma most commonly have an insidious presentation and also have significant medical comorbidity. Time should be taken to ensure that remediable problems are sorted before taking the patient to theatre. Most patients do not need to go to theatre in the middle of the night, and are better served by planned surgery in daylight hours. Not all patients with SDH require operation and conservative 'watch and wait' strategies may be appropriate. Particular issues are:
- History of alcohol use: check clotting, consider alcohol-related medical complications such as alcohol withdrawal and encephalopathy (vitamin B12 and thiamine, avoidance of glucose).
- Dehydration: these patients have often being deteriorating for some time and may not have been eating or drinking properly at home.

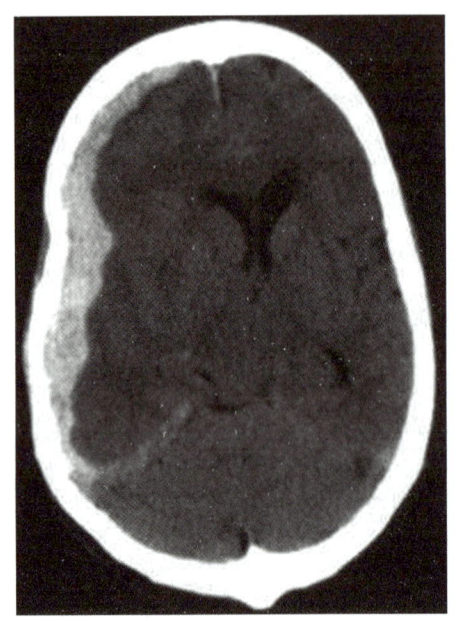

Fig. 7.2 Subdural haematoma. Unenhanced CT scan demonstrating acute SDH with accompanying midline shift to the left. The internally concave haematoma is not limited by the sutures, and extends on to the surface of the tentorium posteriorly.

Surgical approach
Acute traumatic SDH is usually treated with a trauma craniotomy. The management of chronic SDH is affected by surgical preference, extent and age of clot and patient morbidity. There are several options.
- Burr holes (single or multiple). The clot is washed off the brain surface using gentle direct irrigation and flushing, often with a Jacque's catheter. The irrigation continues until the fluid runs clear. A subdural gravity drain is usually left in place after closure.
- Craniotomy with more extensive surgical access. A subdural gravity drain is usually left in place after closure.
- Bilateral SDH are treated similarly.
- In children with open fontanelles, repeated percutaneous trans-fontanelle taps may be used. If this fails, then subdural–peritoneal shunts may be required.

Positioning
Supine with the head turned and the temporal bone uppermost.
- Beware of concomitant cervical spine injury or pathology.
- Appropriate tilting of the theatre table will allow adequate positioning without undue rotation of the neck.

Intra-operative issues
- Patients with known or suspected other trauma should be managed according to trauma guidelines (see Immediate care, p. 340).
- The elderly patient with SDH and multiple comorbidities may not tolerate general anaesthesia particularly well.
  - It may be appropriate to perform burr hole evacuation under local anaesthesia.
- The commonest general anaesthetic technique for evacuation of SDH is to use muscle relaxation and controlled ventilation.
  - Some centres favour spontaneous ventilation with a laryngeal mask airway or similar.
  - Whichever technique is used it is important to avoid marked hypocapnia and hypotension.
- Surgical haemostasis of the scalp edges may be suboptimal due to the need for urgent decompression.
  - Significant blood loss from scalp or other wounds may already have occurred.
- Decompression of the brain may lead to transient cardiovascular instability with hypotension and dysrhythmias.
  - If necessary, short-acting vasopressors can be used.
  - Prolonged cardiovascular instability should lead to consideration of other causes such as scalp bleeding, chest, abdominal or orthopaedic trauma, and spinal cord injury.
- Prolonged cerebral ischaemia or other intracranial injuries may lead to secondary brain injury with oedema. Take a look at the brain when exposed if possible.
- Target the management of cardiorespiratory parameters (PaO_2, $PaCO_2$, MAP etc.) as per TBI guidelines (see Immediate care, p. 340).

Monitoring
- An arterial line is not usually necessary in the absence of significant other injuries or medical comorbidities.
- Temperature should be monitored. These patients are often transferred from peripheral hospitals, and may be significantly hypothermic.
- Check and correct coagulation abnormalities. Remember to recheck the coagulation profile after giving prothrombin concentrate.
- If secondary or other primary brain injury is suspected then postoperative ICP monitoring may be used.

Postoperative care
- Most patients with acute traumatic SDH will have significant associated TBI and other injuries and should be managed postoperatively on ICU.
- Ensure that secondary trauma survey has been completed and documented (see Intracranial pressure, p. 68 and General management, p. 350).
- Patients with chronic SDH can usually be woken at the end of surgery and returned to the neurosurgical ward.
- Emergence from anaesthesia may be prolonged with the combination of advanced age and (recovering) brain injury.

Prognosis
The prognosis is dependent upon the associated pathology.
- Acute traumatic SDH has a poor prognosis (mortality 30–60%), which is probably related to the severity of underlying TBI rather than the SDH itself. Acute traumatic SDH is associated with a worse outcome than other forms of TBI.
  - Mortality for patients aged >80 with acute SDH is >80%.
- Chronic SDH patients may make a full recovery (to pre-SDH function), though some are left with focal deficits. Overall in-hospital mortality for chronic SDH is around 2–4%.

Tips and pitfalls
- Acute traumatic SDH is a severe form of TBI and should be managed as such.
- Be alert to the possibility of other traumatic injuries—hypotension in an adult is rarely a consequence of an SDH alone.
- Do not be pressured in to anaesthetizing frail elderly patients for chronic SDH. If unsure about the appropriateness of surgery and anaesthesia, consultant to consultant discussion should take place.
- Local anaesthesia may be the best option for burr hole evacuation in some patients. It does require someone to remain with the patient however, and very confused patients are unlikely to tolerate this.
- Prothrombin complex concentrates (PCC) are the treatment of choice for reversing warfarin induced coagulopathy.
- Don't forget vitamin K when using PCC otherwise coagulopathy may recur postoperatively.

SUBDURAL HAEMATOMA

Intracranial haematoma

Pathology

Intracranial haematoma may arise from various pathological processes.
- Arterial bleeding from intracerebral vessels (primary haemorrhagic stroke, 10–15% of first strokes).
- Secondary bleeding into thromboembolic stroke:
  - the natural history of a proportion of thromboembolic strokes
  - as a result of thrombolytic therapy for stroke.
- Aneurysmal rupture with intracerebral extension (see, p. 362),
- Arteriovenous malformation rupture (see Intracranial aneurysms and arteriovenous malformations, p. 272).
- Traumatic brain injury (see Pathophysiology, p. 334).
- Bleeding into tumour (primary or metastatic).
- Iatrogenic:
  - thrombolysis (myocardial infarction, stroke, pulmonary embolism)
  - cerebral angiography procedures
  - anticoagulation therapy e.g. warfarin, heparin or clopidogrel.

In most instances the initial bleed is arterial and associated with diseased or abnormal vessels.

- Intracerebral haematoma (ICH) will cause local compressive symptoms related to its location. If sufficiently large, or associated with surrounding cerebral oedema, clinically significant increases in intracranial pressure may occur.
- Most ICH are supratentorial, but posterior fossa and brainstem haematoma are well recognized.
- Recurrent bleeding and clot expansion is common but evidence for preventive therapy in the absence of coagulopathy is currently scarce.

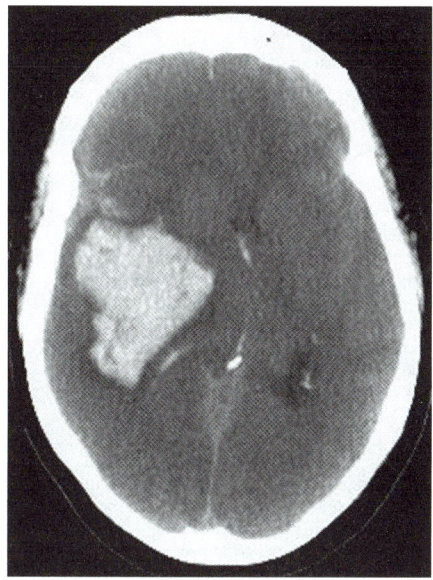

Fig. 7.3 Intracerebral haemorrhage. Unenhanced CT scan. ICH following rupture of a right middle cerebral artery aneurysm. Note the presence of subarachnoid and intraventricular haemorrhage, midline shift with effacement of the ventricular system and cerebral sulci, and generalized loss of grey/white matter differentiation.

Associated conditions
Primary haemorrhagic stroke is associated with hypertension, diabetes, increased age and smoking.

Conditions affecting coagulation and blood vessel mechanics (e.g. anticoagulant therapy, chemotherapy) are associated with increased risk of ICH.

Presentation
Haemorrhagic stroke may be indistinguishable on clinical grounds from thromboembolic stroke, but is often characterized by headache and deterioration in GCS. Presentation is determined by haematoma location and size.
- Focal deficits:
  - arm or leg weakness
  - sensory loss
  - dysphasia
  - visual loss
  - cranial nerve palsies
  - focal seizures.

- Reduction in consciousness:
  - global effect of increased ICP
  - local effects of brainstem haematoma.

Patient population
Most patients with primary haemorrhagic stroke are older reflecting the common underlying pathology.

Pre-operative assessment
Pre-operative assessment should be directed at chronic underlying conditions and acute physiological derangements.
- A small proportion of patients presenting for surgery with ICH will require airway protection before coming to theatre.
- Many patients with ICH will have significant acute systemic hypertension on a background of chronic hypertension.
- There is no clear evidence for the management of blood pressure following ICH.
  - The risk of haematoma expansion caused by elevated blood pressure must be balanced against the risk of ischaemia in both perilesional and normal brain that has autoregulated to chronic hypertension.
  - Although guidelines stress the importance of individualizing treatment based on the patient's normal blood pressure, this is not usually known at the time of admission.
  - Most centres advocate the treatment of systolic and mean arterial pressures >200 and 150 mmHg, respectively.
- Many patients with ICH have pre-existing diabetes or may present with hyperglycaemia.
  - Persistent hyperglycemia >7.8 mmol l^{-1} is associated with a worse prognosis.
  - Most centres will institute insulin therapy if glucose is >10 mmol l^{-1}.

Surgical management
The role of surgical management of ICH is still unclear.
- The International Surgical Trial in Intracerebral Haemorrhage (STICH) showed no overall benefit of surgical evacuation of ICH. However, patients were only included where the surgeon was uncertain about the benefit of surgery.
  - Selected patients with lobar and superficial ICH are thought to be most likely to benefit from surgery and this is currently being investigated in the STICH II trial.
- If supratentorial evacuation is undertaken it is usually performed via a standard craniotomy or minicraniotomy.
- Although there are no trials of surgical management of posterior fossa and brainstem haemorrhage, the outcome is so poor without evacuation that standard practice is to evacuate the clot as a matter of urgency.

Positioning
As for normal craniotomy, dependent on site of haematoma.

INTRACRANIAL HAEMATOMA

Intra-operative issues
A standard neuroanaesthesia technique for craniotomy should be used.
- Hypertension due to laryngoscopy, pinning, skin incision etc. must be avoided with appropriate analgesia and anaesthesia.
- Opening of the dura and evacuation of the haematoma may result in significant swings in blood pressure.
  - Adequate hydration may mitigate some of these changes, but otherwise short-acting vasoactive agents may be required.
- Decompression of posterior fossa and brainstem haematoma can be associated with cardiovascular instability due to effects on the floor of the fourth ventricle.
  - Dysrhythmmia is relatively common in this population, though it is generally short-lived.
- Although modern imaging techniques mean that unexpected aneurysms and AVMs underlying the haematoma are less common, they may still occur.

Monitoring
- An arterial line is generally used due to cardiovascular lability.
- Hypo- and hyperthermia should be avoided.
- Hyperglycaemia should be avoided.
- If patients are coagulopathic (thrombolysis, haemophilia, warfarin) check clotting and liaise closely with haematology.
- Patients with swollen brains usually require postoperative ICP monitoring.

Postoperative care
- Some patients with ICH can be safely woken up, particularly if the pre-operative GCS was only mildly depressed.
- If the brain appears tight at operation, then monitoring on ICU may be more appropriate.
- Patients with posterior fossa and brainstem bleeds are at high risk of sudden deterioration and should be cared for in a critical care unit.

Prognosis
- Overall 30-day mortality of ICH is around 30–50%, though most of these will not be managed operatively. Half of the deaths occur in the first 48 h.
- One-year mortality is around 50% for supratentorial ICH and around 65% for brainstem disease.
- Around 20% of patients with ICH are functionally independent at 6 months.

Tips and pitfalls
- Surgery for ICH is likely to become more common as stroke care becomes more aggressive:
  - treatment of primary ICH;
  - rescue therapy for ICH following thrombolysis.
- Expect and be prepared for cardiovascular instability, particularly with posterior fossa clots.
- Occasionally a straightforward ICH craniotomy will turn into an aneurysm clipping or excision of AVM. Be prepared!

Intracranial aneurysms and arteriovenous malformations (AVMs)

Although neuroradiological treatment of cerebral vascular lesions has become predominant over the last 10 years, open surgery can be required either if a lesion is deemed unsuitable for a neuroradiological approach or if neuroradiological intervention has failed.

Intracranial aneurysms

The majority of aneurysms present with subarachnoid haemorrhage (SAH) following rupture. Giant aneurysms are often identified by imaging undertaken to investigate symptoms of pressure on adjacent structures (e.g. optic chiasm). The presenting signs and pathophysiology of subarachnoid haemorrhage are dealt with in 📖 Subarachnoid haemorrhage, p. 362.

Pre-operative assessment

- The neuroimaging should be reviewed with the neurosurgeon, who should explain the proposed surgical approach. The pattern of subarachnoid blood on CT scan has prognostic significance as to the likely severity of postoperative vasospasm.
- The anaesthetist should evaluate and document conscious level (GCS score), pupillary responses and any motor deficit, in order to facilitate postoperative comparison.
- The cardiovascular sequelae of a presenting SAH should be ascertained. Around 50% of patients have an abnormal ECG, of whom half have ST-segment or T-wave changes. Around one-third of patients have some form of dysrhythmia, though severe arrhythmia is uncommon. The peak incidence is ~day 2. Impaired myocardial function or biochemical evidence of myocardial damage is common (📖 see p. 362).
- Fluid and electrolytes status must be evaluated.
  - Electrolyte abnormalities occur in around one-third of patients following aneurysmal bleeding.
  - Hypokalaemia can be secondary to diuretic administration, intravenous infusions of potassium-free fluids and sympathetic stimulation. Preoperative correction should be undertaken.
- Subarachnoid haemorrhage may result in disordered coagulation; this should be checked and corrected if necessary.

Intra-operative management

- Arterial cannulation and display of the pressure waveform is essential before induction.
- Hypotension and hypertension should both be assiduously avoided and treated. Prevention of surges in arterial pressure is vital: intra-operative rupture can be catastrophic.
- Remifentanil (slow iv bolus or infusion) will reliably obtund the pressor response to laryngoscopy and tracheal intubation. Fentanyl is an alternative.

INTRACRANIAL ANEURYSMS AND AVMs

- Anaesthesia is induced with propofol or thiopental, and neuromuscular blocking drug administered. Full neuromuscular blockade should be ensured before attempts at laryngoscopy.
- Large-bore venous access is needed in case of aneurysmal rupture.
- There is no evidence to suggest that volatile or propofol-based techniques result in better outcome. Remifentanil by manually adjusted or target-controlled infusion is generally used for intra-operative analgesia.
- Cross-matched blood should be available in the theatre suite.
- The anaesthetist must be vigilant for rupture in the course of exposure of the aneurysm. Abrupt changes in haemodynamic variables can be apparent before aneurysmal leakage is apparent to the surgeon.
- As a general rule arterial pressure should be maintained at levels not significantly less than pre-operative values.
- Induced hypotension, once commonplace in neurovascular anaesthesia, is no longer routinely practised on account of concern about the risk of cerebral ischaemia.
- Most aneursyms are secured with application of a single permanent clip.
- Some anatomically difficult aneurysms may necessitate the use of temporary clips either to the aneurysm itself, or to adjacent vessels.
  - The placement of temporary clips may cause localized cerebral ischaemia.
  - Many anaesthetists administer bolus doses of hypnotic (thiopental or propofol) prior to temporary clip application in order to reduce $CMRO_2$. There are theoretical reasons to believe that this may offer some benefit; there is, however, no evidence that this practice alters outcome. Hypotension following administration is a risk and should be promptly treated.
  - There is some suggestion that blood pressure should be raised during temporary clipping, in order to maximize perfusion via the collateral circulation. There is no evidence that this practice improves outcome.
  - The duration of ischaemia is more important and the anaesthetist should record the start and stop times; warning the surgeon if ischaemia is prolonged, e.g. >5 min.
  - However, the 'safe' duration of ischaemia has not been determined and is usually at the discretion of the neurosurgeon.
- If successfully clipped, the aneurysm is no longer at risk of rupture. However, good practice mandates a careful, controlled emergence.
- Antihypertensive therapy (e.g. labetalol in 5–20 mg increments) may be required to control the hypertensive response to tracheal extubation.
- In the event of failure to clip the aneurysm, the surgeon will resort to wrapping the lesion with muslin to offer some reinforcement of the wall and reduction of the risk of rebleeding. In such cases—and for any patient with additional, asymptomatic aneurysms identified on imaging—control of arterial pressure on emergence is particularly important.

Monitoring
- An arterial line is essential.
- Unless there is concern about cardiovascular comorbidity or uncertainty about volaemic status, central venous pressure (CVP) monitoring is not usually necessary. There are theoretical concerns about risks of venous obstruction due to CVC placement. However, CVP monitoring may prove useful if Triple H therapy (📖 see p. 362) is undertaken to treat vasospasm in the postoperative period.
- Evidence does not support the practice of active cooling for cerebral protection.
  - The IHAST study showed no improvement in Glasgow Outcome Score with intra-operative cooling to 33°C vs. normothermia.
- Arterial blood should be sampled in order to establish any disparity between arterial tension and end-tidal CO_2 concentration.
  - Hypocapnia ($PaCO_2$ <4.0 kPa) risks global cerebral ischaemia, and should generally be avoided.
- Placement of a fibre-optic catheter in the jugular bulb (and continuous measurement of saturation by oximetry) can guide treatment of intra-operative cerebral ischaemia. However, this technique has not gained widespread acceptance.

Postoperative care
- In the event of brain swelling (e.g. after intra-operative aneurysmal rupture or protracted ischaemia during clip application) mechanical lung ventilation and sedation should be continued in ICU with ICP monitoring.
- If surgery and the immediate recovery period are uncomplicated, the next 24 h should ideally be spent in a neurosurgical HDU with the facility for continuation of direct arterial pressure monitoring. In the immediate postoperative period, vigilance for decreasing conscious level (indicative of haematoma) is paramount.
- In the ensuing days, vasospasm may be associated with focal neurological signs and obtunded consciousness. Rebleeding, hydrocephalus, seizure activity, sepsis, and electrolyte abnormalities are differential diagnoses requiring exclusion.

Arteriovenous malformations (AVMs)
The most common presentation of an AVM is spontaneous intracranial haemorrhage, although some AVMs may cause symptoms through direct mass effect.

AVMs are usually managed by stereotactic radiosurgery or embolization, but can be excised surgically as a 'tumour' mass, with feeding vessels obliterated.

Peri-operative management
This largely follows the same principles as that for intracranial aneurysm surgery. Particular points to note include:
- AVMs typically cause parenchymal or ventricular haemorrhage, rather than subarachnoid haemorrhage. Vasospasm is, therefore, far less likely.
- The risk of spontaneous intra-operative rupture due to increases in blood pressure is less likely that that seen in aneurysm surgery, as the AVM is able partially to buffer surges in systemic pressure.

- Postoperative hypotension will increase the risk of cerebral ischaemia. The feeding vessels to the AVM that have been sacrificed intra-operatively may also have been supplying normal brain.

Normal pressure perfusion breakthrough (NPPB)
This is sudden development of cerebral oedema or haemorrhage in the absence of another cause and may occur intra- or postoperatively. The existence of this phenomenon has been the subject of much debate, as it is very difficult to exclude the numerous other causes of cerebral oedema and haemorrhage, such as post-retraction oedema and haemorrhage, rupture of an occult part of the AVM or venous outflow obstruction.

Tips and pitfalls
- Although the use of remifentanil has led to reliance on opioid to prevent intra-operative coughing or movement, many anaesthetists feel more comfortable using neuromuscular blocking agents as well, at least until the aneurysm or AVM has been secured.
- Prevention of surges in arterial pressure is vital during aneurysm surgery: intra-operative rupture can be catastrophic.
- There is no 'safe' time period for temporary clipping and it should be kept to as short as period as possible. The risk of ischaemia is not solely related to the time of occlusion, as the position of the aneurysm and collateral vessels are also important.
- NPPB is a rarely the sole cause of cerebral oedema or haemorrhage and should be a diagnosis of exclusion.

EC–IC bypass procedures

Extracranial–intracranial (EC–IC) bypass is the connection of the external carotid artery circulation to the internal carotid artery circulation. The aim is to augment cerebral blood flow and, therefore, parenchymal oxygenation when there is a proximal obstruction to flow in the internal carotid artery circulation. Surgical procedures that achieve EC–IC bypass include:

- Direct bypass procedures:
  - Superficial temporal artery to middle cerebral artery anastamosis.
  - Occipital artery to middle cerebral artery anastamosis.
  - Vein graft anastamosis of external carotid to internal carotid.
- Indirect bypass procedures:
  - Encephaloduroarteriosynangiosis (EDAS). Dural graft containing the middle meningeal artery is placed directly onto ischaemic cerebral cortex to promote revascularization.
  - Encepahalomyosynangiosis. Temporalis muscle is placed on the cortical surface to promote neovascularization.
  - Encephalomyoarteriosynangiosis (EMAS). Temporalis muscle with an identified arterial supply is placed on the cortical surface under a bone flap to promote neovascularization.
  - Multiple burr holes.
  - Omental transposition.

Surgical indications

Adults
- Cerebrovascular disease with focal neurological deficit
- Cerebral artery stenosis with neurological deficit
- Occlusive disease of the circle of Willis
- Giant aneurysms not suitable for clipping
- Moya Moya syndrome (10% associated with cerebral aneurysms).

Children
- Moya Moya syndrome (rarely associated with cerebral aneurysm).

Moya Moya syndrome
- Moya Moya syndrome may be congenital or acquired and causes progressive occlusion of vessels at the skull base and circle of Willis.
- A collateral circulation develops giving rise to the characteristic angiographic appearance of a 'puff of smoke'.
- Patients present initially with transient ischaemic attacks and then strokes.
- The degree and nature of neurological defect will have implications for the level of monitoring and nursing care required postoperatively.
- The congenital form may also affect systemic vessels.
- Cardiac function (baseline ECG) and renal function must be assessed in these children.

Anaesthetic considerations
The anaesthetic technique during EC–IC procedures must maintain cerebral perfusion. If the surgical technique will involve temporary clipping of a cerebral artery then techniques to augment cerebral oxygenation must be used.

General principles
- Maintain normovolaemia.
- Maintain normotension for the patient.
- Avoid vasoconstrictors—intravenous or locally/administered.
- Maintain high normal $PaCO_2$ to avoid cerebrovascular vasoconstriction.
- Mild hypothermia has been advocated for cerebral artery clipping although there is no evidence to show this improves outcome.

Adults
- A careful assessment of the patient's cardiovascular status must be made pre-operatively.
- Invasive monitoring of arterial pressure is mandatory.
- The need for central venous pressure monitoring depends upon the individual patient's cardiovascular status.
- Postoperatively patients should be nursed in an appropriate high-dependency area.

Children
- Children will most commonly undergo an indirect bypass procedure (EDAS or EMAS) which is less complex surgical procedure than direct bypass.
  - Temporary clipping of cerebral vessels will not be necessary.
- Intra-operative analgesia with fentanyl and simple analgesics will negate the need for iv morphine in most patients.
- Invasive monitoring of arterial pressure is not usually required in children undergoing an indirect bypass procedure.
- Postoperatively patients should be nursed in an appropriate high dependency area.

Complications
- Hyperperfusion syndrome—increased cerebral volume secondary to increased flow in a vascular bed with abnormal autoregulation and which is maximally dilated distal to the bypassed stenosis or occlusion. Clinically the syndrome is characterized by cerebral oedema and intracerebral hemorrhage. The syndrome is more likely to occur with high flow grafts (e.g. saphenous vein) than low flow grafts (superficial temporal artery to MCA). Urgent surgical management is required to reduce flow through the graft.
- Graft failure.
- Seizures.
- Haemorrhage.
- Stroke.
- Death.

Tips and pitfalls
- Adults requiring EC–IC bypass often have generalized vascular disease and must be assessed pre-operatively for cardiac and renal impairment.
- Children most commonly undergo indirect bypass procedures and do not usually have widespread vascular disease.
- Hyperperfusion syndrome is a complication of direct bypass procedures and is not seen after indirect bypass procedures.

Carotid endarterectomy

Carotid endarterectomy (CEA) is performed as a prophylactic operation to prevent ischaemic cerebral damage. It is performed in patients at risk from emboli arising from atheromatous plaque at the carotid bifurcation.

Associated conditions
By definition these patients have atherosclerotic disease.
- Most patients will have pre-existing hypertension which may be worsened by recent cerebral ischaemia.
- Ischaemic heart disease is common and may be severe.
- Diabetes mellitus is also a commonly associated condition.

Presentation
There are two groups of patients presenting for CEA:
- symptomatic patients who have transient neurological deficits due to emboli arising from active plaque at the carotid bifurcation;
- asymptomatic patients who have demonstrable disease at the carotid bifurcation but no recent neurological events caused by this.

The role of surgery
- Two large studies provide the evidence in favour of CEA over best medical management.
- For symptomatic patients the benefit of CEA is linked to the degree of carotid stenosis:
  - >70% stenosis: 16% absolute risk reduction (ARR) of peri-operative death or stroke within 5 years;
  - 50–69% stenosis: 4.6% ARR;
  - 30–49% stenosis: no benefit;
  - <30% stenosis: CEA harmful.
- For asymptomatic patients the benefits are less clear.
- Early surgery is associated with the greatest benefit, but also involves operating on a more unstable group of patients. Current guidance is that symptomatic individuals should be operated upon within 2 weeks of presentation.

Pre-operative assessment
The main issues for patients presenting for CEA are concerned with management of blood pressure, ischaemic heart disease, and diabetes mellitus.
- Coronary artery disease is very common, and a significant number of patients will have disease which might otherwise merit angioplasty or revascularization. It is not clear whether CEA should be performed before or after (or even with) coronary artery bypass graft (CABG) in these cases.
- Hyperglycaemia worsens neurological outcome following acute brain injury and diabetics are more likely to have significant vascular disease elsewhere.
- Most medications should be continued during the peri-operative phase, particularly antihypertensives, statins, and aspirin. There is insufficient evidence to provide definitive advice about clopidogrel.

- Any pre-operative neurological deficits must be documented accurately as this will provide a reference for postoperative observations.

Surgical approach

The neck incision is usually a vertical one just anterior to the sternocleidomastoid muscle, over the carotid below the angle of the jaw. The patient's head will be turned away from the operative side, which may become uncomfortable for the patient. Following dissection, the common, external, and internal carotid arteries are clamped. An arteriotomy is performed and the plaque removed. Many surgeons close the arteriotomy with a patch as this reduces the risk of re-stenosis. Patching will prolong the duration of surgical closure. A surgical drain is usually left in place. Eversion endarterectomy is associated with greater cardiovascular lability, probably due to transaction of the carotid sinus nerve.

Conduct of anaesthesia

Local or general anaesthesia?

There are theoretical and practical advantages and disadvantages to both local and general anaesthesia.

The GALA trial, a large (3500 patients) direct comparison between local and general anaesthesia found no differences in peri-operative stroke, death or myocardial infarction. Systematic review of all the randomized studies has failed to find convincing evidence of improved clinical outcomes for either technique.

Local anaesthesia techniques

- Local anaesthesia can be achieved using a combination of local infiltration, superficial and deep cervical plexus blocks.
- Deep cervical plexus blocks carry more risks (subarachnoid and intra-arterial injection, phrenic nerve paralysis) but may be associated with better early analgesia. Cadaver studies suggest that there is connection between the superficial and deep plexuses anyway, provided the local anaesthetic is injected below the cervical fascia. Many practitioners now use only superficial blocks for these reasons.
- Cervical epidural anaesthesia is used by a few centres. It provides good operating conditions, but significant risks of dural puncture, epidural venepuncture and respiratory muscle paralysis.

General anaesthesia techniques

- There is no direct evidence to suggest that any drug or drug combination is better than any other for carotid endarterectomy. Sevoflurane and propofol have theoretical benefits over isoflurane with regard to maintenance of cerebral autoregulation and prompt emergence at the end of surgery.
- Remifentanil is commonly used for intra-operative analgesia.
- Nitrous oxide is associated with increased postoperative myocardial ischaemia in patients undergoing CEA.
- Airway maintenance can be achieved with a supraglottic airway or a tracheal tube. Supraglottic airways may reduce the haemodynamic changes associated with laryngoscopy but access to the airway is

difficult in case of emergency during surgery. They may cause an element of soft tissue distortion which may impede surgical access.

Pain relief
- Postoperative pain relief with paracetamol and weak opioids is usually sufficient.
- NSAIDs should not be added to aspirin and clopidogrel.

Monitoring
- Invasive arterial pressure monitoring should be used for all patients. Venous and arterial cannulae should ideally be placed in the contralateral arm for ease of access.
- Some form of neurological monitoring should be used.

Patients under local anaesthesia
Awake patients can be monitored by assessing various aspects of understanding and responsiveness (cognitive function).
- Simply asking 'Are you alright?' is insufficient.
- Regular assessment of ability to obey commands should be used.
- Squeezing a fluid bag connected to a pressure transducer may allow observation of contralateral motor response without having to go under the drapes.
- Counting backwards from 100 is a commonly used monitor of speech and executive function.
- Any deterioration should be reported immediately to the surgeon.

Patients under general anaesthesia
In addition to standard monitoring, patients should have some form of neurological monitoring, as clinical assessment is impossible. The following monitors are all used, in combination or alone. None of the monitors is perfect.

TCD
TCD serves two purposes during CEA:
- assessment of ipsilateral middle cerebral artery flow velocity (MCAFV) as a surrogate marker of (in)adequate collateral flow around the circle of Willis;
- detection of emboli.

Marked reductions of MCAFV (0–15% of baseline) are associated with postoperative stroke. However, various thresholds of MCAFV (MCAFV <30 cm s^{-1}, clamp/pre-clamp ratio <0.6, >50% reduction in MCAFV) have been shown to be unreliable at detecting ischaemia or identifying patients who would require shunts.

Most postoperative deficits are due to embolic events (with an incidence of 90% during CEA) rather than changes in cerebral haemodynamics. TCD can detect gaseous and particulate emboli either using trained operators or with semi-automatic detection systems. Gaseous emboli can be distinguished from particulate. They usually occur at shunt opening and closure and are not usually clinically significant. Particulate emboli are associated with worsening cognitive function after CEA. A few centres advocate the use of Dextran-40 in patients with a large micro-embolic load in the postoperative period.

Near infrared spectroscopy (NIRS)
Near infrared spectroscopy has been used, but technological limitations, anatomical considerations and poor specificity for detection of ischaemia mean that it is not widely used alone.

EEG
The EEG is changed by ischaemia. However, real-time interpretation of the raw EEG is difficult. Only superficial cortical activity is recorded, so deeper ischaemia may be missed. The BIS™ monitor primarily reflects frontal lobe activity so is not reliable for detecting ischaemia elsewhere.

SSEP
Somatosensory evoked potentials test the integrity of the whole sensory pathway so, theoretically, can detect ischaemia of deeper structures. Unfortunately, in clinical use they are no better than EEG monitoring.

Stump pressure
Following clamping of the common and external carotid arteries the pressure in the internal carotid artery reflects the perfusion pressure of the circle of Willis. Low stump pressures (25–50 mmHg) are reasonably specific for predicting ischaemia, but sensitivity is low.

Blood pressure management

For summary see Table 7.2.

Pre-operative
- The greatest benefit from CEA is seen when it is performed within 2 weeks of presentation—this leaves little time for optimal blood pressure control.
- There is no evidence that reducing blood pressure or delaying surgery influences operative risk but a pre-operative systolic blood pressure >180 mmHg is associated with postoperative stroke and death.
- Although direct evidence is lacking, a pragmatic approach is to postpone surgery and control hypertension in patients with systolic blood pressure consistently >180 mmHg, who do not have severe bilateral disease or frequent neurological events. For patients with severe disease, surgery should probably proceed regardless, in the knowledge that the potential benefits are greater than the risks.
- It is important to estimate the patient's baseline blood pressure. This may require clinical judgement incorporating admission, clinic, ward and anaesthetic room measurements.

Intra-operative
- Intra-operative cardiovascular lability is common, regardless of anaesthetic technique. Some of this is a reflection of the well-known intra-operative lability of the hypertensive patient. In addition the CEA patient undergoes manipulation of the carotid bifurcation, cross-clamping and release, removal of stenosis and possible reperfusion injuries. Inadequate analgesia will exacerbate this problem.
- Some surgeons infiltrate the carotid bifurcation with local anaesthetic in an attempt to reduce instability but the efficacy of this is unproven and local anaesthesia of the carotid sinus nerve is no longer recommended as a routine.

- Excessive hypotension or hypertension should be treated promptly to reduce the risk of myocardial or cerebral injury.
- Arterial blood pressure should be maintained between 100 and 120% of estimated baseline during carotid clamping. This may require fluids, vasopressors or hypotensive agents.

Postoperative
- Postoperative hypertension is seen in ~20% of patients following CEA and hypotension in ~10%. Disturbance of the carotid baroreflex may be part of the cause of hypertension. These changes are often relatively transient, lasting a few hours.
- Hypotension may reduce myocardial perfusion, but excessive increases in blood pressure may risk cerebral hyperperfusion due to improved flow through the carotid artery. Most clinicians aim for normotension by careful titration of vasoactive drugs.
- TCD monitoring of MCAFV may have a role in reducing the risk of hyperperfusion.
- Marked hypertension risks both increased myocardial work and cerebral hyperfusion. Blood pressure should be reduced (carefully) with vasodilators or beta-blockers.

Hyperperfusion syndrome
A small number (1–3%) of patients develop a hyperperfusion syndrome characterized by:
- ipsilateral headache
- hypertension
- seizures
- focal neurological deficits
- high MCAFV (>200% of pre-operative value).

Untreated, these patients are at risk of cerebral oedema, intracerebral or subarachnoid haemorrhage and death. There is little evidence to direct management, but aggressive blood pressure reduction (aiming for a systolic blood pressure <140 mmHg) is often used.

Postoperative care
- Most complications occur in the first few hours after surgery. There is considerable variation between units regarding where postoperative care takes place. Some units send all patients to HDU, others use an extended recovery stay followed by discharge to the ward.
- Patients should be nursed sitting up to improve venous drainage. Monitoring must include airway patency, frequent arterial blood pressure and neurological observations.

The major complications seen are:
- Local haematoma occurs in ~8% of patients, of whom around one-quarter will need to return to theatre. All patients must be observed for signs, and asked to report symptoms of expanding haematoma. If there is any concern, surgical clips (if used) should be removed immediately to decompress the neck, and the patient returned to theatre.

- Cranial nerve injuries occur in ~10% of patients, but are usually transient. These are a consequence of surgical traction or dissection.
- Postoperative stroke is seen in ~4% of patients, though the majority are non-fatal. Most are thromboembolic.
- Postoperative myocardial infarction occurs in ~0.5% of patients.

Tips and pitfalls

- Ensure that antihypertensive agents are continued in the pre- and postoperative period.
- Early communication between surgical and anaesthetic teams is essential, particularly with poorly controlled hypertensive patients, and must continue intra-operatively.
- There is no outcome evidence to support one antihypertensive over another—use what you are most comfortable with. Whatever you use, do so carefully. Rapid boluses are likely to cause problematic swings in blood pressure.
- Measure blood pressure in both arms to estimate baseline blood pressure—there may be clinically significant differences.
- In the event of neurological deterioration under local anaesthesia, dramatic improvements have been seen with administration of 100% oxygen, avoiding the need for shunts.
- Retraction on the angle of the jaw can be uncomfortable for the patient. Subcutaneous local anaesthetic infiltration just under the proximal third of the ramus and anterior to the angle of the jaw as part of the anaesthetic technique can pre-empt this problem.
- If general anaesthesia is used, prophylactic anti-emetics should be given.
- Patients who have taken diuretics prior to surgery may develop significant bladder discomfort, which may cause restlessness and hypertension in the awake patient.

Table 7.1 Comparison of local and general anaesthesia

Technique	Advantages	Disadvantages
Local anaesthesia	Allows continuous awake neurological monitoring Allows for rapid return to theatre for wound exploration	May be stressful for the patient Risk of intra-operative pain Possibly more hypertension during cross-clamping and hypotension after clamp release
General anaesthesia	Allows control of ventilation May be less stressful for patient and/or surgeon Theoretical neuroprotective effects of anaesthetic agents	Requires surrogate markers of neurological function (TCD, EEG, etc.) Possibly more intra-operative hypotension and postoperative hypertension Postoperative nausea and vomiting

Table 7.2 Blood pressure management for carotid endarterectomy

Intra-operative management

Maintain arterial blood pressure within 100–120% of baseline values during clamping.

Interpret these arterial pressure targets according to information available from cerebral monitoring or neurological symptoms.

Postoperative management

If a patient is hypertensive after operation, sit him/her up in bed which can itself reduce arterial pressure and may make the patient more comfortable:
- check for urinary retention;
- check for missed normal hypertensive medication.

Monitor blood pressure for 2–4 h using invasive arterial pressure:
- aim for a target systolic pressure <170 mmHg or within 20% of pre-operative values

Continue invasive monitoring for more than 2 h if vasoactive drugs have been required after surgery.

Monitor neurology.

Recovery room management

Systolic BP >170 mmHg or >20% above baseline:
- labetolol small boluses (10 mg up to 100mg total), +/− infusion;
- hydralizine small boluses (2 mg up to 10mg total);
- GTN infusion;
- observe in HDU for at least 2h after treatment has finished.

Ward management

Systolic BP >170 mmHg or >20% above baseline; no new neurological symptoms; not normally on antihypertensives:
- bisoprolol;
- ramipril.

Systolic BP >170 mmHg or >20% above baseline; no new neurological symptoms; normally on antihypertensives:
- administer normal antihypertensives if not already given;
- add ramipril/bisoprolol/diuretic.

Systolic BP >160 mmHg; new neurological symptoms:
- treat according to recovery room protocol;
- inform senior members of surgical team;
- transfer to HDU for invasive monitoring.

Table 7.2 is a modified version of the protocol used in Leicester Royal Infirmary, UK (courtesy of Dr J.P. Thompson). It is intended as a guide to a systematic approach to management. Other units will have their own local policies.

Chapter 8

Cranial surgery

Cranioplasty *286*
Craniofacial surgery in children *288*

Cranioplasty

Cranioplasty is the repair of a defect or deformity in the cranium. Strictly speaking this includes the replacement of the bone flap at the end of a craniotomy, although the usual neurosurgical interpretation is describing an operation some time after the creation of the defect or using a material other than the original bone.

Indications for cranioplasty
- Defect caused by trauma, tumour or decompressive craniectomy.
- Bone flap not replaced at the end of previous surgery.
- Removal of infected bone after local infection following previous surgery.
- Secondary reconstruction after primary repair of craniosynostosis.

Aims of cranioplasty
- Protection of underlying brain tissue.
- Improvement in cosmetic appearance.
- Prevention of sinking skin flap syndrome (neurological deficits caused by compression of a skin flap by atmospheric pressure).

Procedure
There are several materials available to repair the defect in the cranium:
- Autogenous bone—either the patient's original bone flap which may have been frozen and stored, or bone harvested from another site (e.g. a rib).
- Xenografts, e.g. bovine bone.
- Alloplastic materials: metals such as titanium, acrylics such as polymethylmethacrylate (PMMA) or hydroxyapatite (HA), or a combination such as a titanium mesh covered with PMMA.

Intra-operative management
- Bleeding from scar tissue dissection can be significant.
- Extradural haematoma may complicate the procedure.
- Intra-operative analgesia can be provided with boluses of fentanyl or a remifentanil infusion.
- Postoperative pain is often mild to moderate and oral analgesia is adequate.
  - Pain may be more severe if there is extensive dissection of tissues or attachments to bone.

Tips and pitfalls
- This is usually relatively 'non-invasive' neurosurgery and invasive monitoring is often unnecessary in the absence of cardiovascular comorbidity. Err on the side of caution and place an arterial line if extensive scarring or involvement of the sinuses is expected.
- Infiltration with local anaesthetic solutions containing adrenaline helps reduce skin blood loss and provides some postoperative analgesia.
- In contrast to the use of PMMA in orthopaedic surgery, adverse reactions are extremely rare.

Craniofacial surgery in children

Craniofacial surgery is performed for congenital or acquired conditions affecting the hard and soft tissues of the head and face including:
- craniosynostoses
- craniofacial dysostoses (Crouzon's syndrome)
- orbital dysostosis
- encephalocoeles
- craniofacial clefts.

The commonest condition encountered by the neuroanaesthetist is craniosyntosis. The management of encephalocoeles is discussed in 📖 Neural tube defects, p. 316.

Craniosynstosis

The premature closure of cranial sutures is known as craniosynostosis. It may be associated with severe cranial and facial deformity. The incidence is approximately 1:2000 live births.
- 80% of cases are isolated, idiopathic, single-suture synostoses in healthy children.
- Premature closure of calvarial sutures results in deformity of the skull vault, with characteristic morphological appearances (incidence of suture closure: sagittal > coronal > lamboid and metopic).
- Complex, multiple suture synostoses (facial and cranial) are often associated with other congenital abnormalities and more than 100 syndromes are described. The most common are Crouzon's, Apert's and Pfeizer's.

Abnormal development of the skull and facial bones causes volumetric restriction and may result in raised intracranial pressure, upper airway narrowing and severe exophthalmos.

The aims of surgical correction are to:
- normalize ICP and prevent cerebral and visual impairment
- reduce the complications associated with airway compression
- prevent corneal damage
- resolve feeding difficulties
- improve cosmetic appearance.

Simple cases are operated on in the first year of life, often between 2–6 months. Children with complex craniofacial synostoses may undergo multiple, staged procedures. Surgery is undertaken at specialized centres with well-developed multidisciplinary teams.

Pre-operative assessment
- Assessment will take place in a multidisciplinary clinic, allowing access to specialist opinion and investigation.
- Developmental delay, speech difficulties, and sensory deficits may make communication difficult.
- The aetiology of the craniofacial abnormality directs pre-operative assessment and investigation e.g. cardiology review and echocardiography.
- Look for signs and symptoms of raised intracranial pressure.

- Airway assessment should determine the degree of nasal obstruction and evidence of obstructive sleep apnoea. Feeding difficulties and failure to thrive may be indicative of an obstructed airway.
- Sleep studies and ENT referral may be required pre-operatively (dilatation of the nasal airway and nocturnal CPAP may be helpful).
- Laryngoscopy may be more difficult in the child who has already undergone correction, despite the now apparently 'normal' facies.
- A minority of children require tracheostomy. It is used to improve the airway in children too young for surgery, or in older children with deteriorating upper airway obstruction. Occasionally a tracheostomy is used to provide a secure airway postoperatively.

Positioning
- Careful positioning is required to protect the airway, prevent physical injury, and to provide a good surgical field.
- Extra care should be taken with proptotic eyes.
- Head-up tilt is used to reduce cerebral venous engorgement.
- Positioning may be difficult because of limb and joint abnormalities or contractures.

Intra-operative management
- Inhalation induction is often preferred, as venous access may be difficult secondary to limb and joint abnormalities (syndactly is a commonly associated feature) or multiple previous cannulations.
- Face mask ventilation is often challenging due to facial dysmorphology and difficulty in achieving a seal with conventional face masks.
  - A soft-seal face mask with a deformable rim is often useful.
- Preparation should be made for management of a difficult airway and possible difficult intubation.
  - Asleep fibre-optic intubation via an LMA is a useful alternative to awake FOI in children.
- Tubes may be secured surgically e.g. sutured or wired to the alveolar ridge. As access to the airway will be difficult during surgery, it is imperative to confirm correct tube position through auscultation.
- Major blood loss and the complications of massive transfusion are the predominant risks of craniofacial surgery.
- Blood loss is usually between 50–100% of circulating blood volume, though it may be significantly more and can be lost rapidly and without warning.
- Accurate assessment is difficult, as the loss may be concealed and measured losses are mixed with large volumes of irrigation fluid.
- Scalp infiltration with a local anaesthetic/adrenaline mixture decreases skin blood losses.
- Over 90% of patients require transfusion.
  - Intra-operative cell salvage reduces, but is unlikely to obviate, the need for allogenic transfusion.
  - In an otherwise healthy child a transfusion trigger of 7 g dl^{-1} is acceptable.
- Fentanyl up to 10 µg kg^{-1}, or remifentanil 0.25–0.5 µg kg^{-1} min^{-1}, provide cardiovascular stability.

- Intravenous morphine is administered at the end of surgery.
- Postoperatively, simple analgesics together with oral or intravenous opioid, provide good pain control.

Monitoring
- Invasive monitoring (both arterial and CVP) are commonly employed.
- Core temperature and urine output measurement are mandatory.
- Peri-operative venous air embolism (VAE) may cause circulatory arrest.
  - Transoesophageal echocardiography (TOE) and pre-cordial Doppler ultrasound are sensitive monitors. However, TOE is invasive and difficult to place in children under 10 kg, and interference from diathermy limits the usefulness of Doppler ultrasound.
  - A sudden drop in end-tidal CO_2 is highly suggestive of VAE, and this, together with a high index of suspicion, is the most commonly employed monitor (see Chapter 4).

Postoperative care
- Most children are extubated at the end of surgery if cardiovascularly stable, blood loss has been controlled, and a normal coagulation profile and temperature have been achieved.
- Care is continued in a high dependency area with continued invasive monitoring.
- Children are nursed head-up to reduce oedema.
- Large fluid losses may continue. These must be measured and replaced alongside maintenance fluid requirements.

Tips and pitfalls
- This surgery should only be undertaken in specialist units.
- Surgery is major. Blood loss in excess of one circulating volume is common.
- Peri-operative VAE may cause circulatory arrest.
- Oculocardiac reflex during orbital dissection may cause profound bradycardia.
- The airway is relatively inaccessible during surgery. Secure fixation of the tracheal tube is essential.
- These are very long operations; meticulous attention to positioning is required.

Chapter 9

Spinal surgery

Cervical spine surgery *292*
Lumbar surgery *298*
Spinal cord masses and vascular malformations *302*
Spinal injury *308*
Baclofen pump implantation *314*
Neural tube defects *316*
Spinal haematoma and abscess *320*

Cervical spine surgery

Cervical laminectomy offers decompression of the cervical cord and roots via a posterior approach. Patients are generally in middle to old age and usually have degenerative disease.

Indications
- Cervical myelopathy
- To protect the cord against minor trauma
- Relief of radicular arm pain.

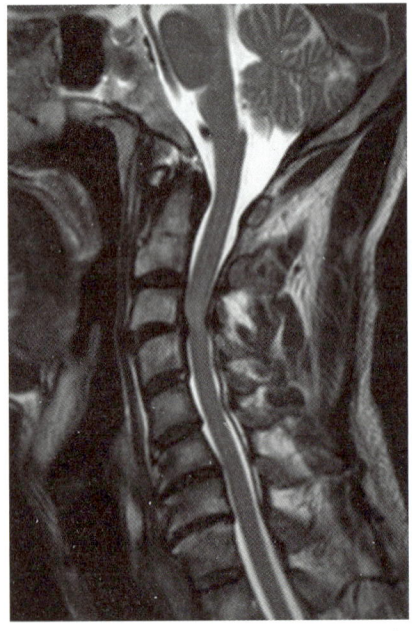

Fig. 9.1 Cervical spine stenosis. Sagittal T2-weighted image showing degenerative change in the cervical spine with stenosis at the C3/C4 level. Note the accompanying cord signal increase at the level of the stenosis indicating associated cord injury.

CERVICAL SPINE SURGERY

Pre-operative assessment
- The neck should be assessed in terms of mobility, stability, and exacerbation of symptoms on neck movement, particularly pain or neurological symptoms such as L'hermitte's sign whereby extension or flexion of the neck causes 'electric shock' symptoms down the limbs or body due to spinal cord compression.
- The airway should be assessed concurrently for any other features that may suggest a difficult intubation.
- Indications for awake fibre-optic intubation:
    - abnormal anatomy making airway access difficult, e.g. flexion deformities of the neck, abnormal facial anatomy, poor mouth opening
    - instability of the cervical spine
    - exacerbation of neurological symptoms on neck movement.
- Respiratory function should be evaluated (if necessary by pulmonary function testing if the patient is unable to exercise). Patients may have lost accessory muscles of respiration as a result of myelopathy and may be difficult to extubate postoperatively.
- Inability to exercise may also mask relatively severe cardiovascular disease. There should be a high index of suspicion of this; echocardiography may offer further evaluation.

Intra-operative management
- If awake fibre-optic intubation is not deemed necessary then anaesthesia is induced with a combination of opioid and an intravenous anaesthetic agent, and muscle relaxation may be given either by intermittent boluses or infusion.
- Intravenous access should be accessible once the patient is prone. A second cannula in the foot is often useful, particularly if relaxant and opioid infusions are being used.
- Intra-arterial pressure monitoring is necessary as blood pressure is often labile when turning prone and during decompression of a tightly held spinal cord.
- Blood loss is usually in the region of 100–500 ml; it can be significantly more if multiple levels are being decompressed.
    - Epidural venous bleeding may be sudden and profuse.
    - High level laminectomy (C1/2) may be associated with more blood loss.
- The procedure usually takes 1–3 h.
- Graduated compression stockings should be worn pre- and postoperatively and intra-operative intermittent pneumatic calf compression devices should be used. Prophylactic anticoagulation is usually started on the first postoperative evening, although this varies between surgeons.

Positioning (see also p. 162)
- Care must be taken when positioning the patient prone to avoid unnecessary or extreme neck movement.
- Hypotension must be promptly treated to avoid endangering an already compromised cord.

- Patients are usually positioned either on a Montreal mattress or on soft bolsters under the chest and iliac crests.
  - Care should be taken to avoid pressure on the upper abdomen by the chest bolster as associated hepatic ischaemia has been described.
  - Venous drainage must not be impeded by the lower bolster to avoid raised pressure in the epidural venous plexus and decreased venous return to the heart.
- The head is best held slightly flexed in Mayfield head pins, which prevents undue pressure on the face in the prone position.
- Particular care must be taken of the eyes if the head is resting on the horseshoe support.
- Over-flexion of the head should be avoided as this risks obstruction of venous drainage and engorgement of the tongue which may result in postoperative airway obstruction.
- Arms are positioned by the side to avoid nerve damage.
- The knees may be flexed against a knee support to allow head-up tilt to minimize venous bleeding.
- Care should be taken with the degree of head-up tilt in a hypovolaemic patient to reduce the risk of air embolism.

Postoperative management
- The airway should be reassessed prior to extubation if there is any suspicion of oedema from positioning.
- A cervical collar is not usually required.
- Pain relief afterwards is provided by oral or intravenous strong opioids.
- NSAIDs are avoided for the first 24–48 h.
- Rapid postoperative mobilization is encouraged if possible.
- Extensive comorbidity may necessitate ITU or HDU admission.
- Postoperative haematoma formation may result in cord compression.

Tips and pitfalls
- Beware of profound hypotension on prone positioning if cardiac reserve is poor.
- Cardiovascular instability may occur (particularly bradyarrhythmias) if the cervical cord is manipulated.
- The patient with a severe myelopathy may not be able to use a PCA handset.
- Intra-operative cord damage during surgery may result in tetraplegia or respiratory compromise postoperatively.
- New onset neurological impairment postoperatively should be investigated promptly.

Anterior cervical discectomy
These patients are usually younger than those undergoing cervical laminectomy and may have sustained damage as a result of sporting injuries. Once the intervertebral disc has been removed the surgeon may choose either to leave the space empty, insert various bone grafts, prosthetic grafts or an artificial disc (arthroplasty). The latter are increasingly being used in the hope of avoiding abnormal stresses on adjacent levels leading to accelerated degeneration.

Indications
- Decompression and relief of radicular arm pain or myelopathy
- Restoration of normal cervical lordosis
- Improvement in cervical spine stability
- Treatment of severe neck pain.

Pre-operative assessment
- As for cervical laminectomy the airway must be assessed in terms of neck movement and stability. Awake fibre-optic intubation may occasionally be necessary.
- Respiratory and cardiovascular systems may be compromised as a result of cord compression and should be carefully evaluated.

Intra-operative management
- If awake fibre-optic intubation is not required anaesthesia is induced with a combination of an opioid and intravenous induction agent; muscle relaxant drugs may be given by bolus or infusion.
- Two large-bore cannulae are placed, one often in the foot.
- Intra-arterial pressure monitoring is often employed.
- The surgical approach is usually from the right side of the neck so the tracheal tube should be secured to the left side of the mouth.
- A throat pack is not necessary and may distort the anatomy in the neck. The X-ray opaque line may also obscure the anatomy during on-table X-ray.
- The procedure usually takes 1–2 h and blood loss should be less than 100 ml.
- If the spine is to be fused, bone graft may be taken from the iliac crest.
- Disc replacement (arthroplasty) has no particular additional anaesthetic considerations.

Positioning
- The procedure is carried out supine.
- Care should be taken when moving the patient; if the neck is unstable the patient should be log rolled.
- X-rays are required to confirm the appropriate vertebral level and an operating microscope is often used.

Postoperative management
- If the neck has been fused the airway should be assessed again prior to extubation in case re-intubation should be required.
- A soft collar is sometimes used for patient comfort and reassurance.
- Pain relief afterwards is provided by oral or intravenous opioids.
- NSAIDs are usually avoided for the first 24–48 h.
- Rapid postoperative mobilization is encouraged.

Tips and pitfalls
- Be wary of damage to surrounding structures including trachea, oesophagus, thyroid, blood vessels (jugular vein or carotid artery), nerves (vagus, sympathetic chain and recurrent laryngeal), thoracic duct (during operations on the lower levels on the left), and pleura (lower levels).

- Tracheal tubes may be kinked or bent against the wall of the trachea when the retractors are in place. Repositioning of retractors may be necessary.
- Haematoma formation in the neck may result in catastrophic airway compromise.
  - Voice change is a warning sign
  - Urgent re-opening of the wound may be required
  - Tracheostomy may be required in emergency situations
- Local anaesthesia of a bone graft donor site will provide useful analgesia.
- Local anaesthesia placed at the surgical site may result in a temporary phrenic nerve paresis.

Posterior fossa upper cervical decompression (PFUCD)

This procedure is most commonly carried out in patients with a symptomatic Chiari malformation (herniation of cerebellar tonsils through the foramen magnum) causing syringomyelia. Four types are described.
- Type I. Extension of the cerebellar tonsils into the foramen magnum, not involving the brainstem. This is the most common form and may be congenital or acquired. It may be asymptomatic.
- Type II. Arnold–Chiari malformation. Extension of both cerebellar and brainstem tissue into the foramen magnum. It may be accompanied by a myelomeningocele.
- Type III. Herniation of the cerebellum and brainstem. May be accompanied by part of the fourth ventricle causing severe neurological defects.
- Type IV. Cerebellar hypoplasia. The cerebellar tonsils are located further down the spinal canal and parts of the cerebellum are missing.

Other indications
- Impulse headache (coughing, sneezing or laughing resulting in tonsillar impaction).
- Resection of arachnoid scarring which is obstructing CSF drainage. This may result from previous attempts at PFUCD, haemorrhage, infection or trauma.

Pre-operative assessment
- Patients may be otherwise well and present with pain and headache or may be unwell with a decreased conscious level, limb weakness, raised intracranial pressure, poor respiratory function, and cardiovascular disturbance.
- Bulbar function should be assessed.
- Vomiting may cause electrolyte disturbances.

Intra-operative management
- The cervical spine is not usually unstable and so awake fibre-optic intubation is not necessary unless dictated by other factors.
- Anaesthesia is usually induced with an intravenous agent and opioid and a muscle relaxant given by bolus or infusion.
- Induction should take account of possible raised intracranial pressure and swings in ICP or blood pressure should be avoided.

- Two large-bore cannulae are required, with one usually in the foot.
- Intra-arterial pressure monitoring is required.
- Measures to avoid increasing ICP should be employed intra-operatively including controlled ventilation, adequate oxygenation, and ensuring adequacy of venous drainage.
- Cerebral perfusion pressure must be maintained with vasopressors in the presence of raised ICP.
- The procedure usually takes 2–4 h depending on the indication. Blood loss varies; bleeding from the epidural venous plexus may be sudden and profuse and cell salvage may occasionally be required.
- Graduated compression stockings should be worn pre- and postoperatively and intra-operative intermittent pneumatic calf compression devices should be used. Prophylactic anticoagulation is usually started on the first postoperative evening, although this varies between surgeons.

Positioning
- Positioning is similar to that for cervical laminectomy with care to avoid excessive neck flexion and venous engorgement.
- The sitting position may be used but this should not be attempted outside specialist centres. Proponents claim it gives excellent surgical access but there is high risk of venous air embolism, hypotension, pneumocephalus, and paradoxical embolism.

Postoperative management
- Ideally the patient should be nursed in an HDU as there is a risk of cord oedema and respiratory compromise.
- The procedure is often painful and PCA analgesia is required if the patient is able to operate the handset.
- NSAIDs are usually avoided in the first 24–48 h.
- Early mobilization is encouraged if possible.
- Symptoms of raised ICP should have been alleviated but there may still be some neurological deficit and full neurological observations should be continued.

Tips and pitfalls
- Arrhythmias, commonly bradycardia, may occur as the cervical cord is decompressed. This usually responds to withdrawing the surgical stimulus rather than requiring pharmacological intervention.

Lumbar surgery

Surgical procedures on the lumbar spine are common and may be performed by either neurosurgeons or orthopaedic surgeons. The exact differentiation between neurosurgery and orthopaedic spinal surgery depends on local factors and particular staff appointments.

In general, orthopaedic spinal surgeons tend to care for patients requiring corrective surgery (e.g. for scoliosis), stabilization for tumour, degenerative conditions (spondylolisthesis) or fractures and operations for mechanical low back pain, whilst intramedullary and intradural lesions are dealt with almost exclusively by neurosurgeons. Both groups undertake decompressive surgery for disc protrusions and epidural masses such as abscesses and haematomas (see p. 320). Laminectomy for epidural masses is covered elsewhere (see p. 300).

Most lumbar spine surgery is to release compression from a disc or the ligamentum flavum (or a combination) pressing on nerve roots.

Indications
- Relief of radicular leg pain
- Neurological deficit (such as motor weakness in the distribution of a nerve root) including cauda equine syndrome
- Radicular claudication
- Prevention of worsening pain or neurological symptoms.

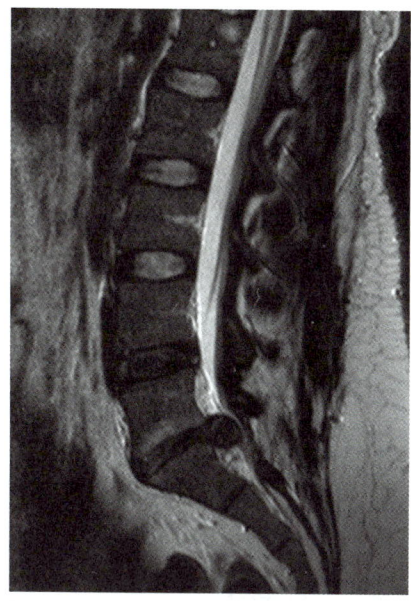

Fig. 9.2 Cauda equina compression. Sagittal T2-weighted MRI showing a large L5/S1 disc protrusion causing compression of the thecal sac and cauda equina.

Surgical procedures

Microdiscectomy and laminectomy with discectomy

Microdiscectomy is an approach to removing smaller disc fragments without a full, open laminectomy. The anaesthetic isuues are the same. Larger fragments or patients with an element of stenosis (see p. 300) require a laminectomy.

- Small disc prolapses cause symptoms by pressing on the nerves as they pass through the lateral parts of the epidural space and leave via the foramina.
  - The whole disc does not enter the epidural space, just a small fragment or bulge.
  - The pain from an acute prolapse may be exquisite.
- Larger, more central prolapses may present with cauda equina syndrome.
  - This causes autonomic dysfunction due to interruption of the sacral parasympathetic outflow and may affect bladder and bowel function.
  - To prevent a permanent deficit these patients require urgent decompression.

Laminectomy for spinal stenosis
Spinal stenosis describes a spectrum of pathology which results in narrowing of the spinal canal. This may be due to degenerative disc bulge combined with overgrowth of bone such as the facet joint or as a result of thickening of the ligamentum flavum, and leads to a generalized compression of the dural sac and spinal nerves.
- In the lumbar region it usually presents insidiously with:
  - general deterioration of motor function of the legs
  - exercise-induced radicular pain or fatigue (mimicking vascular claudication)
  - paraesthesia.
- Removal of the lamina and spinous processes relieves the compression without leading to instability of the bony structures and most patients do not require instrumentation.

Pre-operative assessment
- Many patients with disc prolapses are young and healthy or have isolated minor degenerative disease of the spine.
- Older patients may have extensive osteoarthritis—including other areas of the spine such as the cervical levels. In these patients tracheal intubation may be difficult.
- Patients with lumbar spinal stenosis tend to be older and have more extensive spinal degenerative disease. Cardiovascular comorbidities are more common and these patients may be less tolerant of prone positioning.

Peri-operative management
- Due to the position and length of surgery (especially more extensive procedures) general anaesthesia is used for the majority of operations.
- Subarachnoid anaesthesia has been used for single-level lumbar disc surgery.
- Surgeons may request that the blood pressure is lowered to reduce blood loss and improve visualization. While this dilemma is more common during corrective, multiple-level spinal surgery or vertebrectomy for tumours, the risk of the potential for spinal ischaemia should be borne in mind. Elderly patients with comorbidities may have less robust spinal perfusion and are at particular risk.
- Wide-bore intravenous access should be accessible once the patient is prone.
- Intra-arterial pressure monitoring is necessary for extensive procedures and in those with significant cardiac disease. Single-level spinal surgery (e.g. discectomy) in an otherwise healthy patient does not require an arterial line.
- Blood loss is usually in the region of 50–500 ml; it can be significantly more if multiple levels are being decompressed. Epidural venous bleeding may be sudden and profuse and cell salvage may be used. The procedure usually takes from 45 min for a single-level discectomy to 2–4 h for an extensive laminectomy.

Positioning

- The usual position for posterior lumbar surgery is the prone position but it can be performed in the lateral position (e.g. discectomy in the pregnant patient). This is covered in more detail in 📖 Positioning, p. 162.
- The usual prone position is on bolsters or a Wilson frame, but the knee-chest position can be used.
- The head is normally placed on a horseshoe ring or other suitable support.
- A patient placed in the prone position and undergoing spinal surgery is at risk of venous air embolism (📖 see Air embolism, p. 142).
- Pressure on the abdomen, pressure points over the iliac crests and axillae, and around the face (especially the eyes) must be avoided (📖 see Positioning, p. 162).

Postoperative management

- The degree of postoperative pain is related to the amount of bone that is excised.
- Microdiscectomy may be performed with little or no bone removal and some patients may go home on the day of surgery.
- The treatment of a large or central disc protrusion or laminectomy requires a more extensive exposure and this necessitates opioids for several days after surgery and PCA morphine is often used.
- Intra-operative and postoperative analgesia includes strong opioids in combination with paracetamol and NSAIDs.

Tips and pitfalls

- Major surgery, at multiple levels or for tumours, is often associated with considerable blood loss. Cell-salvage techniques may be applicable.
- Before you start the anaesthetic, check with the surgeon the exact position required and the type of support to be used when placing the patient prone.
- While subcutaneous local anaesthetic may alleviate incisional pain, deeper structures will not be adequately analgesed.
- Prolonged prone spinal surgery has been associated with postoperative visual loss (📖 see Positioning, p. 162).

Spinal cord masses and vascular malformations

Tumours and vascular malformations that affect the brain may also be found in the spinal cord. They may occur throughout the length of the cord and may be:
- extradural
- intradural but extrinsic to the cord
- intrinsic within the substance of the cord

Symptoms usually arise from compression or disruption of the integrity of the cord or from abnormal blood flow. The extent of symptoms will depend on the nature of the lesion and also on the vertebral level and patients may present with varying degrees of disability.

Tumours

Spinal cord tumours account for approximately 15–20% of CNS tumours.
- Although they can occur anywhere, the thoracic region is most common.
- Many spinal tumours are histologically benign and surgery may be curative.

Intramedullary
- Ependymoma is the most common (around 50%)
- Astrocytoma (more common in children)
- Haemangioblastoma.

Intradural
- Most commonly these are meningioma, schwannoma or neurofibroma
- A small proportion of neurofibromas are malignant and associated with a very poor prognosis.

Extradural
- Extradural components of nerve sheath tumours
- Menigioma
- Metastases.

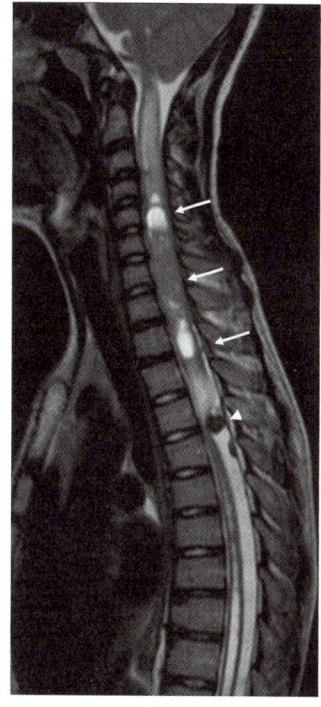

Fig. 9.3 Thoracic intramedullary lesion. Sagittal T2-weighted MRI in a patient with neurofibromatosis type II. A heterogeneous mass expands the cord from C4 to T3 (white arrows). A small meningioma at the T4/T5 level results in high-grade cord compression (arrow head). Note the cord oedema above and below the intramedullary tumour, and the syrinx formation in the cord below the compressive lesion.

Vascular malformations

Arteriovenous malformations and dural arteriovenous fistulae (AVF) are congenital abnormal connections between the arterial and venous circulation. They present in similar fashion to tumours, though many are asymptomatic and diagnosed following imaging for other reasons.
- There is a risk of haemorrhage which presents with sudden onset of spinal cord neurology.
- More commonly they present with progressive myelopathy.
- Symptoms may be due to abnormal blood flow (hyperaemia, steal, oligaemia), venous congestion and oedema rather than a mass effect of the AVM/AVF itself.

Pre-operative assessment
- The level of the lesion should be determined as this will guide positioning. Existing neurology should be clearly documented.
- If the tumour is in the cervical region, the neck should be assessed for any exacerbation of symptoms on moving the head or neck. Appropriate airway management is then planned.
- If the tumour is in the cervical region the respiratory muscles may be compromised and pulmonary function should be evaluated.
- Poor respiratory function may necessitate ITU admission postoperatively. Similarly, inability to exercise may mask cardiovascular disease. There should be a high index of suspicion in patients with risk factors for cardiovascular disease.
- Postoperative ITU care should be considered in patients with high cervical cord lesions regardless of pre-operative status, as there is the potential for damage to the cord or postoperative oedema causing respiratory embarrassment.

Surgical management

Tumour
Laminectomy or laminoplasty is performed at the relevant level followed by tumour resection.
- The aim of surgery is to limit progression of the disease without causing further injury.
- The extent of tumour resection is strongly influenced by findings at operation (discrete vs. diffuse tumour) and intra-operative response of the patient to dissection.

Vascular malformation
The aim of surgery for vascular malformations is to interrupt the feeding arterial vessel without affecting normal spinal cord blood supply.
- Embolization by interventional radiologists is the treatment of choice.
- Surgery is reserved for lesions untreatable by embolization.

Positioning
- Positioning is dictated by the level of the lesion.
- Cervical or upper thoracic cord lesions are usually accessed with the patient placed prone on a Montreal mattress or on bolsters with the head held in Mayfield head pins.
- Lower thoracic or lumbar lesions may be best accessed with the patient on a Wilson frame or in the knee-chest position.
- Close liaison with the surgeon is necessary pre-operatively so that intravenous and arterial lines may be appropriately positioned to allow easy intra-operative access.
- Care should be taken with pressure areas particularly when positioning the arms if the patient is in knee-chest or on the Wilson frame to avoid brachial plexus injuries.

Intra-operative management
- Standard induction with an opioid and an intravenous induction agent is appropriate if there are no concerns about airway management and the cervical cord.

- Wide-bore intravenous access should be accessible once the patient is prone.
- Intra-operative analgesia is usually provided by an opioid infusion such as remifentanil.
- Muscle relaxant may be given by bolus or infusion with appropriate monitoring.
- Care should be taken to maintain an adequate perfusion pressure; areas of the cord infiltrated by tumour may be particularly vulnerable to ischaemia.
- Patients are usually receiving dexamethasone pre-operatively and a further bolus (16 mg) should be given at induction.
- During the laminectomy there is the potential for significant blood loss from the epidural venous plexus.
- Intermittent pneumatic calf compression devices should be used, as patients do not usually receive pre-operative LMWH.
- The procedure often takes in the region of 4 h but may be longer if the tumour is extensive or particularly adherent to the cord.

Monitoring
- Intra-arterial pressure monitoring should be employed.
- A urinary catheter should be inserted for intra- and postoperative use.
- CVP monitoring may be useful if the tumour is particularly vascular or the laminectomy is expected to generate significant blood loss. This may be achieved by a peripherally inserted central catheter (PICC) or CVC.

Postoperative management
- Patients are often required to remain flat or with a maximum of 30° head-up:
  - to protect the cord whilst autoregulation may be disturbed
  - to minimize the risk of CSF leak.
- Analgesia is required for the laminectomy and is usually via intravenous opioids such as a PCA.
- NSAIDs should be avoided.
- Patients who have high cervical cord lesions are best nursed on HDU postoperatively as there is the risk of cord oedema. Patients with lumbar and thoracic lesions often go back to the general neurosurgical ward if otherwise well.

Tips and pitfalls
- Spinal cord monitoring is not often employed as it lacks specificity for cord damage and often only confirms that damage has already been done.
- Stimulation of the cord during tumour dissection may cause profound haemodynamic changes.
- These usually respond to cessation of the stimulus but their occurrence must be communicated to the surgeon as they may herald cord damage.
- Ideally the anaesthetist should be situated where both the monitors and the video display of the surgical field can be seen. This will enhance communication about problem areas of dissection.

Spinal injury

Although different centres vary with regards to who manages acute spinal injury, the common coexistence of significant head and spinal trauma means that neuroanaesthetists should be aware of the particular problems posed by bony and neural spinal injury.

Pathology
Bony and cord injury do not have to occur together; either can exist without the other.

Bony/ligamentous injury
- Approximately half of all spinal fractures occur in the cervical region.
  - In sports-related cord injury the cervical region is affected in two-thirds of patients.
- Spinal fractures occur in around 40% of multiply-injured patients.
- Fractures at C1 and C2 are the commonest spinal fractures (25%).
- 10% of cervical fractures are associated with another fracture in the spinal column.

Spinal cord injury
- Spinal cord injury can be due to compression, contusion, or penetrating injury.
- The onset may be at the time of injury, or delayed as a result of uncontrolled movement in an unstable spine or haematoma.
- Secondary cord injury can occur at any time from hypoxia, hypoperfusion/ischaemia or oedema (analogous to traumatic brain injury).
- Cord injury can be complete, with loss of all neurological function below the level of injury, or incomplete, with a varying degree of function preserved and, importantly, a better prognosis for recovery.
- Further life-threatening injuries, e.g. head injury, pulmonary contusions, and pneumothorax are common in patients with spinal cord injury.

Associated conditions
- Relatively high-energy trauma is the commonest cause of spinal injury.
- Underlying disorders as tumours, infection, ankylosing spondylitis, and rheumatoid arthritis can lead to spinal fractures and/or spinal instability compromising the cord without major trauma.

Presentation
- Significant cord disruption in the upper cervical region (C1–C3) is usually fatal due to brainstem injury and acute respiratory failure.
- Serious neurological complications are commoner in patients with lower cervical spine injuries than with higher C1/2 injuries due to the narrower spinal canal at these levels.
- Pharyngeal haematoma in upper cervical spine injuries can compromise the airway and may warrant early intubation.

SPINAL INJURY

- About a third of patients with a severe cervical fracture are tetraparetic, half of the patients with a lumbar spine injury are paraparetic.
- Normal X-rays do not rule out a spinal injury, as ligamentous injury can also result in instability.
  - Neurological symptoms and signs should always raise suspicion of the instability, prompting further specialist imaging (CT, MRI).
- The majority of cord injuries occur at C5/6.
- Around a third of patients with cervical spine injury have significant brain injury.

Patient population
- Traumatic spinal cord injuries typically affect young, predominantly male (4:1), healthy adults, and are commonly caused by RTAs, falls, and sports injuries.
- Patients presenting with pathological spinal fractures due to underlying disorders are usually older.

Preoperative assessment
Initial assessment of emergency patients should follow ATLS guidelines. In addition to the general points for pre-operative assessment, anaesthetists need to be aware that multiple organ systems can be affected, depending on the level of injury.

Respiratory
- Lesions at the level of C4 will cause complete, and those at C5 partial diaphragmatic paralysis.
- Lesions at the level of C6–T1 will cause a reduction in tidal volume due to intercostal paralysis, also resulting in an inefficient cough.
- Abnormal tracheal reflexes may lead to bradycardia during tracheal suctioning and intubation when sympathetic reflexes are lost.

Cardiovascular
- Sudden hypertension and dysrhythmia is the immediate response to cord injury.
- This is often followed by hypotension and a fall in heart rate due to loss of sympathetic function in lesions above T5 (spinal shock).
  - This can exacerbate the effects of hypovolaemia/blood loss due to lack of compensatory mechanisms.
  - Patients may require inotropic support to maintain adequate cardiac output.
  - The period of spinal shock may range from days to weeks.
  - Recovery from the acute phase is usually incomplete with postural hypotension becoming a permanent problem.

Temperature
Hypothermia is a common problem but hyperthermia can occur as well, as the ability to control temperature has been lost due to inability to sweat or vasoconstrict, and patients are poikilothermic.

Gastrointestinal and urinary
- Paralytic ileus can occur in patients with high cervical lesions. Any resulting metabolic abnormality has to be addressed.

- Gastric distension, constipation, and urinary retention need to be anticipated.

Autonomic function
- Spinal shock is characterized by the loss of autonomic pathways below the level of injury and can last for several weeks.
- Autonomic dysreflexia: with an uncoordinated return of reflexes, visceral stimulation can later lead to an exaggerated autonomic response with pyrexia, hypertension and bradycardia/arrhythmias, vasodilatation above, and vasoconstriction below the level of injury. This may result in myocardial ischaemia and cerebral haemorrhage.

Motor system
- Paralysis with absent reflexes is seen initially in levels below the lesion.
- Spasticity occurs weeks to months following the injury. This has implications for the use of suxamethonium.

Purpose of surgery
Surgery for spinal injury may be undertaken for a variety of reasons.
- Stabilization of an unstable spine without cord injury.
- Stabilization of an unstable spine with prior complete cord injury.
  - To allow earlier mobilization.
- Stabilization of an unstable spine with prior incomplete cord injury.
  - To reduce the risk of further injury and to allow earlier mobilization.
- Removal of compressive fragments.
  - Performed more urgently in the hope of reducing injury.

The decision on whom to operate, how and when, is complex and should be taken after assessment of patient wishes, comorbidities, and extent of spinal and other injuries.

Psychology
Patients with cord injury will be making decisions about treatment in the wake of dramatically life-changing trauma. They may show a whole range of emotions and attitudes.
- The anaesthetist must provide a consistent, empathetic approach.
- Patients' questions should be answered honestly and sensitively.
- Patients with high lesions, or at significant risk of tetraplegia (with or without ventilator dependence) may wish to discuss issues around resuscitation and long-term care. It is wise to involve an experienced clinician in these decisions.

Surgical approaches
- Traction devices (i.e. a halo) may be required as temporary stabilizing measure or definitive treatment (e.g. reduction of cervical fracture/dislocations and indirect cord decompression).
  - If the patient is awake and cooperative, this will usually be applied under local anaesthesia.
- Definitive surgery for fixation of the vertebral column may be a semi-elective procedure.
- Timing of surgery needs to take into account other injuries, e.g. head injury and cerebral oedema or chest trauma with contusions and coagulopathy, especially in polytrauma patients.

SPINAL INJURY

- If a prolonged ITU stay is anticipated, anterior cervical surgery should precede tracheostomy as the presence of the latter increases the infection rate and cervical stability facilitates nursing care of the unconscious patient.
- Cervical stabilization will be performed using an anterior or posterior approach. Discussion between the anaesthetist and surgeon regarding the appropriateness of oral vs. nasal intubation is required.
- The majority of thoracolumbar fractures can be stabilized by posterior surgery.
- In some instances thoraco-abdominal approaches with thoracotomy and diaphragmatic section are required.
- Vertebral body resection (corpectomy) can produce extreme haemorrhage, aggravating the physiological challenges imposed by the surgical approach.

Positioning

Patients may be positioned supine or prone.
- Whichever position is used, meticulous attention to maintenance of spinal alignment is required and requires support from the surgical team.
- The process of positioning on the operating table demands a sufficient number of trained staff to assist with this.
- Pressure area care is vital for these patients as they may have long-term sensory loss which increases the risk of skin breakdown.

Intra-operative management

The aim of anaesthesia for the injured or potentially injured cord is the same as for the injured brain, namely prevention of secondary injury (see General management, p. 350).
- Hypoxia, hypotension, and hyperglycaemia should all be avoided.
- There are numerous techniques of anaesthesia described but there is no evidence that volatile-based techniques have a different outcome to TIVA techniques.
- Remifentanil infusions are often used.

Airway management
- Intubation for initial resuscitation will usually involve a rapid sequence induction for general anaesthesia maintaining in-line stabilization.
- Traction devices for temporary or definitive treatment as a sole procedure will typically be applied under local anaesthesia.
- In patients scheduled for semi-elective procedures, a rapid sequence induction will usually not be required.
  - Suxamethonium is relatively contraindicated in spinal cord lesion older than 24 hours for up to a year following injury, as this can result in marked potassium release.
- Full neck immobilization with a hard collar limits neck movement and mouth opening: the anterior part of the collar should be removed to facilitate intubation, but only once manual immobilization has been secured.

- The surgeon can provide valuable information regarding the degree of instability (e.g. level, instability with flexion or extension) and cord compromise in the patient.
- Different options for tracheal intubation can be considered including:
  - Awake fibre-optic intubation. Experience in this technique and a cooperative patient are required. It allows assessment and documentation of the patient's neurologic status after intubation and prior to the start of the operation.
  - Conventional laryngoscopy. The anaesthetist should not aim to achieve the best possible view of the cords but instead use aids such as the gum elastic bougie to intubate with minimal disturbance of the patient's head and neck position while manual in-line stabilization is provided. Conventional laryngoscopy with a patient in skull traction can lead to significant cervical positional distortion. Traction must be removed before direct laryngoscopy and be replaced by manual in-line stabilization.
  - Fibre-optic intubation through a laryngeal mask using an Aintree airway exchange catheter facilitates intubation with minimal neck movement; experience in the use of this technique is required. Pressure on the posterior pharyngeal wall should be avoided to prevent dislocation of the unstable spine.
- Meticulous care and attention to detail, and a careful, considered approach are important, whatever technique is used.
- Documented injury to the spinal cord as result of anaesthetic management of these patients is extremely rare. There is no evidence for superiority of one technique over another.
- In most cases, the injured cervical spine is safest in neutral or modest extension; unsupervised flexion should be avoided.
- The only exception is cervical fracture in ankylosing spondylitis where the patient's usual posture is often flexed and should be reproduced during the intubation procedure.

Cardiovascular
- Blood pressure should be kept high-normal to maintain cord perfusion. Autoregulation of cord blood flow may be affected by injury.
- Due to loss of sympathetic output in high lesions, the effects of blood loss may be exaggerated, as the patient lacks the ability to compensate through increases in heart rate and vasoconstriction.
- Fluids need to be administered in judicious amounts as overload can lead to pulmonary oedema.
- Vasoactive drugs may be required to maintain an adequate blood pressure.

Other issues
- Temperature control is important, as the extensive surgical exposures in spinal surgery and lengthy operations make patients prone to hypothermia.
- Pre-operative administration of high-dose steroids (e.g. methylprednisolone) is no longer recommended in spinal cord-injured patients.

Monitoring
- Routine non-invasive and invasive monitoring is used including arterial blood pressure and central venous pressure measurement in patients with high lesions.
- Core temperature should be measured.
- A urinary catheter should be inserted.

Postoperative management
- Patients with polytrauma, complex cases, long procedures and major blood loss will usually require postoperative care on HDU or ITU.
- Elective sedation and ventilation may be indicated to manage cord oedema especially in patients with cervical spine injuries.
- Postoperative airway obstruction can be caused by haematoma or oedema at the site of injury/operation in cervical lesions.
- Re-intubation can be more difficult following extensive fusion of the cervical spine, and delayed extubation should be considered.

Prognosis
- While incomplete sensory and motor deficits can improve rapidly, complete neurological deficits show very little improvement over time. The mortality of isolated spinal cord injury within the first year is up to 7%.
- Once spinal shock resolves, spasticity sets in and leads to an improvement in respiratory function with a higher muscle tone in the intercostals muscles, less passive movement of the rib cage, and easier patient care/possibly mobilization, depending on the level of the lesion.
- Respiratory complications are frequently seen in these patients.
- DVT and pulmonary embolism are common.
- Urinary tract problems often require further surgery.
- Osteoporosis and decubitus ulcers are a concern in patients with long-term sequelae, as is the development of chronic pain.

Tips and pitfalls
- Arrhythmias, commonly bradycardia, may occur as the cervical cord is manipulated and decompressed. This usually responds to withdrawing the surgical stimulus rather than requiring pharmacological intervention.
- Be clear about what the purpose of surgery is.
- There is no 'right' way to achieve tracheal intubation; use the technique most appropriate to the patient and your expertise.

Baclofen pump implantation

Baclofen pump implantation is indicated for the treatment of hypertonia where treatment with oral baclofen and other drugs is not sufficient or is associated with unacceptable side effects. The indications for baclofen pump implant currently include:
- cerebral palsy
- dystonias
- multiple sclerosis.

Baclofen pumps are used in both children and adults.

Surgical process

The insertion of a baclofen pump is a two-stage process:

Baclofen test

The purpose is to assess the effect of intrathecal baclofen and to inform the decision to proceed to pump implantation.
- The test procedure involves percutaneous placement of an intrathecal catheter.
  - Catheters are generally placed in the lumbar region.
  - The indications for a cervical catheter include severe scoliosis and previous spinal surgery.
- All children require general anaesthesia and muscle relaxation for catheter placement to allow the surgeon to assess the extent of fixed contractures.
- In adults general anaesthesia may be required but sedation or local anaesthesia alone is often sufficient.
- Test doses are only given following recovery from anaesthesia. Some operators give increasing doses of intrathecal baclofen whilst some prefer to give a single bolus.
- The intrathecal catheter is subsequently removed.

Baclofen pump implantation

If the test dose has been successful in decreasing spasticity, a baclofen pump is subsequently implanted.
- Under general anaesthesia a baclofen pump is sited in the anterior abdominal wall. An intrathecal catheter sited and tunnelled subcutaeneously to connect with the pump.
- Surgery is usually performed in the lateral decubitus position.

Pre-operative assessment

The range of aetiologies and medical therapies in patients presenting for baclofen pump implantation is wide, necessitating careful pre-operative assessment. There should be a high index of suspicion for:
- sleep apnoea
- gastro-oesophageal reflux
- decreased upper airway reflexes.

Intra-operative management
- Inhalational or intravenous induction.
- Intubation and ventilation is preferred due to risks of reflux and potential for unexpectedly prolonged procedures.
- Intra-operative analgesia: fentanyl 2–3 µg kg^{-1} (max 5 µg kg^{-1}), paracetamol, NSAID (e.g. diclofenac) and wound infiltration with a long-acting local anaesthetic.
- Hypothermia will develop rapidly in many children during pump implantation. Temperature monitoring is mandatory and equipment to maintain normothermia should be in place.
- Postoperative analgesia should be based around regular simple enteral analgesics. Rescue analgesia, if needed in recovery, can be provided with fentanyl boluses. Long-acting opioids are only occasionally required.
- GABA$_B$ agonists such as baclofen enhance the analgesic effect of morphine. The risk of decreased conscious level and respiratory depression is increased if long-acting opioids are used (e.g. morphine).

Complications
The half-life of intrathecal baclofen is variable, ranging from 1–8 h. An inadvertant baclofen overdose may produce side effects that are likely to be prolonged including:
- depressed conscious level
- respiratory depression
- bradycardia and cardiovascular instability.

The management of complications should be directed at supportive measures including close monitoring and airway support as necessary. Lumbar drainage and physostigimine have been suggested for baclofen overdose, but supportive measures are usually sufficient.

Tips and pitfalls
- Consider benzodiazepines if postoperative analgesia is difficult and muscle spasm is a feature of the pain.
- Beware of the risk of delayed respiratory depression if morphine is used peri- or postoperatively.

Neural tube defects

The neural tube is formed by the end of the fourth week of gestation and is the embryological precursor from which the central nervous system develops. Abnormalities in its development can result in a spectrum of congenital abnormalities ranging from the minor which can be considered part of normal variation in the general population (e.g. spina bifida occulta) to those which result in stillbirth (e.g. anencephaly).

Approximately 75% of neural tube defects (NTD) occur in the lumbosacral region, but they may arise at any point from sacrum to cranium.

Large defects are becoming less common in countries routinely promoting increased folate intake in early pregnancy. Improved antenatal diagnosis may also be contributing to this trend.

Spinal malformations
- Spinal dermal sinus
  - Represents the final point of ectoderm and neural tube separation.
  - In some cases the dermal sinus may be connected to the dura by a fibrous band and may also be associated with tethering of neural tissue to the dura.
  - Tethering of neural tissue results in progressive neurological deficits as the child grows and the spinal cord is prevented from migrating cephalad.
- Spinal dermal fistula
  - Fistula connecting the external skin and the subarachnoid space.
  - Occurs rarely.
  - May lead to recurrent meningitis.
- Spina bifida occulta
  - Failure of fusion of the vertebral arches.
  - Present in ~10% of the population
  - No clinical symptoms.
  - A marked sacral dimple with or without a tuft of hair may be present.
- Meningocele
  - Failure of fusion of vertebral arches.
  - The defect is filled with a sac containing meninges and CSF.
  - Variable degree of neurological symptoms.
- Meningomyelocele
  - Failure of fusion of vertebral arches.
  - The defect is filled with a sac containing neural tissue (spinal cord or nerve roots).
  - Often associated with neurological deficit.
  - May be covered by skin or a thin membrane.
  - Rupture of the covering increases the risk of neurological injury.
- Myeloschisis
  - Failure of the neural folds to meet and fuse to form the neural tube.
  - Neural tissue in the affected area has no covering and is a flattened mass.
  - Associated with neurological deficit.

Cranial malformations

Theses occur predominantly in the midline and are usually associated with malformations of the meninges or brain.
- Encephalocele: small bony defect containing meninges and CSF only.
- Meningoencephalocele: larger bony defect containing meninges and brain.
- Meningohydroencephalocele: large bony defect allowing herniation of meninges, brain and part of the ventricular system.

Associated conditions
- Arnold–Chiari Malformation Type II
  - Herniation of medulla and cerebellum into the foramen magnum causing obstruction of CSF circulation and resulting hydrocephalus.
  - Commonly associated with meningomyelocele and myeloschisis
- Diastematomyelia
  - Spinal cord separated in to two halves each with its own covering of dura.

Anaesthetic considerations

Implications for the anaesthesia technique used are dependent on the malformation being treated and the magnitude of surgery being planned.

Minor malformations (e.g. encephalocele or untethering of spinal cord)
- Young child; precautions to maintain normothermia.
- Prone positioning.
- Risk of postoperative apnoea in neonates and children <3 months of age.
- Analgesia: fentanyl 2–3 µg kg^{-1} intra-operatively (maximum 5 µg kg^{-1}). Simple oral analgesics postoperatively.
- Urinary catheter for any procedure requiring operation involving neural tissue (including release of tethered spinal cord).

Major defects (e.g. myelomeningocoele, myeloschisis)

Intra-operative considerations
- Patients are usually operated on in the first days of life. Consideration must be given to the general requirements for safe neonatal anaesthesia.
- Positioning for induction. If there is no skin covering the defect, neural tissue must be protected. This can be achieved by use of an assistant to support the child supine during laryngoscopy or by the use of bolsters or a head ring to ensure there is no pressure on neural tissue. Laryngoscopy in the left lateral position is possible but often difficult.
- Induction of anaesthesia can be intravenous or inhalational followed by tracheal intubation.
- Intra-operative analgesia with a short-acting opioid (e.g. fentanyl) is usually sufficient. Postoperative analgesia can usually be achieved with simple oral analgesics.
- Non-invasive monitoring is sufficient in almost all cases.
- All patients will require a urinary catheter.

Postoperative considerations
- Risk of apnoea if <3 months of age.
- Risk of apnoea is increased in the presence of Arnold–Chiari II malformation.
- Impaired ventilation may occur with tight closure of skin over a large defect.
- Risk of hydrocephalus requiring ventriculo-peritoneal shunt insertion.

Tips and pitfalls
- Exposure of patients to latex should be limited because of the potential for long-term urinary catheterization and likely need for repeated surgical procedures in later life.
- Suxamethonium is *not* contraindicated solely by the presence of a neural tube defect.
- Blood loss may become significant during closure of large defects.

Spinal haematoma and abscess

Acute compression of the spinal cord due to abscess or haematoma is rare. The outcome is probably improved by prompt management, so a high index of suspicion, access to appropriate diagnostic facilities and surgical decompression is essential.

Pathology

Abscess
Spinal epidural abscesses are usually located in the thoracic or lumbar region.
- In ~2/3 of cases there is an identifiable source of infection.
- Infection may be contiguous (e.g. discitis, osteomyelitis, retroperitoneal sepsis) or remote (e.g. endocarditis, dental abscess, urinary or skin sepsis).
- Trauma precedes ~15–35% of epidural abscesses, suggesting that in some cases the abscess is a secondarily infected haematoma.
- A proportion of epidural abscesses occur after neuraxial intervention, e.g. surgery, epidural or spinal anaesthesia.
- S. aureus is the most common causative organism found, followed by E. coli and mixed anaerobes.
- When small, abscesses may cause local pain and tenderness without neurological impairment; fever and signs of sepsis are common.
- Larger abscesses cause neurological injury through direct spinal cord or root compression and venous thrombosis.
- Some abscesses present as chronic granulomata, mimicking extradural tumours.

Haematoma
Spinal epidural haematoma are rare and may occur at any level of the spine.
- There is almost always a clear cause: bleeding diathesis, trauma or surgical/anaesthetic intervention.
- Presentation is similar to epidural abscess with local pain and tenderness and progressive neurological symptoms dependent on the site of the abscess or haematoma.
- Cauda equina compression presents with bladder and bowel dysfunction, cord compression with sensory disturbance and motor weakness at the relevant level.
- Late presentation following neuraxial blockade is relatively common due to misattribution of leg weakness to persistent block.

Population

Haematoma
The male to female ratio is 4:1, with a bimodal age distribution (childhood and late middle age). The overall incidence is estimated at around 0.1 per 100 000 person years, of which ~50% are spontaneous.

Although spontaneous haematoma may occur, risk factors include:
- Bleeding diathesis
- Invasive procedures on neuraxis
  - Surgery
  - Spinal and epidural blocks
- Neuraxial trauma

Abscess
- Risk factors for epidural abscess are similar to those for haematoma with the addition of immunosuppression:
  - Steroids
  - Diabetes
  - Intravenous drug abuse
  - Malignancy.
- The overall incidence of epidural abscess is unclear but is estimated at around 1 case per 100,000 person years. Most occur in middle to older age.

Diagnosis and investigation

Diagnosis is made by MRI in patients with suggestive symptoms and signs. CT is not an adequate investigation, so if MRI is not available locally, the patient may need to be transferred to a unit that can perform urgent MRI.
- There is some evidence that early decompression improves outcome. If abscess or haematoma is suspected MRI must be performed urgently.
- Small haematoma or haematoma in very unfit patients may be managed conservatively.

Pre-operative assessment

- The principles of pre-operative assessment are the same as for other urgent laminectomy (see Cervical laminectomy, p. 292, and Lumbar surgery, p. 298). In addition, the anaesthetist should be alert for signs and symptoms of sepsis.
- A search for the septic focus should be made, which may include echocardiography. However, these should not delay surgical decompression.

Intra-operative management

- The intra-operative management and positioning of these patients is the same as for laminectomy (see Cervical laminectomy, p. 292, and Lumbar surgery, p. 298).
- There is a potential for greater blood loss, due to inflammation around the abscess.
- Cell salvage should be avoided in infected cases.

Postoperative management

- The airway should be reassessed prior to extubation if there is any suspicion of oedema from positioning or from cervical sepsis.
- Postoperative analgesia is provided by oral or intravenous opioids.
- NSAIDs are avoided.
- Extensive comorbidity may necessitate ITU or HDU admission.
- Neurological function should be recorded in the early postoperative phase, though delayed recovery is possible.

Tips and pitfalls

- Beware of profound hypotension on prone positioning if cardiac reserve is poor or if the patient is septic.
- Check with the surgeon about which antibiotics to give and when.

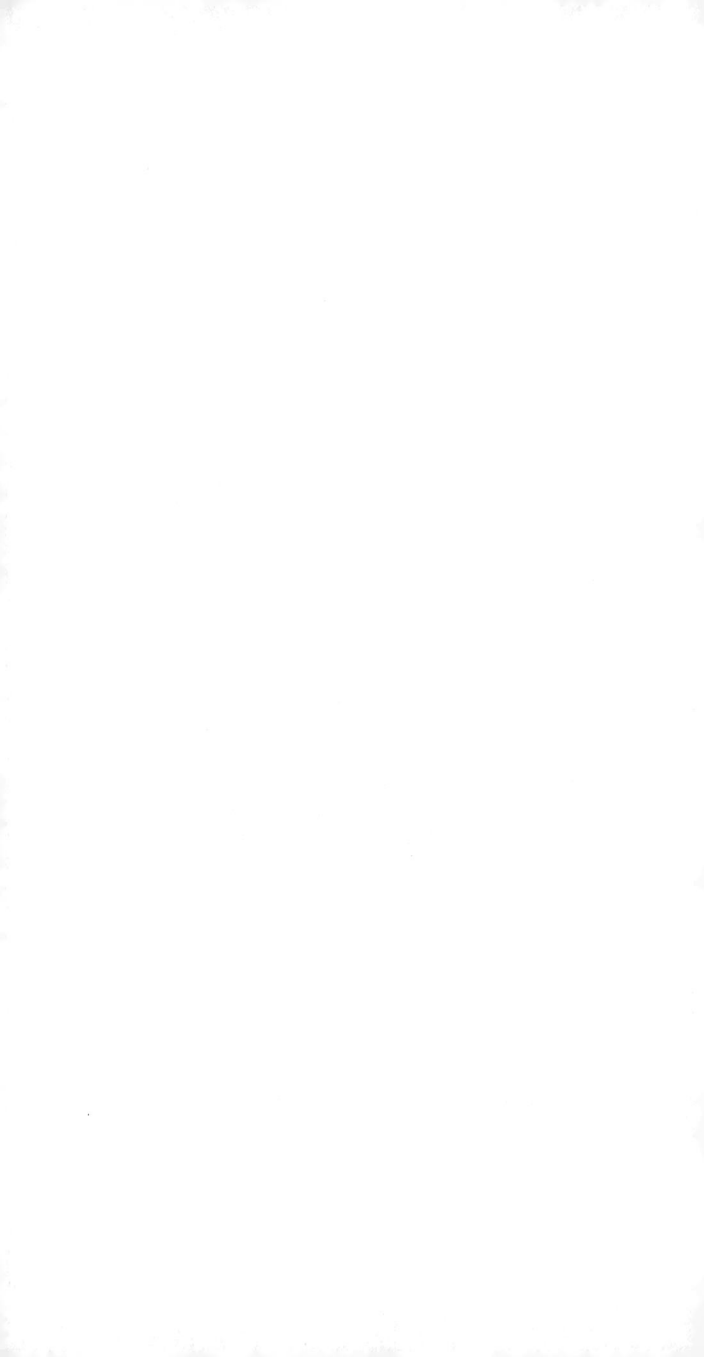

Chapter 10

Neurodiagnostics and interventional procedures

Anaesthesia for neuroradiology *324*
Anaesthesia for MRI and CT scans *330*

Anaesthesia for neuroradiology

Since the publication of the International Subarachnoid Haemorrhage Trial (ISAT), the involvement of the neuroanaesthetist in interventional neuroradiology (INR) has increased as a greater number of intracranial aneurysms are treated endovascularly. Other interventional radiology procedures (both therapeutic and diagnostic) are likely to become more frequent in the future and the underlying principles are much the same as those for endovascular coiling.

Interventional radiology procedures
- Coiling of intracerebral aneurysms
- Embolization of arteriovenous malformations (AVM), fistulae (AVF), and tumours (both intracranial and spinal)
- Angioplasty
- Vertebroplasty and kyphoplasty.

Key anaesthetic issues
- The anaesthetist may be isolated and remote from immediate support.
- Need for intrahospital transfers.
- Management of peri-procedure anticoagulation.
- Management of sudden procedure-specific crises.
- Requirement for rapid emergence from anaesthesia to allow early neurological assessment.
- Radiation safety issues.

Coiling of intracerebral aneurysms

Preoperative assessment

The majority of patients will have suffered an acute SAH and coiling is usually undertaken within the first 48 hr after the bleed.

The decision of 'if, when and how' to treat SAH can be difficult. The team has to balance the risk of rupture and ischaemic vasospasm against the risks of the procedure. There is evidence to support the early use of endovascular management of SAH. Early clipping of aneurysms risks technically challenging surgery—a problem obviated by the endovascular approach. However, this means the neuroanaesthetist will be expected to anaesthetize patients for coiling that would not have been considered fit for neurosurgery. In addition, these cases may be undertaken at weekends, posing a challenge to the emergency anaesthetic team.

If there is clinical evidence of cerebral vasospasm, intracranial neurovascular access can be challenging. This vasospasm may be exacerbated by manipulation of the intravascular catheter, which may result in more complex postoperative management.

The systemic complications of SAH and their management are discussed in Systemic complications of brain injury, p. 370.

Patient positioning
- The screening table is narrow, without patient sides and maybe slow or unable to adopt the Trendelenberg position. It is advisable to anaesthetize the patient on a standard tipping trolley and transfer to the screening table after induction.

ANAESTHESIA FOR NEURORADIOLOGY

- INR procedures may last several hours and pressure areas must be protected.
- Newer radiology equipment may offer 3D reconstruction techniques, using rotational image acquisition. A large, bulky C-arm rotating at speed through greater than 180° is well-equipped to disrupt an anaesthetic by impacting on breathing circuits, infusion lines and anaesthetic machines.

Anaesthetic techniques

There is no clear consensus on the best technique. There is a move towards general anaesthesia as opposed to sedation techniques due to the requirement for reliable patient immobility to optimize image quality. Sedation techniques are indicated when neurological assessment is required during the procedure.

General anaesthesia

The anaesthetist should employ an anaesthetic technique which follows the same principles of neuroanaesthesia as described in 📖 General principles of anaesthesia, p. 110.

- Due to presence of an unprotected cerebral aneurysm that is at risk of rupture, the haemodynamic response to laryngoscopy should be controlled and patient coughing or movement on intubation avoided.
- Popular techniques include the use of sevoflurane in oxygen and air or a propofol infusion, combined with an infusion of remifentanil or intermittent fentanyl.
- Nitrous oxide is avoided as there is an additional risk of microbubbles with the use of pressurized catheter flushing systems and during injection of contrast agents.
- Due to the risk of aneurysmal rupture caused by patient movement whilst the microcatheter tip is in the aneurysm, a continuous infusion of a muscle relaxant is recommended.
- To decrease the risk of thromboembolic complications associated with the placement of the coils, heparin is given (~70 iu kg^{-1}) with the target of a 2–3 times prolongation of the baseline activated clotting time (ACT).
- Blood pressure management can be problematic. Generally the procedure is non-stimulating, so blood pressure tends to be low during the procedure unless active measures are taken to maintain it. Because of the risk of cerebral vasospasm, hypotension should be avoided. Conversely, hypertension should be avoided until the aneurysm is protected.

Monitoring

- Invasive blood pressure monitoring is mandatory as arterial pressure can change dramatically without warning. An arterial cannula also facilitates blood sampling for monitoring of anticoagulation.
- A urinary catheter is mandatory. Patients receive a significant crystalloid load due to the continuous flushing system of the femoral artery catheters.

Radiation safety

All staff working in the X-ray treatment room need a minimum basic understanding of radiation safety and safe working practices. There are three sources of radiation: direct from the emitting tube; leakage through collimators which limit the beam; and scattering from reflection off the patient and surrounding surfaces. Anaesthetists with lead protection, working away from the beam, should receive exposure well within recommended limits.

General complications of interventional radiology

- Overt haemorrhage at the puncture site or less obvious groin or retroperitoneal haematomas are a significant risk because of the combination of large bore femoral arterial sheaths and the administration of heparin.
  - The use of percutaneous vessel-sealing devices such as the Angioseal® reduces the risk of haemorrhage.
- Contrast media may trigger adverse reactions, although the newer non-ionic agents are associated with a lower incidence of reactions, which tend to be of mild to moderate severity.
- The reported incidence of contrast-induced nephropathy (CIN) varies between 5 and 50%. Risk factors are:
  - high dose of contrast
  - hypovolaemia
  - diabetes mellitus
  - pre-existing renal disease.
- The risk of CIN is minimized by the maintenance of euvolaemia and a normal renal perfusion pressure.
  - There is no conclusive evidence to support the use of N-acetylcysteine as prophylaxis against CIN.
- Intracranial vessel injury and dissection may follow catheter manipulation.

Complications specific to endovascular coiling

Aneurysmal rupture

Aneurysmal rupture and further SAH may occur at any time during the procedure. Presentation varies from mild, subtle changes in the patient's condition to sudden catastrophic deterioration.

- The radiologist may notice extravasation of contrast.
- The anaesthetist may observe an increase in arterial pressure, with or without changes in heart rate, in keeping with a Cushing's response to an increase in ICP.
- If a sedation technique has been used, general anaesthesia should be induced immediately—a potentially challenging scenario.
- Heparin should be reversed with protamine (1 mg per 100iu heparin).
- The anaesthetist should anticipate dramatic haemodynamic changes and institute appropriate therapy.
- Changes in ICP can be mitigated by administration of mannitol and the maintenance of normocapnia.
- The radiologist will attempt to rapidly fill the aneurysmal sac with coils. A post-procedural CT scan may reveal acute hydrocephalus (requiring

ventricular drainage) and the extent of subarachnoid haemorrhage or intracerebral haematoma.

Vascular occlusion
- Vasospasm during embolization may be ameliorated by direct intra-catheter injection of vasoactive drugs such as nimodipine, glyceryl trinitrate and papaverine, or by cerebral angioplasty.
  - These vasoactive drugs may sometimes have systemic effects though these are usually mild and short-lived.
- The intraluminal clot formed after embolization may encroach beyond the neck of the aneurysm and inhibit distal blood flow necessitating pharmacotherapy, e.g. platelet aggregation inhibitors such as abciximab. This will increase the risk of spontaneous haemorrhage elsewhere.
- Coils may become displaced and cause a distant occlusive event. This may necessitate further anticoagulation and coil removal, either endovascularly or by emergency craniotomy.

Emergence and recovery from anaesthesia
- The aim is to achieve rapid return of consciousness and ability to obey commands, to facilitate early neurological assessment.
- Attention should also be given to the control of arterial pressure. Commonly there is a hypertensive surge during extubation—antihypertensive drugs should be given to mitigate against this effect, especially if the aneurysm remains unprotected following unsuccessful treatment.
- Postoperative management, ideally in an HDU environment, should include regular neurological assessment and monitoring for signs of haemodynamic instability.
- Continuous intravenous infusion of heparin may be required if there have been thrombo-embolic complications.

Embolization of arteriovenous malformation (AVM), arteriovenous fistula (AVF), and tumours
This involves selective catheterization and them embolization of vessels feeding the nidus using a variety of techniques: N-butyl cyanoacrylate, Onyx® (a proprietary embolic agent), balloons and coils. Following reduction in the size of the nidus, further treatment may include radiotherapy or surgery. Apart from anaesthetic considerations as discussed above, the anaesthetist may be asked to provide controlled hypotension during embolization to reduce blood flow through the AVM. Following the embolization regional cerebral hyperaemia may follow the re-establishment of normal flow in areas related to the AVM. See Intracranial aneursysm and AVMs, p. 272.

Pre-operative embolization of vascular tumour
Vascular tumours, for example meningioma or glomus tumours, may be embolized before surgery to reduce intra-operative haemorrhage. Tumour feeding vessels are selectively catheterized and embolized using polyvinyl alcohol (PVA) particles. The potential benefit of reduced intra-operative haemorrhage during surgical excision needs to be balanced against the risks of the procedure including tumour swelling or haemorrhage.

Tips and pitfalls
- Do not underestimate the ability of the radiology equipment to obscure, disrupt, and dislodge anaesthetic equipment.
- Although remifentanil is a good drug for providing haemodynamic stability, interventional radiology is generally unstimulating, so hypotension is a risk. Some anaesthetists prefer to use fentanyl or alfentanil to cover stimulating periods.
- Aneurysmal sac rupture is a stressful time for the radiologist. Calmness from the anaesthetist is essential.
- All radiology departments will have safety procedures, which should be observed. If in doubt, ask the radiographer.

Anaesthesia for MRI and CT scans

There are a number of anaesthetic considerations that are common to both MRI and CT, however the MRI environment produces additional challenges for the anaesthetist and will be discussed in more detail.

Issues for the anaesthetist are:
- Patient factors
- Environmental factors in the MRI suite
- Anaesthetic factors.

Patient factors

The MRI and CT scanners attract a challenging subset of patients.
Planned lists consist of:
- Paediatric patients:
  - assessment of intracranial tumours
  - complex neurological conditions
  - inability to cooperate, e.g. autism.
- Adults:
  - anxiety states, e.g. claustrophobia
  - inability to cooperate, e.g. learning difficulties.

There is less call on the MRI scanner out-of-hours, but the emergency workload for the CT scanner is significant, especially for hospitals providing neurosurgical services.
- This workload consists of assessment of patients with head injury, which will include seriously ill patients with multiple trauma and patients transferred from ICU.
- Emergency CT scan is increasingly being requested for early assessment of acute stroke.
- Some patients will be obtunded and may require tracheal intubation and general anaesthesia to protect their airway and facilitate immobility.

Environmental factors

In an MRI scanner superconducting magnets generate a high-intensity magnetic field, between 0.5 to 2 Tesla (1 Tesla = 10,000 Gauss).

Although magnetic fields and radiofrequency energy are considered not to be a risk to biological tissues, the magnetic field exerts a potent force on ferromagnetic objects, which are attracted into the central bore of the scanner. Strict safety precautions are necessary to safeguard both patients and staff. In practice this means that the anaesthetist should appreciate the 5 and 50 Gauss lines around the scanner.

Within the 5 Gauss zone staff and the patient will be screened for loose items such as pens, watches, scissors, credit cards. Similarly, internal objects such as metallic fragments in the eye, aneurysmal clips, and pacemakers must be excluded. Within the 50 Gauss zone the attractive force becomes more significant and again, these items must be excluded.

ANAESTHESIA FOR MRI AND CT SCANS

Another concern is the potential for a hypoxic atmosphere in the scanner room. This can arise if the superconducting magnet 'quenches', i.e. the coolant (usually helium) is dumped, depressing ambient oxygen concentration. Scanner rooms usually contain a low oxygen concentration alarm.

The gradient coils give rise to high-intensity acoustic noise, which is unpleasant for the patient. Ear plugs are mandatory to minimize patient distress and avoid risk of temporary or permanent hearing loss.

Anaesthetic monitoring
The magnetic field interferes with monitoring in a number of ways.
- Inadequately shielded electronic equipment will not function correctly within the field.
- Induction of stray currents in cables and ECG wires interferes with the signal and risks burns to the patient.
- Manufacturers of anaesthetic monitoring have developed MRI-compatible monitors which can be within the MRI room.
- Carbon fibre leads are used for ECG monitoring and a fibre-optic cable connects the pulse oximeter.
- The monitors are shielded to prevent electromagnetic interference.
- A slave monitor can be sited in the control room.

Anaesthetic equipment
- Infusion pumps are problematic: they are susceptible to the strong magnetic fields and may function inaccurately or be damaged.
- Non-essential infusion devices should be removed prior to entering the MRI scan room.
- Required infusions may be safely continued by siting pumps outside the high-strength magnetic zone and using extended connector lines.
- MRI-compatible anaesthetic machines are available and can safely be positioned near the scanner.
- MRI-compatible aluminium gas cylinders must be used—a standard gas cylinder is potentially lethal if placed within the high-strength magnetic field.

Anaesthetic factors
- An immobilized patient is required for good-quality image acquisition from both CT and MRI scanners.
- The patient is relatively inaccessible during scanning.
- The anaesthetist is remote from the patient.
- There is a risk of adverse reactions to contrast media.

General anaesthesia may be maintained using either an inhalational technique or intravenous infusion technique.
- As described above, the MRI scanner demands care from the anaesthetist when using an infusion device.
- The airway needs to be maintained, either using a tracheal tube or laryngeal mask airway.
- Anaesthesia utilizing a laryngeal mask airway in a patient breathing spontaneously is the most popular technique when raised intracranial pressure is not an issue.
- Neonates can often be managed by feeding before the examination and wrapping up warmly. Most will sleep through the scan.

- Many patients, especially children, may be satisfactorily managed by using sedation techniques.
- These should be given according to local guidelines. In some centres this is provided by anaesthetists, while other centres have developed specialist nursing teams to provide paediatric sedation safely.

Tips and pitfalls
- The same standard of monitoring is required for general anaesthesia in the MRI suite as anywhere else. Do not accept substandard monitoring.
- Familiarize yourself with the MRI suite and the equipment before working there alone. Much of the monitoring is unique to MRI.
- Do not be tempted to work in the CT or MRI suite without suitably trained and experienced assistance.
- Double check yourself and others for ferrous objects before entering the MRI suite. Pagers and credit cards are commonly forgotten about.
- Do not press the MRI emergency stop button unless there is an absolute reason.

Chapter 11

Acute brain injury

Pathophysiology *334*
Immediate care *340*
Transfers *346*
General management *350*
Cerebral protection *356*
Subarachnoid haemorrhage *362*
Systemic complications of brain injury *370*
Status epilepticus *374*
Death *378*

Pathophysiology

Traumatic brain injury (TBI) is common and affects around 400 people per 100,000 population each year with an incidence of death of around 6–10 per 100,000 per year. Most TBI is classified as mild, but around 10% is moderate or severe. TBI is the leading cause of death in children aged 1–15 and in adults less than 45 years.

The relative incidence of the primary causes of TBI varies between countries and with patient age. Road traffic collisions and alcohol-related trauma are the leading causes in young adults (alcohol is associated with ~65% of all TBI in adults). Around 80% of head injuries occur in males, and 50% occur in children. Twenty per cent occur in people >65 years old and they are more likely to present following a fall. Penetrating injuries are more common in war zones and in areas with high rates of gun-shot injuries.

Primary injury

The initial mechanical insult imposes compressive and shearing forces on the brain (see Figure 11.1). Vessels are better able to withstand these forces than nerve tissue, so focal injuries such as contusions tend to occur on a background of diffuse neuronal injury. This initial injury is not necessarily lethal on its own—one-third of patients who die following TBI have talked or obeyed commands after injury. These mechanical insults result in a cascade of events which may result in both local and distant cell death:
- Impaired regulation of cerebral blood flow (CBF) and metabolism
- Increased cell membrane permeability
- Cellular oedema
- Anaerobic metabolism and lactic acid accumulation
- Depletion of ATP-stores and failure of membrane ion pumps.

A secondary cascade then ensues:
- Terminal membrane depolarization
- Release of excess amounts of excitatory neurotransmitters (e.g. glutamate, aspartate)
- Activation of NMDA and AMPA receptors and voltage-dependent Ca^{2+} and Na^+ channels.
- Ca^{2+} activation of intracellular catabolic processes, leading to necrosis or apoptosis.

Although axons may be disrupted (axotomy) at the time of initial injury, most axotomy occurs days after injury. This suggests that it is a programmed event, which may be amenable to therapeutic intervention.

Secondary injury

A series of pathological processes initiated at the time of injury may then follow which results in a wider area of cell death than the initial injury. The area of brain tissue surrounding the primary injury is at most risk (the 'penumbra'). Management of TBI is aimed at minimizing the effects of these secondary insults.

Cerebral blood flow

Following TBI, CBF is disturbed. Globally, CBF tends to follow a triphasic pattern.

- Immediately following injury, CBF is reduced.
- The second phase (days 1–2) is characterized by relatively high CBF.
- A vasospastic phase may follow with high MCA FV but low CBF.

Changes in cerebral blood flow are temporally and spatially heterogenous; areas of low CBF may coexist with areas of high CBF. CBF changes are multifactorial:

- CBF may be appropriately low or high, coupled to low or high $CMRO_2$.
- Blood flow-metabolism coupling may be impaired leading to hyperaemia or oligaemia.
- Autoregulatory failure may lead to low CBF in the presence of systemic hypotension:
  - This may develop immediately or over time.
  - Different areas may have different autoregulatory behaviours
  - Carbon dioxide reactivity is better preserved than pressure regulation. Injudicious use of induced hypocapnia may result in cerebral ischaemia.
- Vessel calibre may be reduced through mechanical displacement or compression (contusion, intracranial hypertension).
- Vessels may be occluded by debris, thrombus or leucocytes.
- Vasospasm occurs through a variety of mechanisms:
  - Enhanced prostaglandin-induced vasoconstriction
  - Endothelin release
  - Reduced availability of nitric oxide
  - Reduced cGMP levels
  - Free radical formation

It is important to note that hyperperfusion and oligaemia can only be diagnosed if CBF and $CMRO_2$ are measured in the same region at the same time.

Cerebral metabolism

After TBI cerebral metabolism (oxygen and glucose consumption) is temporally and spatially heterogenous.

- The use of substrates may also be altered as reflected in tissue phosphocreatine levels and lactate/pyruvate ratios.
- Lower metabolic rates are associated with a worse outcome, reflecting the severity of initial metabolic injury and mitochondrial dysfunction.
- Hypermetabolism may also occur due to large membrane ionic fluxes. If CBF does not increase enough, secondary ischaemia will ensue.

Cerebral oxygenation

The end result of inadequate CBF compared with $CMRO_2$ is global or focal cerebral hypoxia. Infarction occurs at tissue PO_2 <1.5 kPa.

Excitotoxicity

The initial insult and secondary events result in excessive release of neurotransmitters, particularly glutamate.

- NMDA and AMPA receptor activation leads to large Na^+, Ca^{2+} and K^+ fluxes. This may trigger catabolic processes directly, such as necrosis, apoptosis and blood–brain barrier disruption.
- Increased Na^+/K^+ ATPase activity increases the metabolic demands on the cell, which in turn may lead to further ischaemia.

- Excitotoxicity and inadequate anti-oxidant activity may also lead to accumulation of reactive oxygen species, which in turn may trigger inflammation and apoptosis.

Oedema
Cerebral oedema after TBI is common. As with CBF and $CMRO_2$ it is spatially and temporally hetergeneous with various causes.

Vasogenic oedema is a consequence of impaired blood–brain barrier function and autoregulatory behaviour. This results in the transfer of ions, proteins and water from the intravascular to the extracellular space.
- Generalized and temporary loss of blood–brain barrier function may occur immediately following head injury.
- Areas of contusion may have prolonged disturbance of blood–brain barrier function.
- Coupled with a loss of autoregulation, this may make some patients more likely to increase ICP when systemic blood pressure increases.

Cytotoxic oedema may be a consequence of cellular membrane failure and absorption of extracellular osmotically active substances, which leads to expansion of intracellular volume (particularly the glia).
- Increased uptake of neurotransmitters by astrocytes may also lead to intracellular accumulation of Na^+ and water.

Cytotoxic oedema is more common than vasogenic oedema. Both forms of oedema increase the distance between capillary and neuronal tissue, which may result in areas of tissue ischaemia despite adequate cerebral oxygen delivery.

Regardless of the cause, if compensatory mechanisms are exhausted, increased brain volume may result in dangerous degrees of intracranial hypertension (Intracranial pressure and CSF, p. 22).

Inflammation
Both primary and secondary injuries can initiate and maintain an inflammatory reaction in injured and adjacent tissue. Immune and glial cells are activated through release of chemokines, cytokines, prostaglandins, and free radicals. This may lead to adherence of activated leucocytes to the endothelium and subsequent tissue infiltration. Ultimately astrocytes produce scar tissue in the affected areas. These processes start within the first few hours after injury, but may take several weeks to complete.

Cell death
Severe mechanical or ischaemic injury results in cell necrosis following metabolic failure. Inflammatory processes remove the cellular debris, replacing it with scar tissue.

Apoptosis (programmed cell death) occurs in response to primary and secondary injuries, and is characterized by a well-regulated sequence of events ultimately leading to cell death, but not scar formation. Although apoptosis may be initiated very soon after injury, it is a more prolonged process, and may offer potential therapeutic targets.

Functional and anatomical issues
Some areas of the brain are more at risk of injury than others. Mechanical and anatomical factors mean that contusions are most common in the frontal lobes and tip of the temporal lobe. Loss of specific neural

pathways may result in significant functional impairment following TBI, despite only small volumes of ischaemic damage.

Outcome

Outcome after TBI is dependent upon several factors.

- *Mode of injury*: pedestrians and cyclists do worse than vehicle occupants in motor vehicle accidents.
- *Gender*: for the same severity of injury, women have a worse outcome than men.
- *Age*: worse outcome correlates with increasing age.
- *Glasgow Coma Scale*: GCS on presentation is a significant prognostic factor (see Table 11.1).

Table 11.1 Outcome 1 year after TBI, assessed using the Glasgow Outcome Scale

Initial severity	Initial GCS	Good recovery (%)	Moderate disability (%)	Severe disability (%)	Dead or vegetative (%)
Mild	13–15	45	28	20	8
Moderate	9–12	38	24	22	16
Severe	3–8	14	19	29	38

- *Genetics*: there is evidence that the ε4 allele of apolipoprotein E is associated with a worse outcome.
- *Pupils*: bilaterally fixed pupils after resuscitation in severe TBI are associated with around 80% poor outcome (vegetative or dead) compared with 30% poor outcome for severe TBI and bilaterally reactive pupils.
- *CT findings*: worse appearance on CT is associated with worse outcome. The Marshall classification, based on CT appearance, is prognostic (see Table 11.2).

Table 11.2 The Marshall classification

Category	Definition	Approximate frequency (%)	Outcome (%) Unfavourable (severe disability, dead vegetative)	Favourable (good recovery, mild disability)
Diffuse injury I	No visible intra-cranial pathology on CT scan	7–12	38	62
Diffuse injury II	Cisterns are present with midline shift <5 mm and/or lesion densities present. No high- or mixed-density lesion >25 ml, may include bone fragments and foreign bodies.	24–33	65	35
Diffuse injury III	Cisterns compressed or absent with mid-line shift 0–5 mm. No high- or mixed-density lesion >25 ml	10–21	84	16
Diffuse injury IV	Mid-line shift >5 mm. No high or mixed-density lesion >25 ml	2–4	94	6
Evacuated mass lesion	Any lesion surgically evacuated	38–48	77	23
Non-evacuated mass lesion	High- or mixed-density lesion >25 ml, not surgically evacuated	4–5	89	11

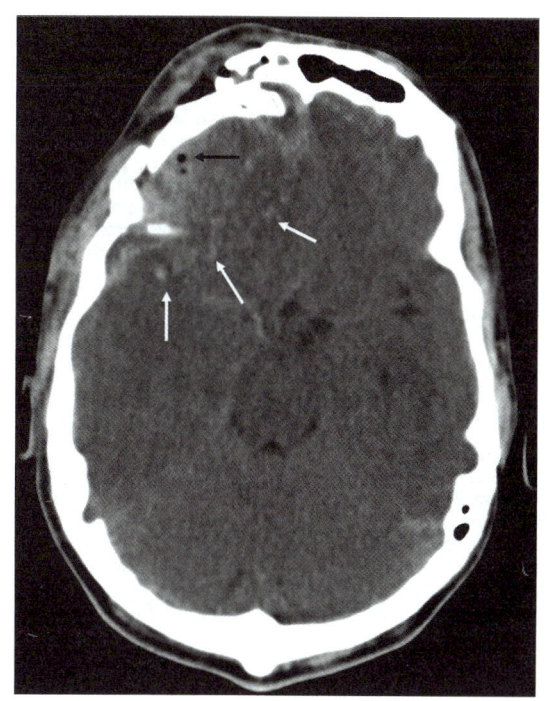

Fig. 11.1 Head injury. Unenhanced CT scan. Depressed right frontal fracture, extra-axial haemorrhage containing locules of gas (black arrow) and multiple small right frontal haemorrhagic contusions (white arrows).

Minor and moderate TBI also carries significant morbidity, with almost 50% of survivors experiencing some significant sequelae (📖 see Systemic complications of brain injury, p. 370) lasting at least several weeks.

Cause of death
Death following TBI occurs for a variety of reasons:
- In the immediate phase it may due to cerebral ischaemia, hypoxia due to airway or respiratory pathology, or haemorrhage as a consequence of trauma.
- Later deaths are most commonly due to other injuries, infection or cerebral ischaemia.
- Cerebral ischaemia may be diffuse, or localized to critical regions.
- A common terminal event is brainstem ischaemia due to brain swelling leading to compression of the brainstem during transtentorial herniation (coning).

Summary
The causes of neurological injury following TBI are diverse and heterogenous in space and time, both within and between patients. The distinction between primary and secondary injury is blurred, but later insults can worsen the extent of the initial injury.

Immediate care

There is little that medical care can do to affect the mechanical insult that causes traumatic brain injury (TBI) in the first place. However, the cascade of events which is started at that moment may be affected, for better or worse, by the care the patient subsequently receives.

There are very few high-quality trials demonstrating positive impact of specific interventions. There is reasonable evidence that providing care for TBI patients in centres with sufficient experience and expertise in brain trauma management is associated with improvements in mortality.

By definition, TBI patients are trauma patients, and initial assessment should follow the same basic principles as for any trauma patient.

Airway and cervical spine

Patients with low conscious levels following TBI will not be able to protect and maintain their own airway. Although tracheal intubation may be the definitive solution, in the short term, simple manoeuvres such as jaw thrust or an oropharyngeal airway may be life-saving. Nasopharyngeal airways should be avoided due to the risk of basal skull fractures, potentially resulting in intracranial positioning. Triggers for tracheal intubation are listed in Table 11.3.

Cervical spine (5%) and cord (2.5%) injury are relatively common in patients with severe TBI. Caution must be exercised with airway manipulation. However, this must not override the provision of a clear airway.

- Tracheal intubation is a means to an end, not an end in itself.
- There is no direct evidence associating tracheal intubation with improved outcome.
- Current guidance suggests GCS ≤8 as a threshold for intubation and ventilation. This should be interpreted in clinical context. Some patients with GCS >8 will not be able to maintain or protect their own airway. The benefits of emergency anaesthesia and potentially difficult intubation must outweigh the risks.
- Planned tracheal intubation is preferable to emergency intubation.
  - Most patients requiring intra- or inter-hospital transfer are likely to require tracheal intubation.

Table 11.3 Triggers for intubation and ventilation

Inability to maintain and protect own airway regardless of conscious level.
Inability to maintain adequate oxygenation with less invasive manoeuvres.
$PaO_2 < 13$ kPa.
Inability to maintain normocapnia.
Spontaneous $PaCO_2$ <4.0 kPa or >6.0 kPa.
Irregular respiration.
GCS ≤8.
Patients undergoing transfer with:
Deteriorating conscious level (≥ 2 point on motor scale).
Significant facial injuries (unstable facial fractures; copious bleeding into the mouth or pharynx, e.g. basal skull fracture).
Seizures.

Breathing

Hypoxia (SpO_2 <90% or PaO_2 <7.9 kPa) is associated with a worse outcome after TBI for several reasons:
- Severity of hypoxia may be a marker of TBI severity.
- Hypoxia is a surrogate for hypoventilation and hypercapnia.
- Hypoxia acts a secondary insult to at risk areas of brain.

Regardless of the cause, hypoxia must be avoided and treated.
- Subjects able to maintain their own airway should be given supplemental oxygen to maintain adequate arterial oxygenation (>13 kPa).
- Subjects unable to maintain their own airway or adequate arterial oxygenation despite oxygen therapy may need tracheal intubation, paralysis, positive pressure ventilation and sedation.
- Current guidance suggests aiming for PaO_2 of >13 kPa. (Table 11.4)

Marked hypercapnia and hypocapnia are both associated with worse outcome following TBI. Hypercapnia results in increased cerebral blood volume, which in turn *may* cause large increases in intracranial pressure. Hypocapnia reduces cerebral blood flow, which may increase the volume of ischaemic brain.
- Patients who are unable to maintain normocapnia may need tracheal intubation, paralysis, positive pressure ventilation and sedation.
  - Patients with a spontaneous $PaCO_2$ of <4.0 kPa or >6.0 kPa require assisted ventilation.
- Current guidance suggests aiming for $PaCO_2$ of 4.5–5.0 kPa.

Circulation

Systemic arterial hypotension is common in patients with TBI. Both early (resuscitation phase) and late (treatment phase) hypotension are independently associated with worse outcome; this includes single episodes of hypotension and intra-operative events.

- Avoidance of hypotension is probably more important than the agent used to support blood pressure.
- Studies supporting the use of low-volume trauma resuscitation specifically excluded TBI subjects.
- Hypertonic saline (e.g. 250 ml of 7.5% saline) is used by some centres as an initial resuscitation fluid.
  - There are no prospective data to suggest that use of hypertonic saline improves outcome, though surrogate measures such as ICP do improve.
- There are no data to suggest that outcome is improved by any one vasoactive drug compared with another.
- Targets for arterial blood pressure vary between countries, but MAP ~80–90 mmHg is generally quoted (Table 11.4).
- Head injury alone rarely causes hypotension except where there is significant scalp bleeding, or large intracranial haematoma in infants.
  - Other causes of hypotension must be sought and excluded.
- Treatment of cardiovascular instability due to other causes such as bleeding takes priority over direct head injury interventions.
- Systemic hypertension and bradycardia are classic signs of coning. Urgent intervention to reduce ICP is required.

Disability

Accurate recordings should be made during resuscitation of any changes in GCS, motor function and pupil size and reaction. Prompt reversal of hypoxia and hypotension may result in rapid improvement of conscious level and papillary signs. There are national guidelines detailing which

Table 11.4 Physiological targets for care immediately after severe head injury

Physiological measure	Target
Mean arterial blood pressure (adults)	>80 mmHg
Mean arterial blood pressure (children)	40–60 mmHg (<3 months)
	45–75 mmHg (3 months–1 year)
	50–90 mmHg (1–5 years)
	60–90 mmHg (6–11 years)
	65–95 mmHg (12–14 years)
PaO_2	>13 kPa
$PaCO_2$	4.5–5.0 kPa (minimum 4 kPa if clinical signs of high ICP)

patients require emergency or early CT scan (Table 11.5) and discussion or transfer to a neurosurgical centre (Table 11.6).

With the advent of fast multi-slice CT scanners, the threshold for scanning the cervical spine in patients where clinical examination is unreliable is low. Cervical spine imaging must include the cranio–cervical and cervico–thoracic junctions, which are the commonest sites of injury. Traditional 3-view plain X-ray series miss 40–50% of fractures.

Patients with persistent low GCS, unreactive pupils or other signs of high ICP may require short-term measures to reduce ICP and hence the risk of 'coning'.

- Blood pressure control: treatment of hypotension may result in a reduction in intracranial pressure.
- Oxygenation: reversal of hypoxia may also lead to a reduction in ICP.
- Mannitol: there is little evidence that routine use of mannitol for TBI improves outcome. However, it does reduce ICP temporarily and may be used if coning is thought to imminent or present.
- Hypertonic saline: as with mannitol, evidence for outcome benefit is lacking, but may be used for acute elevations of ICP.
- Hyperventilation: routine hyperventilation is associated with a worse outcome, presumably due to an increase in ischaemic brain volume.
- Short-term hyperventilation may be of use if coning is thought to be imminent or present.
- Normoglycaemia: hyperglycaemia is associated with worse outcome after TBI. There is little evidence for the best blood glucose concentrations to aim for, but observational studies suggest that concentrations of <10–11mmol l^{-1} are associated with improved outcome. There is no evidence supporting very tight control, and hypoglycaemia is deleterious to the injured brain.

Table 11.5 UK guidance for CT scan after head injury

Urgent CT brain completed within 1 hour of request
GCS <13 on initial assessment in the emergency department.
GCS <15 at 2 h after the injury.
Suspected open or depressed skull fracture.
Any sign of basal skull fracture (haemotympanum, 'panda' eyes, CSF leakage from the ear or nose, Battle's sign).
More than one episode of vomiting in adults; three or more episodes of vomiting in children.
Post-traumatic seizure.
Coagulopathy (history of bleeding, clotting disorder, current treatment with warfarin) providing that some loss of consciousness or amnesia has been experienced; patients receiving antiplatelet therapy may be at increased risk of intracranial bleeding, though this is currently unquantified—clinical judgement should be used to assess the need for an urgent scan in these patients.
Focal neurological deficit.
CT brain completed within 8 hours of injury
Amnesia for events more than 30 min before impact (the assessment of amnesia will not be possible in preverbal children and is unlikely to be possible in any child aged under 5 years).
Age 65 years or older, providing that some loss of consciousness or amnesia has been experienced.
Dangerous mechanism of injury (a pedestrian struck by a motor vehicle, an occupant ejected from a motor vehicle or a fall from a height of greater than 1 metre or five stairs) providing that some loss of consciousness or amnesia has been experienced.

Table 11.6 Triggers for discussion with neurosurgeon

New, surgically significant abnormalities on imaging.
Persisting coma (GCS ≤8) after initial resuscitation.
Unexplained confusion which persists for more than 4 h.
Deterioration in GCS score after admission (greater attention should be paid to motor response deterioration).
Progressive focal neurological signs.
Seizure without full recovery.
Definite or suspected penetrating injury.
Cerebrospinal fluid leak.

Transfer to neurosurgical unit

Some patients will require transfer to a local neurosurgical unit. This is discussed fully later in this chapter.
- All patients with severe TBI (GCS ≤8) should be transferred to a neurosurgical unit, regardless of whether an operable lesion is present.
- Cardiovascular instability should be adequately treated prior to transfer.
- For some conditions, such as an acute extradural haematoma, transfer should be expedited.

Tips and pitfalls

- Alcohol intoxication is a common cause of reduced consciousness. It is also a risk factor for TBI. Never assume that alcohol is the sole cause of impaired consciousness.
- Other differential diagnoses for reduced consciousness following trauma should always be considered:
  - Hypoglycaemia
  - Drug overdose
  - Spontaneous intracranial haemorrhage
  - Stroke
  - Convulsions
- There is no evidence to support the use of high-dose corticosteroids for the treatment of traumatic brain injury (see General management, p. 350).
- The risk–benefit ratio of all interventions must be carefully considered. Rushing to intubate a patient should not result in surges of blood pressure, hypoxia or hypercapnia.
- Intra- and inter-hospital transfers should provide the patient with the same level of care as if they were not being transferred.

Transfers

Abbreviated transfer guidelines are printed in the appendix at the back of this book.

Patients with brain injury may require transfer both within and between hospitals for clinical and non-clinical reasons. During the transfer, the patient will be isolated from the normal clinical environment and staff and faces additional hazards. Poorly performed transfers may worsen patient outcome. Various organizations have published guidelines on safe transfer. All of these emphasize the need for well-trained staff, adequate planning, (both at hospital and patient level) appropriate equipment and regular audit and review of transfer provision.

Indications

Inter-hospital
- Lack of intensive care beds in primary hospital
- Specialist treatment or investigations unavailable in the referring hospital
- Repatriation to local healthcare facility.

Intra-hospital
- Neuroimaging such as CT or MRI
- Neuroradiological procedures, such as aneurysm embolization
- Operative intervention in theatre
- Movement from one clinical area to another for ongoing care, e.g. resuscitation room to intensive care, or intensive care to general ward.

Principles

The principles are identical for any type of transfer. One systematic approach to transfers is based on the ACCEPT principle:

Assessment
- Neurosurgical patients may have multiple injuries or be critically unwell due to secondary injury, or sepsis.
- Individuals involved in transfers may have had no previous contact with the patient, so a thorough handover and re-assessment is mandatory. It is important to resist the temptation to act purely as a courier. Throughout the transfer, the standard of care the patient receives should be of the same high level as that provided prior to departure. This requires adequate knowledge of the patient's history and clinical condition.

Control
- A team leader for the transfer should be nominated.
- This leader should make sure the necessary tasks for a safe transfer are completed, in addition to ensuring continuation of clinical care.

Communication
- There are multiple individuals involved in transfers all of whom need to be kept informed.
- These include responsible consultants (both surgical and critical care) at the primary and receiving hospitals, relatives and ambulance control.

- A written record of the transfer is important: for ongoing clinical care in the receiving hospital; for audit and service improvement; and for medico-legal reasons in the event of adverse events.

Evaluation
- The transfer of a patient constitutes a treatment, and is not without risk. Careful evaluation is necessary to determine:
  - whether the transfer is appropriate for the patient
  - the urgency of the transfer.
- The urgency of the transfer will determine which personnel should accompany the patient, and what method of transportation will be used.

Preparation and packing
Preparation includes the stabilization of the patient and the organization of transfer personnel and equipment
- Patient preparation:
  - airway maintenance is essential. If there are any concerns regarding this, tracheal intubation should be performed prior to transfer
  - spinal immobilization and eye protection where appropriate
  - drug infusions should be rationalized—few patients require more than 3 infusions
  - hypothermia during a transfer is common, and efforts should be made to minimize heat loss, e.g. by 'mummy wrapping'.
- Personnel preparation:
  - the UK Intensive Care Society recommends that accompanying doctors should have had specific transfer training and have completed training in an acute care specialty. They should be competent in resuscitation, airway care, ventilation, and other organ support
  - all transfer team members should have adequate protective clothing, a mobile telephone and contact telephone numbers at both the transferring and receiving unit.
- Equipment preparation:
  - a full selection of airway and intubation equipment
  - twice the estimated amount of oxygen needed should be carried
  - a self-inflating bag for manual ventilation
  - a minimum of 2 iv cannulae, that are easily accessible
  - adequate amounts of maintenance and emergency drugs, such as sedatives, muscle relaxants, and inotropes
  - portable suction device
  - monitors should be fully charged and syringe drivers should have spare battery units
  - NIBP pumps rapidly deplete monitor batteries (and are also prone to movement artefact) so invasive monitoring is usually preferable
  - capnography is mandatory for all mechanically ventilated patients
  - ECG, arterial blood pressure, SpO_2 and temperature monitoring are required for all patients
  - all tubes, cannulae and catheters must be securely fastened and checked before transfer.

Transportation:
- The mode of transport is determined by numerous factors, both clinical and geographic

- Inter-hospital transfers are most commonly by road ambulance, although fixed-wing aircraft may be considered for journeys of greater than 150 miles
- The extra speed of transfers by air has to be offset against the logistical difficulties of access to the patient and the need for vehicular transfers at the beginning and end of the journey.
- Specific 'transfer trolleys' may be available, but these may be compatible with a limited number of ambulances only.

Specific issues for the brain-injured patient

Airway and breathing
Tracheal intubation and controlled ventilation should be used for patients with:
- GCS ≤8
- Significantly deteriorating GCS (e.g. fall in motor score ≥2)
- Loss of protective pharyngeal reflexes
- Hypoxaemia (PaO_2 <13 kPa on oxygen)
- Hypercapnia ($PaCO_2$ >6 kPa)
- Spontaneous hyperventilation causing $PaCO_2$ <4.0 kPa
- Bilateral fractured mandible
- Copious bleeding into the mouth (e.g. from skull base fracture)
- Seizures.

Appropriate sedation, analgesia and muscle relaxation should be used. Aim for PaO_2 >13 kPa and $PaCO_2$ 4.5–5.0 kPa. More aggressive, short-term hyperventilation to control ICP should be accompanied by an increased FiO_2. Blood gases should be checked prior to departure: $ETCO_2$, FiO_2 and SpO_2 monitoring should continue throughout transfer.

Circulation
Hypotension is associated with worse outcome after brain injury.
- Mean arterial pressure should be maintained ≥80 mmHg.
- Any causes of hypotension should be identified and treated prior to transfer.
  - hypovolaemia is tolerated poorly during transfer so normo- or mild hypervolaemia should be aimed for, along with a haematocrit over 30%.
- Major haemorrhage should be stopped and significant clotting derangements treated
  - if transfusion blood is likely to be required, blood should be cross-matched and taken with the patient in the ambulance.
- Sedative-induced hypotension may be treated judiciously with inotropes and vasopressors.
- Urine output should be monitored by urinary catheter.

Disability (neurology)
- Pupil size and reactivity should be checked prior to departure. It is often impossible to check pupils whilst restrained by a seat-belt during transfer. If concerned the attendant should stop the ambulance.
- If underway, ICP monitoring should continue during transfer, and CPP targets should be the same as prior to departure.

- If possible the patient should be positioned with 20° head-up tilt, whilst maintaining spinal immobilization if appropriate.
- A patient who has had a seizure may be loaded with phenytoin or other anticonvlusants prior to departure.

Tips and pitfalls
- Size D cylinders contain 340 and size CD 460 litres of oxygen. Most front line ambulances have two size F cylinders, each of which contains 1360 litres of oxygen.
- Ensure a road atlas is available if transferring by road ambulance. Satellite navigation devices may fail.
- Before you set off check that you, and the crew, know exactly where you are going and where to go once you arrive at the destination hospital. If in doubt, request that someone meets you at an obvious place on arrival.
- In acute, time-critical, transfers for neurosurgical emergencies, do not forget to take copies of imaging investigations.
- Infusion pumps are preferable as gravity-fed drips are unreliable in moving vehicles.
- If interventions are necessary during a road transfer, the ambulance should first be stopped in a safe place.
- If you would not be happy to care for the patient alone in the hospital then you should not transfer the patient alone.
- Skilled assistance can be literally life-saving.

General management

The aim of intensive care management in acute brain injury is to minimize the secondary injuries that may occur by optimizing cerebral perfusion and oxygenation. Although cerebrovascular accidents account for the vast majority of patients presenting with acute brain injury, the intensive care population is heavily biased towards those with traumatic brain injury (TBI). The principles of management are broadly the same.

Despite the relative high prevalence, poor outcomes and huge costs to society of TBI the evidence base regarding management is limited. Research is difficult due to the diversity and dynamic nature of TBI and a lack of collaborative research. For this reason, practice varies across the world, and is often based on expert opinion rather than good-quality evidence. One of the most widely used sources is the US Brain Trauma Foundation series of reviews.

Where patients should be cared for?

An estimated 40% of severe TBI patients are managed in non-neurosurgical centres in the UK—this may either be due to a poor predicted outcome or because neurosurgical centres cannot accommodate patients that do not require neurosurgical intervention. There is continuing debate as to whether such patients fare worse than similar patients managed in specialist centres.

Patients with TBI should be transferred to a neurosurgical centre if they meet the following criteria:
- Severe head injury (GCS ≤8)
- Focal neurological signs
- Needing invasive ventilation or ICP monitoring.

Key principles in the management of TBI

There are no studies which demonstrate conclusively that any single intervention improves outcome following TBI. Improvements in outcome in recent years are probably a reflection of improvement in adherence to key principles and the general management of the critically ill. The five key principles in the management of TBI are:

Normotension
- Maintain SBP ≥120 mmHg, MAP 70–90 mmHg, CVP 5–10 mmHg with a combination of intravenous fluids and vasopressors (norepinephrine).
- Hypertension may worsen vasogenic oedema
  - β-blockers are the agent of choice for treatment as they do not cause cerebral vasodilatation.

Normoxia
- Maintain SaO_2 ≥95%, PaO_2 >13 kPa.
- Hypoxaemia (SaO_2 <90%) is associated with a worsened outcome.
- PEEP may impede cerebral venous return and increase ICP. High levels in patients with both TBI and lung injuries can be problematic.

Normocapnia
- Maintain $PaCO_2$ between 4.5–5.0 kPa.

- Hyperventilation causes cerebral vasoconstriction, thus reducing CBV and ICP. It has been used for many years in the treatment of TBI despite growing evidence that it is harmful.
- Based on expert opinion, many treatment algorithms for TBI suggest mild hyperventilation to a $PaCO_2$ of 4.0–4.5 kPa in patients with a raised ICP. This should be done with caution and in conjunction with some measure of cerebral oxygen delivery-consumption (e.g. jugular bulb saturation, brain tissue oxygen tension).
- Hyperventilation to $PaCO_2$ <4.0 kPa, should only be used for short periods (<30 min), as a temporizing measure to decrease ICP.
- Hypercapnia causes cerebral vasodilatation and increased ICP. Thus permissive hypercapnia (frequently used in a lung protective ventilation strategy) should be avoided
  - clinical judgement is required when these two requirements conflict.

Normothermia
- Maintain temperature ≤37 °C.
- Avoid hyperthermia as it increases cerebral metabolic oxygen requirement which can worsen brain ischaemia.
- The use of hypothermia in the management of TBI is discussed in 📖 Cerebral protection, p. 356.

Normoglycaemia
- Maintain blood sugar between 4–8 mmol l^{-1} with insulin infusions and by avoiding the use of dextrose containing intravenous fluids.
- In the presence of reduced cerebral blood flow, hyperglycaemia can result in increased anaerobic metabolism and worsening cerebral intracellular acidosis.

General management
- Patient positioning: 15–20° head up:
  - this improves cerebral venous return without compromising cerebral perfusion pressure
  - it may also reduce the risk of ventilator-acquired pneumonia.
- Clearing the cervical spine is problematic in the unconscious patient and local protocols should be in place. The spine should be cleared as soon as possible as immobilization hinders nursing care.
- Maintenance fluid: 0.9% saline or Hartmann's solution. Aim for plasma Na$^+$ 145–155 mmol l^{-1} and serum osmolarity 320 mOsm l^{-1}. Treat hypernatraemia with nasogastric or rectal water.
- Feeding: early (preferably enteral) feeding. Start within 72 h and aim for full feed by day seven.
- Prophylactic antibiotics are not recommended. The risk of pneumonia is high (70%) in TBI (aspiration, ventilator-associated pneumonia, associated pulmonary trauma).
- DVT prophylaxis

- there is a 15–20% risk of DVT in patients with TBI; there is also a significant risk of haematoma/contusion expansion in the first few days following injury
- mechanical prophylaxis (graduated lower limb compression stockings or intermittent pneumatic compression) should be used for the first 72 h, followed by LMWH thereafter.
- Stress ulcer prophylaxis
  - there is ~10% risk of stress ulcers (Cushing's ulcer) in these patients
  - routine prophylaxis is recommended (e.g. ranitdine, sucralfate).
- Chest physiotherapy, turning, eye care, laxatives etc. should be instituted as with all intensive care patients.

Sedation and analgesia

Sedation and analgesia are used to minimize $CMRO_2$ and to allow continued invasive ventilation. A multi-drug approach is recommended to minimize drug dosages and to allow titration to specific effects. There is no good evidence that one combination of drugs is better than another. Muscle relaxants may be added to assist artificial ventilation or to reduce afferent nervous activity.

- A combination of a benzodiazepine (midazolam) plus an opioid (morphine, fentanyl or remifentanil) plus propofol is normally used.

Advantages
- Minimize pain and the response to noxious stimuli that might increase ICP.
- Decrease $CMRO_2$ and improve oxygen supply–demand ratio.
- Facilitate ventilation.
- Anticonvulsant (benzodiazepines, propofol, thiopental).

Disadvantages
- Impair neurological examination. 'Sedation holds' may counteract this.
- Adverse haemodynamic effects (hypotension).
- Drug accumulation.
- Paradoxical raised ICP and tachyphylaxis (opioids).
- Muscle relaxants must not be used as replacements for adequate sedation and analgesia.

Barbiturate coma (thiopental) is used for patients with intracranial hypertension refractory to other treatments.

- Electroencephalogram monitoring should be used to ensure burst suppression.
- Thiopental has significant cardiodepressant effects leading to hypotension.
- Drug accumulation leads to very prolonged emergence times following barbiturate coma.
- Etomidate is not used because of adrenal suppression and theoretical concerns about worsening cerebral oxygen delivery.

Neuro-specific management

Various protocols exist for TBI management each of which aims to maintain cerebral perfusion whilst minimizing iatrogenic injury. The most widely used are variations of the 'Rosner' protocols, which aim to maintain cerebral perfusion pressure by maintaining adequate systemic arterial

GENERAL MANAGEMENT

pressure whilst keeping ICP down. An example of such a management guideline is shown below.
- Maintain CPP >60 mmHg and ICP <20–25 mmHg
- Surgical:
  - haematoma/SOL evacuation, CSF drainage
  - decompressive craniectomy (unilateral or bifrontal)—rescue procedure in patients with raised ICP refractory to other treatment; the impact of decompressive craniectomy on outcome is currently under evaluation (see Decompressive craniectomy, p. 254).
- Medical:
  - *Osmotic agents to decrease ICP*: mannitol or hypertonic saline
  - *Anticonvulsants*: phenytoin; seizures increase $CMRO_2$ and ICP; no benefit from prophylactic use
  - *Neuromuscular blockade* (atracurium): prevent the adverse effects on ICP of coughing, straining and shivering
  - ❶ *Corticosteroids*: **not recommended in TBI**. decrease brain oedema, CSF production, and free radical production.

TBI management protocols

Protocol-led TBI management improves outcome. Several protocols are used that incorporate the principles and elements discussed above. The most widely used protocols target ICP and CPP (see Figure 11.2), as first described by Rosner in 2005, although other protocols claim (similar) excellent results.

CPP management protocols (Rosner)
- Aim to maintain CPP 60–70 mmHg by manipulation of factors that affect MAP and ICP (CPP = MAP − ICP).

Lund protocol
- Aim to decrease cerebral oedema by decreasing $CMRO_2$ and CPP.
- Plasma oncotic pressure is normalized with albumin and blood pressure normalized with α and β-adrenorecptor anatagonists. Vasopressors, mannitol and crystalloids are avoided.
- Intracerebral microdialysis monitoring of cerebral energy metabolism is used to optimize treatment.

Protocols that use multi-modality monitoring
- These include modalities such as jugular bulb saturation, transcranial Doppler ultrasound, single-photon emission computed tomography and brain tissue oxygen monitoring.

Monitoring
- Invasive BP and CVP haemodynamic monitoring in all patients.
- ICP and CPP:
  - ICP is an independent predictor of outcome and absolute ICP control is associated with improved outcome
  - Useful in patients who are sedated and ventilated in whom neurological assessment is limited. See Intracranial pressure, p. 68.

- EEG: primarily used to detect subclinical seizures or in conjunction with barbiturate infusions for burst suppression. It has been used to detect focal cerebral ischaemia.
- Imaging: repeated CT scans are useful in patients with raised ICP to identify or exclude causes that may be amenable to surgery.
- Near infrared spectroscopy (NIRS)—this is a research tool which provides a non-invasive measure of regional cerebral oxygenation.
- The following additional monitoring modalities have no clear benefit with respect to mortality and morbidity. Multimodal monitoring involves using a combination of these (see p. 86).
  - *Transcranial Doppler* —used to demonstrate hyperaemia or decreased cerebral perfusion in patients with increased ICP. Only allows global assessment of large blood vessel flows.
  - *Jugular bulb saturation* (maintain between 50–75%)—global assessment of cerebral oxygen uptake. Can be used to calculate global CBF from the arteriovenous difference in saturation.
  - *Intraparenchymal cerebral microdialysis*—can be used to measure cerebral glucose, lactate, pyruvate, lactate/pyruvate ratio, and glutamate concentrations.
  - *Brain tissue oxygen tension*—used to maintain tissue oxygenation tension >1 kPa.

Tips and pitfalls
- Meticulous attention to the five key principles of normoxia, normocapnia, normoglycaemia, normothermia, and normotension is paramount.
- Hyperventilation or a bolus dose of propofol (or thiopental) will rapidly lower ICP for a limited period.
- Mannitol should always be considered in a patient with signs of brainstem compression, with or without ICP monitoring.
- Early spinal clearance in TBI patients is recommended to facilitate general patient care.
- Don't forget the secondary and tertiary survey in TBI patients to prevent missed injuries.
- Neurocritical care logistical planning should include steps necessary to expedite CT scanning of TBI patients (e.g. proximity to scanner, pre-prepared transfer equipment, rapidly accessible suitably trained staff etc.).

GENERAL MANAGEMENT

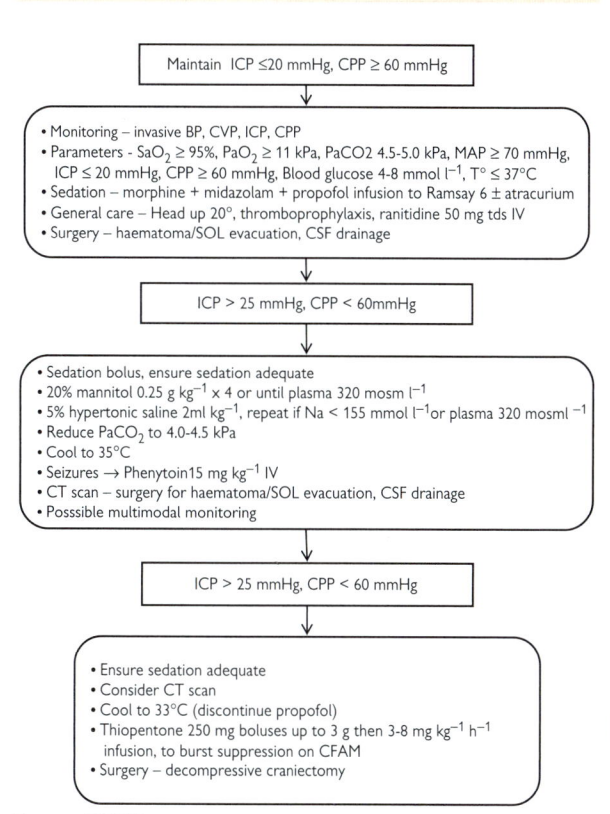

```
┌─────────────────────────────────────────────┐
│ Maintain ICP ≤20 mmHg, CPP ≥ 60 mmHg        │
└─────────────────────────────────────────────┘
                     ↓
```

- Monitoring – invasive BP, CVP, ICP, CPP
- Parameters - SaO_2 ≥ 95%, PaO_2 ≥ 11 kPa, $PaCO_2$ 4.5-5.0 kPa, MAP ≥ 70 mmHg, ICP ≤ 20 mmHg, CPP ≥ 60 mmHg, Blood glucose 4-8 mmol l^{-1}, T° ≤ 37°C
- Sedation – morphine + midazolam + propofol infusion to Ramsay 6 ± atracurium
- General care – Head up 20°, thromboprophylaxis, ranitidine 50 mg tds IV
- Surgery – haematoma/SOL evacuation, CSF drainage

```
┌─────────────────────────────────────────────┐
│ ICP > 25 mmHg, CPP < 60 mmHg                │
└─────────────────────────────────────────────┘
```

- Sedation bolus, ensure sedation adequate
- 20% mannitol 0.25 g kg^{-1} × 4 or until plasma 320 mosm l^{-1}
- 5% hypertonic saline 2ml kg^{-1}, repeat if Na < 155 mmol l^{-1} or plasma 320 mosml^{-1}
- Reduce $PaCO_2$ to 4.0-4.5 kPa
- Cool to 35°C
- Seizures → Phenytoin 15 mg kg^{-1} IV
- CT scan – surgery for haematoma/SOL evacuation, CSF drainage
- Posssible multimodal monitoring

```
┌─────────────────────────────────────────────┐
│ ICP > 25 mmHg, CPP < 60 mmHg                │
└─────────────────────────────────────────────┘
```

- Ensure sedation adequate
- Consider CT scan
- Cool to 33°C (discontinue propofol)
- Thiopentone 250 mg boluses up to 3 g then 3-8 mg kg^{-1} h^{-1} infusion, to burst suppression on CFAM
- Surgery – decompressive craniectomy

Fig. 11.2 ICP/CPP management algorithm.

Cerebral protection

Cerebral protection can be defined as any strategy designed to minimize injury by:
- Reduction in cerebral metabolic rate:
  - this may reduce ischaemia by improving oxygen supply demand ratios and/or
  - reduce intracranial pressure through a coupled reduction in cerebral blood volume.
- Reduction in excitotoxin release
- Reduction in free radical/oxidative damage

This section will review temperature management and drug therapies specifically used for this purpose.

Temperature control

Raised brain or core temperature is associated with worse outcome following acute brain injury. Although there are mechanistic explanations which suggest that high temperature is itself harmful, it may also be the case that patients with a worse outcome have more pyrexial episodes. Temperature control for the injured brain falls into two categories, namely: prevention of pyrexia and induced hypothermia.

Prevention of pyrexia

An increase in brain temperature results in an increase in $CMRO_2$ and CBF which may worsen brain ischaemia. In patients with acute brain injury, normothermia should be maintained. Pyrexia can be avoided/ameliorated by:
- Careful use of induced warming devices.
- Paracetamol or NSAIDS
  - there is little evidence of effectiveness of these drugs but they are commonly used.
- Use of cooling devices (internal or external).

Induced hypothermia (32–34 °C)

There are several mechanisms by which induced hypothermia could improve outcome following brain injury:
- Reduction in $CMRO_2$ therefore minimizing ischaemia if CBF is low and also reducing ICP through a coupled reduction in CBV
- Reduced release of excitotoxins
- Reduced severity of blood–brain barrier opening.

The use of induced hypothermia in TBI is widely practiced, but remains controversial. A Cochrane review in 2004 and four other meta-analyses have failed to support its use.
- There is experimental evidence suggesting that cooling may have mechanisms of benefit, but direct evidence from trials is lacking.
  - a lack of benefit has been demonstrated both in traumatic brain injury and for intra-operative cooling for surgical treatment of cerebral aneurysm.
- Cooling decreases ICP but hypothermia may impair cerebral oxygenation.

- Animal experimental studies have shown that temperature reduction can prevent and minimize neurological damage.
- TBI patients that are hypothermic on initial presentation have a poorer outcome.
- Outcomes are worse in children cooled within 8 h and continued for 24 h.
- There is some evidence to suggest that induced hypothermia in TBI may be beneficial if maintained for ≥48 h and that although it does not improve mortality, it may improve outcome scores.

Cooling after cardiac arrest

Unlike TBI, systemic cooling following a cardiac arrest has been shown to improve outcome. The inclusion criteria for the trials were slightly different but the evidence suggests that survival and favourable neurological outcomes rates can be improved in comatose patients following out of hospital cardiac arrest who are cooled to 32–34°C promptly for 12–24 h. Criteria for cooling are:

- Witnessed cardiac arrest
- Initial cardiac rhythm of VF from a presumed cardiac cause
- Age 18–75 years
- <15 min from time of collapse to resuscitation by emergency personnel
- <60 min from collapse to the return of spontaneous circulation
- SBP >90 mmHg or MAP ≥60 mmHg, SpO_2 ≥85%

Cooling techniques

Pharmacological
- Paracetamol
- NSAIDs
- Selective cyclo-oxygenase inhibitors.

Systemic
- Surface cooling: air or water-circulating blanket, wet packs and fans
- Intravascular venous cooling catheter
- Cooled (4°C) intravenous fluids
- Extracorporeal methods.

Side effects of systemic cooling:
- Shivering
- Immunosuppression
- Increased risk of ventilator-associated pneumonia and hospital-acquired infections
- Impaired platelet function and coagulation
- Diuresis
- Electrolyte imbalance
- Aggravated hyperadrenergic state.

Direct cerebral
There are experimental direct cooling techniques that are not as effective as systemic cooling, but avoid the systemic side effects.
- Cooled nasal air flow with head fanning
- Cooling caps and cooling neck collars
- Intravascular cold carotid perfusion
- Direct irrigation of the brain surface.

Drug therapies for cerebral protection

The purpose of clinical management following acute brain injury is to minimize the secondary injury that occurs by optimizing cerebral perfusion and cerebral oxygenation whilst minimizing iatrogenic injury. This section will discuss drug therapies intended to directly reduce brain injury.

There are no pharmacological agents that have been shown to provide cerebral protection (minimizing the secondary brain injury) in acute brain injury, although there are several agents with theoretical benefits.

Anaesthetic agents

Anaesthetic agents suppress neurotransmission and therefore reduce cerebral energy requirement. This could potentially be useful in the ischaemic brain.

Barbiturates (thiopental)
- Barbiturates have been used in the management of TBI since they were shown to reduce ICP in 1937.
- Barbiturates reduce $CMRO_2$ (75%) and ICP, increase CPP and suppress seizures. They are free radical scavengers and antioxidants.
- In TBI, thiopental is used for the treatment of refractory raised ICP and can either be administered as a bolus dose or as an infusion.
- Although there is evidence of pre-ischaemic protection in animals and humans, there is little evidence of sustained benefit in humans
  - some centres advocate bolus administration of thiopental prior to temporary clipping of aneurysms (see Intracranial aneurysms and AVMs, p. 272).
- There are several problems associated with thiopental infusion:
  - with prolonged infusion, the half-life of thiopental becomes dependent upon metabolism not redistribution; emergence times are prolonged (hours to days)
  - cardiovascular depression and collapse requiring increased use of vasoactive drugs
  - respiratory depression necessitating mechanical ventilation
  - immune suppression
  - hepatic dysfunction
  - hypernatraemia secondary to the large Na^+ load
  - sudden cardiovascular collapse and hyperkalaemia upon withdrawal.

Etomidate
- Similar beneficial effects to barbiturates but with less cardiovascular depression.
- *Disadvantages*: may worsen brain ischaemia by inhibiting nitric oxide synthetase, significant adrenocortical suppression, less evidence of benefit that for barbiturates.

Propofol
- Similar beneficial effects to barbiturates.
- Some evidence for post-ischaemic protection in animals.
- *Disadvantages*: not yet fully tested, cardiovascular instability, high lipid load, should be avoided in hypothermic patients. Some evidence of increased rates of jugular venous desaturation during craniotomy.

Volatile agents
- Volatile agents have been shown to reduce $CMRO_2$, inhibit excitatory neurotransmission, potentiate inhibitory receptors, inhibit Ca^{2+} channels and protect against global and ischaemic injury in animals.
- A clear benefit has not been shown in clinical practice compared with other therapies.

Ketamine
- Ketamine is a *N*-methyl-D-aspartate receptor antagonist, and as such has theoretical neuroprotective properties.
- Ketamine has been shown to protect against focal ischaemia in animals but there are no clinical data to support its use.

Lidocaine
- Reduces $CMRO_2$ by inhibiting apoptosis, reducing ischaemic transmembrane ion shifts, modulation of leukocyte activity, and reduction of ischaemic excitotoxin release.
- No large clinical trials support its use.

Corticosteroids
Corticosteroids reduce cerebral oedema around brain tumours. There is no evidence of benefit in traumatic brain injury, stroke or following cardiac arrest.
- *Disadvantages*: Glucocorticoids are immunosuppressive. They may worsen global ischaemia by causing hyperglycaemia.

Calcium antagonists
Nimodopine has been shown to be of benefit following SAH. Theoretically it could prevent Ca^{2+} flux into cells and decrease lactic acidosis. No benefit has been demonstrated following TBI to prevent vasospasm.

Magnesium is a calcium antagonist that also antagonizes NMDA receptors and glutamate release but again there is no demonstrated benefit in TBI.

Glutamate antagonists
Glutamate is an excitatory neurotransmitter, implicated in brain injury and acts via the NMDA and AMPA receptors. Competitive (selfotel) and non-competitive (dizocilipine dexanibol, aptiganel) glutamate receptor antagonists have been shown to have no benefit.

Antioxidants
Mitochondirial dysfunction following brain injury may lead to increased lipid peroxidation via increased oxygen free radicals. Neither superoxide anion scavengers (e.g. pegorgotein) nor lipid peroxidation inhibitors (21-aminosteroids—lazaroids) have been shown to be of benefit.

Tromethamine (THAM)

THAM is a weak base which can enter cells and decrease intracellular acidosis. There is some preclinical evidence of benefit in traumatic brain injury, but no clinical data to support its use.

Tips and pitfalls
- There are no proven 'magic bullets' for cerebral protection.
- Improvements in outcome from head injury are probably related to improved protocols and general intensive care.
- Induced hypothermia has been shown to be of benefit in adults in a subset of cardiac arrest survivors only.
- Successful induction of hypothermia requires a clear policy on how this is to be achieved and managed.

Subarachnoid haemorrhage

Primary subarachnoid haemorrhage accounts for ~5% of all strokes. Even with modern management, the mortality of patients in good grade groups is ~8%. The care of these patients can be categorised broadly into three domains: prevention of re-bleeding; prevention and treatment of medical complications; and prevention and treatment of neurological complications.

The commonest cause of subarachnoid haemorrhage is trauma. see Pathophysiology, p. 334, and Immediate care, p. 340.

Epidemiology

The estimated incidence of SAH is around 10 per 100,000 population per year. It occurs most frequently in the fifth decade, though any age can be affected. The underlying causes of spontaneous SAH are:
- Ruptured cerebral aneurysm (85%)
  - anterior (carotid) circulation (80–90%)
  - posterior (vertebro-basilar) circulation (10–20%)
- Unknown (peri-mesencephalic) (10%)
- Other (5%)
  - arteriovenous malformations
  - dissections/vasculitis/tumours

Prognosis

A significant number of patients die before, or shortly after receiving medical attention.
- Survival in patients in good grade groups is over 90%
- Of the early survivors, 25–30% are dead or dependent at 1 year
- Prognosis is strongly associated with clinical grade and the amount of blood visible on CT (see Figure 11.3).

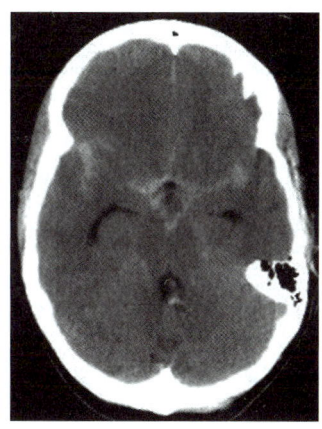

Fig. 11.3 Subarachnoid haemorrhage. Unenhanced CT scan. SAH secondary to ruptured intracranial aneurysm, with hyperdense blood seen in the basal cisterns and right insular cistern. A small amounbt of blood is visible in the 4th ventricle, and the temporal horns are dilated indicating the presence of hydrocephalus.

Pathophysiology

A variety of genetic, environmental and lifestyle factors interact to support the formation of aneurysmal outpouchings of basal cerebral arteries. Identified risk factors include:
- Smoking
- Hypertension
- Moderate to high alcohol consumption.

Small aneurysms are less likely to rupture than large (5–10 mm diameter) (Laplace's law). Unruptured, so-called giant aneurysms may form which may produce significant mass effect.

At the time of rupture, the CSF becomes in continuity with the arterial system, and, briefly, ICP will approach MAP. This is probably the cause of the initial headache and/or loss of consciousness.

- The blood may remain subarachnoid
- The bleed may also cause intracerebral or intraventricular haematoma
- This extravascular blood may result in local mass effect, meningeal irritation, vasospasm, obstruction to CSF flow through interventricular pathways and reduction in CSF reabsorption
- Cerebral metabolism and autoregulation are also disturbed
- Extracranial complications may also interact with the intracranial disease to worsen outcome.

Presentation

The classical presentation of SAH is a sudden severe, occipital headache which may or may not be associated with brief or prolonged loss of consciousness.

- Meningism (stiff neck, photophobia), seizures, focal neurological deficits, and isolated cranial nerve palsies may all occur.
- A small number of patients will present with mass effect (causing cranial nerve palsies) or incidentally when investigations reveal intracranial aneurysms.

Classification

Various classifications have been described for standardization of clinical assessment and prognosis. The most widely used scale is the World Federation of Neurological Surgeons (WFNS) grading. The Hunt and Hess and Fisher gradings are not widely used now and are largely of historical interest. See Boxes 11.1, 11.2 and 11.3.

Box 11.1 WFNS grading scale

Grade	GCS	Motor deficit
I	15	Absent
II	13–14	Absent
III	13–14	Present
IV	7–12	Absent/present
V	3–6	Absent/present

Motor deficit excludes cranial nerve palsies but includes dysphasia

Box 11.2 Hunt and Hess grading scale for subarachnoid haemorrhage

Grade	Description
I	Asymptomatic or mild headache, slight nuchal rigidity
II	Moderate to severe headache, nuchal rigidity, no neurologic deficit other than cranial nerve palsy
III	Drowsiness, confusion or mild focal neurologic deficit
IV	Stupor, moderate to severe hemiparesis
V	Coma, decerebrate posturing

Box 11.3 Fisher CT grading scale

Grade	CT findings
1	No clot seen
2	Diffuse layer of subarachnoid blood (<1 mm thickness)
3	Localized clot or >1 mm thickness subarachnoid blood
4	Intracerebral or intraventricular clot with or without visible subarachnoid blood

Investigation

Patients with suspected subarachnoid haemorrhage require investigations with three complementary purposes:
- Confirm the diagnosis
- Identify complicating factors
- Identify the cause of SAH.

Confirming the diagnosis
CT is the diagnostic modality of choice for patients with classical symptoms and signs.
- Many centres now used contrast-enhanced CT for all suspected SAH patients followed by reconstructive CT angiography.
- Early CT is necessary since 2% and 7% of SAHs are missed at 12 and 24 h, even with modern technology.
- For patients with negative CT but strong suspicion of SAH, lumbar puncture demonstrating either non-clearing bloody CSF or xanthochromia is the second line investigation.

Identifying complicating factors
Local practice may vary, but a core set of investigations for SAH includes:
- FBC: anaemia may be pre-existing and may affect cerebral oxygen delivery
- Coagulation: abnormal coagulation is a consequence of SAH
- U&E: hyponatraemia following SAH is relatively common
- Glucose: hyperglycaemia is relatively common, due to the physiological stress response
- Magnesium: hypomagnesaemia is common and associated with poor outcome
- ECG: the commonest abnormalities seen are changes in T and U waves, prolongation of the QTc interval and ST segment depression
- Chest X-ray: pulmonary aspiration and pulmonary oedema may occur.

Identifying the cause of SAH
- CT angiography has high specificity and sensitivity for detection of aneurysms. It can be used to guide decision-making about endovascular or surgical approaches.
- Four-vessel angiography is still the gold standard for delineating the precise anatomy.
- A proportion of patients will have more than one aneurysm and it can be difficult to be certain which one has ruptured.

Prevention of rebleeding

Rebleeding has a significant detrimental effect on outcome following SAH. 2–4% of patients rebleed in the first 24 h and 15–20% rebleed within the first two weeks. The outcome of patients who are WFNS grade IV–V is largely dependent upon the initial bleed.

There are two treatment options:
- Endovascular obliteration of the sac using detachable metal coils (coiling) (see Coiling of intracerebral aneurysms, p. 324)
- Surgical closure of the aneurysm neck using metal clips (clipping) (see Intracranial aneurysms, p. 272)

The chosen option for any one patient is based on various factors:
- Trial evidence and guidelines
- Local expertise and opinion
- Patient factors: clinical grade, co-morbidities etc.

The ISAT trial of 2143 patients demonstrated 24% death or dependence at one year with coiling vs 31% with clipping. Although these data appear strongly in favour of coiling, those in favour of clipping argue that:
- Only 22% of screened patients were randomized
- Few patients were high risk
- 95% of treated aneurysms were small and in the anterior cerebral circulation
- Incomplete occlusion was more common in the coiling group
- Long-term rebleed rates are unknown.

Since publication of ISAT radiological expertise has improved greatly. Many centres now view coiling as the treatment of choice. Surgical clipping is still the treatment of choice for some aneurysms:
- Anatomically not possible to coil
- Patients requiring craniotomy for evacuation of haematoma
  - insertion of EVD does not preclude coiling as first option.

Prevention and treatment of medical complications

Cardiovascular

SAH is associated with acute and marked systemic and pulmonary hypertension, cardiac arrhythmia, ECG abnormalities, temporary and permanent myocardial dysfunction, and pulmonary oedema. The underlying cause is believed to be excessive sympathetic discharge following SAH resulting in vasoconstriction and myocardial calcium overload.
- 25–100% of patients may have ECG abnormalities.
- Elevated troponin levels are found in ~20% of patients and elevated CK-MB levels are found in ~35%.
- Left ventricle (LV) dysfunction can be demonstrated in ~25% of patients.
- The degree of cardiac dysfunction correlates most closely with neurological severity rather than ECG abnormalities.

There is no consensus on the optimal management of SAH associated myocardial injury/dysfunction. It does not appear to associate directly with outcome and is usually temporary. However, the degree of myocardial injury probably predicts cardiovascular instability
- Pulmonary oedema occurs in around 10% of patients.
  - it responds well to CPAP and positive pressure ventilation and is usually relatively transient.

Following SAH, patients are typically relatively immobile and have an increased risk of DVT/PE.
- Once the aneurysm is protected, pharmacological DVT prophylaxis should be instituted in addition to mechanical measures.

Pulmonary
Aspiration at the time of presentation or associated with reduced level of consciousness is relatively common. Once the aneurysm is protected aggressive respiratory physiotherapy can be used safely.

Renal
Electrolyte disturbances are common following SAH. Hyponatraemia, hypokalaemia, hypocalcaemia, and hypomagnesaemia should all be sought and treated. Mannitol, diuretics, and intravenous fluid therapy may exacerbate these problems.

Hyponatraemia occurs in around 30% of patients following SAH. In addition to iatrogenic causes, cerebral salt wasting and syndrome of inappropriate ADH secretion (SIADH) may occur (see Systemic complications of brain injury, p. 370).

Prevention and treatment of neurological complications

Vasospasm
Angiographically demonstrable narrowing of cerebral arteries occurs in ~70% of patients. Clinically detectable effects (delayed ischaemic deficits) occur in ~30%. Typically it occurs 3–12 days after the first bleed and may persist for ~2 weeks.

The precise mechanism of injury associated with vasospasm is unclear and is probably multifactorial. Theories include:
- Alterations in the contractile/relaxation behaviour of arterial smooth muscle (biochemical or structural)
- Vasoconstrictive effects of blood and blood breakdown products
- Immune-mediated vasoconstriction
- SAH-induced neurotoxicity.

Vasospasm may also cause an increase in ICP due to compensatory vasodilation of reactive resistance vessels distal to the spastic segment.

Diagnosis of vasospasm can be clinical, radiological or based on (semi) continuous monitoring.
- Clinical: new neurological deficits should be assumed to be vasospasm unless there is evidence for another cause. Deficits may be subtle, and may not occur in the territory of the feeding artery.
- Radiological: angiography may demonstrate the characteristic of constricted vessels. Angiography carries a small but real risk of neurological morbidity so is not normally used for routine monitoring.
- Multimodal monitoring: various aspects of multimodal monitoring have been assessed for prediction of vasospasm:
  - TCD flow velocities, absolute (>120 cm s^{-1}) or relative (3–6 times carotid flow)
  - microdialysis has demonstrated abnormalities before other evidence of cerebral ischaemia is apparent; in theory this would allow early institution of treatment
  - cerebral oxygenation assessed by invasive tissue probes, or indirectly by SjVO$_2$ can be used as a marker of onset of ischaemia.

Nimodipine

Outcome following SAH improves with the use of nimodipine. Current recommendations are that all patients should receive 60 mg nimodipine 4 hourly (oral or nasogastric [NG]). Intravenous infusions can be used, but cause more hypotension. (Administer via a central line starting at 0.5 mg h^{-1} titrated up to a maximum of 2 mg h^{-1} if blood pressure remains stable.) The beneficial effects of nimodipine are probably through neuroprotective effects rather than vasodilation.

Triple-H therapy

The purpose of triple-H therapy (hypertension, hypervolaemia, haemodilution) is to improve cerebral blood flow by increasing CPP and reducing blood viscosity. There is no consensus on how this should be achieved, precisely what the targets are and for how long it should continue. Although neurological deficits resolve in up to 70% of patients with this technique there is no good evidence of improvement in outcome and it may worsen mortality. It is relatively contraindicated in those with partially or completely unprotected aneurysms and those with significant myocardial dysfunction.

- Typical targets are: systolic BP 160–200 mmHg, CVP 8–12 mmHg and [Hb] 8.0 g dl^{-1} or haematocrit 30–35%.

Balloon angioplasty and intra-arterial papaverine

In patients with new neurological deficits unresponsive to medical therapy and demonstrable vasospasm in an appropriate vessel, balloon angioplasty can be performed. Distal vessel disease can be treated with intra-arterial papaverine. Radiological improvement does not always associate with clinical improvement.

Hydrocephalus

Intracranial hypertension may occur due to obstruction of CSF drainage, either between the ventricles or at the level of the arachnoid granulations.

- Sudden deterioration in consciousness following SAH is usually due to re-bleed, seizures or high ICP. A CT is therefore required.
- Temporary treatment is with an EVD. This may need conversion to a V-P shunt at a later date.

Seizures

Seizures following SAH are relatively unusual occurring in <5% of patients. Prophylactic anticonvulsants are not routinely used.

Tips and pitfalls

- Simple things matter for these patients. Meticulous attention to prevention of medical complications is important.
- Interventional radiology may be less of a systemic insult than craniotomy, but the patient with SAH is still a high-risk patient.
- Sudden onset of deterioration in a patient with SAH may be due to seizure, rebleed or hydrocephalus. Urgent investigation, usually by repeat CT, is required.

Systemic complications of brain injury

Mortality and morbidity after acute brain injury of any kind is not only determined by the nature of the original insult, but also by the development of medical complications. That such complications occur is not surprising when one considers that the brain controls most of the body's systems via hormonal, autonomic, biochemical or neural biofeedback mechanisms. Anatomical or physiological disruption of these central systems will inevitably result in dysfunction of their target organs.

Airway and respiratory complications

Decreased level of consciousness is the hallmark of brain injury.

- Once the GCS falls to ≤8, the ability to maintain and protect the airway is compromised to the extent that airway obstruction may occur leading to hypoxaemia and hypercapnia. This may result in secondary brain injury.
- Impaired airway protection may also occur at higher GCS if there is specific damage to those areas of the brain that control swallowing and the gag reflex so that aspiration of gastric contents and subsequent pneumonia may occur.
- Patients with a GCS of ≤8 should undergo tracheal intubation, those with a higher GCS who cannot protect their airway should undergo elective tracheostomy and both groups of patient will require nasogastric intubation.
- In severely head injured patients requiring long term ventilation, the incidence of pneumonia is 35–50% with a mortality of up to 50%.

Additional risk factors for pneumonia in brain injury

- Associated chest trauma
- Prolonged positive pressure ventilation
- Induced hypothermia
- Barbiturate coma for control of ICP
- Steroid therapy for intracranial tumours.

Neurogenic pulmonary oedema

This is an acute onset pulmonary oedema generally occurring 4–12 h after brain injury, but may be delayed.

- It is often associated with damage to the brainstem and medulla and may be mediated by release of catecholamines causing acute myocardial depression and ischaemia as a result of transient extreme hypertension and tachycardia.
- The chest X-ray appearance mimics that of ARDS.
- Mechanical ventilation, PEEP and inotropic support are generally required.
- Resolution may be rapid or take several days.

SYSTEMIC COMPLICATIONS OF BRAIN INJURY

Cardiovascular complications

Sympathetic hyperactivity (autonomic dysfunction syndrome)
Acute brain injury is followed by an initial period of sympathetic hyperactivity resulting in tachycardia and hypertension.
- Various ECG changes may be seen including U waves, inverted T waves, notched T waves and Q-T interval abnormalities.
- Myocardial 'stunning' may be so severe as to require intra-aortic balloon pump therapy.
- Subendocardial damage may be seen in the heart up to 50% of brain injured patients at post mortem.
- Hypertension may occur to the point where, in the presence of failure of cerebral autoregulation, increased cerebral blood flow and cerebral perfusion pressure may lead to the formation of cerebral oedema.
- In general systolic hypertension should not be treated unless:
  - >200 mmHg
  - there is evidence of myocardial ischaemia
  - the brain injury is the result of spontaneous SAH from an aneurysm that remains unprotected.

Deep vein thrombosis (DVT)/pulmonary embolism (PE)
DVT occurs in ~15–20% of patients with acute brain injury on an intensive care ward; fatal PE is reported in ~1–3%.
- Mechanical prophylaxis, usually by intermittent calf compression or graduated compression stockings, is a minimum standard.
- Prophylaxis with enoxaparin remains controversial since the evidence on the balance of risks is unclear.
- An inferior vena cava filter can be used when DVT develops and anticoagulation is contraindicated.
- There is no consensus on when anticoagulation is safe following head injury.

Coagulopathy
There is 10–35% incidence of clotting abnormality in head injury and 8% incidence of disseminated intravascular coagulation (DIC).
- Coagulopathy is triggered by release of brain thromboplastin.
- Peak incidence is at 2–4 days following injury.
- Maturation (enlargement) of cerebral contusions can occur as a result.

Electrolyte disturbances
These may occur for a variety of pathological or iatrogenic reasons.

Hypernatraemia
- Resuscitation or maintenance fluids with 0.9% saline or high sodium enteral feeds
- Repeated doses of mannitol or furosemide for cerebral oedema
- Traumatic diabetes insipidus (DI)
- DI following brainstem death
- Barbiturate coma with sodium thiopental (high sodium load).

Hypokalaemia
- Sympathetic hyperactivity with cathecholamine release
- Increased aldosterone production.

Hyponatraemia
Hyponatraemia is the most common electrolyte disturbance complicating acute brain injury and may occur from several causes.

Syndrome of inappropriate antidiuretic hormone secretion (SIADH)
SIADH is responsible for ~12% of episodes of hyponatraemia observed after brain injury.
- There is both increased ADH and aldosterone.
- ADH increases re-absorption of water and causes dilutional hyponatraemia.
- Diagnosis requires:
  - low serum sodium (<135 mmol l^{-1})
  - low serum osmolarity (<280 mosmol l^{-1})
  - high urinary sodium (>20 mmol l^{-1})
  - urine osmolarity > serum osmolarity
  - normovolaemia
  - no other cause of hyponatraemia present
- Correct chronic hyponatraemia slowly (<8 mmol 24 h^{-1}) because of risk of central pontine myelinosis.
- SIADH is generally self limiting with fluid restriction.

Cerebral salt-wasting syndrome (CSWS)
The precise cause is unknown but is probably due to increased brain naturetic peptide formation.
- Occurs 1 week after brain injury and resolves in 3–4 weeks.
- Need to differentiate from SIADH as treatment is rehydration with 0.9% saline rather than fluid restriction.
- Urinary sodium generally >40 mmol l^{-1}.
- Urinary sodium excretion (Urine Na mmol l^{-1} x Urine volume l 24 h^{-1}) is high in CSWS but normal in SIADH.
- If CSWS fails to respond to normal saline replacement, fludrocortisone therapy may be required.

Pituitary and hypothalamic complications
Brain injury of sufficient severity to damage the pituitary and hypothalamus often causes death. Less severe injuries are associated with increased ACTH release, raised serum cortisol and abnormal diurnal cortisol levels. Pituitary dysfunction should be suspected if fractures of the sella turcica are present.

Diabetes Insipidus
Neurogenic DI results from failure to release vasopressin/ADH from the posterior pituitary. DI results in large volumes of dilute urine with low specific gravity which is hypo-osmolar compared with simultaneous serum osmolarity.
- Uncorrected DI leads to hypotension, dehydration and hypernatraemia.
- Desmopressin acetate (DDAVP) should be administered if urine output is more than 200 ml h^{-1} for 4 h in the presence of diagnostic urine biochemistry.

Hypopituitarism

Hypopituitarism is less common than DI because complete destruction of the gland or hypothalamus is necessary.
- Symptoms are often delayed
  - low levels of ACTH and TSH may conceal DI until steroid replacement therapy is started.
- There is no evidence to support the use of high-dose glucocorticoids in traumatic brain injury.
- The role of physiological steroid replacement in patients with subclinical hypoadrenalism is controversial.
- Growth hormone levels are reduced.
- DI may occur early after transphenoidal hypophysectomy
  - this is usually self-limiting and can be managed with increased water intake. (See Pituitary tumours, p. 200.)

Metabolic complications

Brain injury may double $CMRO_2$. Blood in the CSF is pyrogenic and energy expenditure increases by ~10% for each 1°C increase in temperature.
- Patients with high ICP should be cooled to normothermia.
- Hyperglycaemia may occur and normoglycaemia should be maintained.

Gastrointestinal complications

Acute gastric and oesophageal erosions

In common with other intensive care patients, acute oesophageal, gastric, and duodenal erosions are common.
- H_2 receptor antagonists or proton pump inhibitors should be prescribed.

Other complications

Other complications relate to long-term alteration of consciousness and include susceptibility to infection from invasive lines, pressure area care, mouth care and the need to avoid flexion contractures and footdrop.

Tips and pitfalls

- Systemic complications will cause morbidity and mortality. Meticulous attention to prevention may improve outcome.
- Although there is no consensus on how to reduce the risk of VTE in patients with brain injury, individual units should have their own guidelines to ensure that the issue is considered for all patients.
- High-dose glucocorticoids are not recommended for acute brain injury. The role of physiological steroid replacement is controversial.

Status epilepticus

Definitions
Status epilepticus (SE) is an acute medical emergency with a mortality of ~20%. Unless the seizure is stopped and airway and ventilation maintained, irreversible brain damage may occur.

There are various non-exclusive definitions of SE:
- A seizure that persists for more than 30min or recurrent seizures between which the patient fails to regain consciousness
- Continuous generalized convulsive seizure which lasts for more than 5 min
- Two or more seizures between which the patient does not regain consciousness.

Refractory SE may be defined as:
- A seizure that persists for more than 2 h
- Two or more recurrent seizures per hour without improvement in conscious level between seizures, which do not respond to therapy with 'first line' anti-epileptic therapy such as benzodiazepines or phenytoin.

Refractory SE generally requires intubation, ventilation and termination of seizure activity with general anaesthetic agents.

Non-convulsive SE can also occur, with persistent electrical seizure activity, despite absent or fragmentary associated movements.

Pathophysiology
SE occurs when there is a failure of the normal inhibitory neuronal mechanisms or excessive excitatory neuronal activity. The major inhibitory neurotransmitter is γ-aminobutyric acid (GABA) produced in GABAergic neurons and targeting several different types of GABA receptors. The excitatory neuro transmitter glutatamate, acting via N-methyl-D-aspartate (NMDA) receptors, seems to be important in the propagation of seizure activity. Once seizures become prolonged, excessive NMDA-mediated excitation seems to be a more intense driver of epileptiform activity than inadequate GABA inhibition. Brain damage, particularly in the cortex, thalamus, and hippocampus occurs as a result of NMDA receptor activation increasing intracellular calcium levels. In addition, secondary brain damage may occur as a consequence of associated hypoxaemia, hyperthermia, and hypotension.

Aetiology
The underlying causes are diverse, but can be subdivided into three groups, which have approximately equal representation:

Exacerbation of an underlying idiopathic seizure disorder

First presentation of a seizure disorder

Brain injury: structural, metabolic or toxic.
- Traumatic brain injury.
- Central nervous system infection:
  - meningitis, abscess, encephalitis.
- Central nervous system tumours.
- Cerebral hypoperfusion:
  - ischaemic or haemorrhagic stroke
  - prolonged systemic hypotension or hypoxaemia.

- Toxicity:
  - drugs: cocaine, theophylline, isoniazid
  - alcohol withdrawal.
- Metabolic disorders:
  - hypo/hypernatraemia, hypercalcaemia, hypoglycaemia.
  - hepatic encephalopathy.
- Epileptiform encephalopathies.

Diagnosis

The initial clinical features are those of generalized tonic-clonic convulsions associated with autonomic dystonia resulting in hypertension, sweating, hyperglycaemia, hypersalivation and hyperthermia (generalized convulsive SE).

Initially, CBF and $CMRO_2$ increase in parallel. After ~30 min there is a decrease in cerebral blood flow, failure of autoregulation and systemic hypotension. The tonic-clonic fits diminish in intensity and often only small amplitude twitches of the face, hands or feet remain. Occasionally only minor jerking movements of the eye or tongue are seen and the clinical diagnosis may be missed particularly if the patient is already sedated and ventilated on ICU. Later there may be no signs of any motor activity but an EEG shows ongoing epileptiform electrical activity (non-convulsive SE). In this stage the EEG often shows increasing periods of relative electrical silence with periodic discharge rather than the almost merging electrical discharges seen in the earlier stages of the disease.

- Non-convulsive SE can still cause brain damage so sedated and ventilated patients need to be monitored continuously with an analysing cerebral function monitor (CFAM) to ensure that anti-epileptic drug therapy is effective.
- Once stable, patients should have a brain CT or MRI to exclude structural triggers of SE. Lumbar puncture is required to exclude infective triggers.
- In non-convulsive SE specific investigations are required to exclude metabolic encephalopathy, drug reactions and the rare epileptiform encephalopathies such as NMDA receptor antibody encephalitis.

Systemic effects of generalized convulsive status epilepticus

- Hypoxaemia and hypercapnia
- Hyperthermia (both central and secondary to muscle activity)
- Hypertension (early)/hypotension (late)
- Hyperglycaemia (early)/hypoglycaemia (late)
- Tachycardia and arrhythmias
- Leucocytosis
- Raised intracranial pressure
- Increased CSF protein
- Rhabdomyolysis, hyperkalaemia and lactic acidosis
- Neurogenic pulmonary oedema.

Treatment

Initial assessment and management

- Assess airway, breathing, circulation and GCS.

- Give 100% oxygen and decide on the need for immediate intubation and ventilation.
- Obtain intravenous access and take blood for baseline investigations including creatinine kinase levels and an immediate blood glucose.
- Correct hypoglycaemia if present.
- Monitor pulse, blood pressure and pulse oximetry.
- Obtain arterial blood gases.
- Hypoxaemia, hypercapnia and coma indicate the need for elective intubation and ventilation—ongoing fitting *per se* does not mandate intubation if the airway can be maintained.
- If intubation is required then it should be achieved following intravenous induction of general anaesthesia (which may stop the fits initially).
  - if fits have been prolonged, then hyperkalaemia may have occurred so suxamethonium is best avoided and a rapidly acting non-depolarizing muscle relaxant such as rocuronium used.
- Aspiration pneumonia is always a risk and a nasogastric tube should be inserted.
- If the patient is hyperthermic, surface cool to normothermia.
- Aim for normotension, normovolaemia, normocapnia, normoglycaemia, normal oxygenation, and normal electrolyte status.

Seizure control

The goal is to achieve rapid cessation of seizure activity without causing respiratory or cardiovascular failure or worsening a decreased level of consciousness. Drug therapy should be instituted in a step-wise fashion.

- Intravenous benzodiazepines e.g. diazepam 0.2 mg kg^{-1} at 5 mg min^{-1} up to a total dose of 20 mg or lorazepam 0.1 mg kg^{-1} at 2 mg min^{-1} up to a total dose of 10 mg
  - increased doses of benzodiazepines increase the risk of respiratory depression.
- If benzodiazepines stop the seizures, give phenytoin to prevent recurrence
  - iv phenytoin 15–20 mg kg^{-1} (maximum infusion rate: adults <50 mg min^{-1}; children, 1 mg kg^{-1} min^{-1}).
- Persisting seizure activity may require more phenytoin: 5 mg kg^{-1} to a maximum of 30 mg kg^{-1} may be required
  - monitor BP and ECG during infusion and stop or slow the rate if hypotension or arrhythmia occurs.

Persisting seizures following this treatment (refractory SE) indicate a need for intubation and ventilation and more aggressive seizure therapy.

- Propofol 1–2 mg kg^{-1} intravenously followed by 2–5 mg kg^{-1} h^{-1} as an infusion
  - prolonged propofol infusions may rarely cause severe metabolic acidosis, rhabdomyolysis, hyperlipidaemia, and cardiovascular collapse particularly in children.
- Midazolam infusions 0.1–1 mg kg^{-1} h^{-1} may also be used in isolation or in combination with propofol.
- Thiopental 3–5 mg kg^{-1} intravenously followed by 1–5 mg kg^{-1} h^{-1} as an infusion
  - prolonged thiopental infusions may result in hypotension and hypernatraemia and a long duration of emergence from coma. They

should only be used if propofol and midazolam infusions fail to control the seizures.
- Avoid infusions of muscle relaxants as these mask the motor effects of seizure activity. Only use for severe muscle activity that causes lactic acidosis or interferes with adequate mechanical ventilation.
- Additional anti-epileptic drugs such as sodium valproate, topiramate or lamotrigine may also be given.
- Ketamine infusions should be reserved for those cases that do not respond to any of the above treatments.

Monitoring seizure activity
All intubated and ventilated patients should be monitored by CFAM. (see Electrophysiological monitoring, p. 72).
- Sedation may be titrated to achieve burst suppression on the CFAM but there is no evidence that this end point improves outcome.
- Following burst suppression continued sedation can result in brainstem anaesthesia with a very low voltage raw EEG signal on CFAM and sluggish pupillary responses. Sedation must be stopped if this occurs.
- Stop propofol, midazolam or thiopental infusions after 12 h of no seizure activity on CFAM once adequate loading doses of other anti-epileptic drugs have been given and therapeutic blood levels achieved.
- Restart the infusions if seizure activity recommences on CFAM and repeat the cycle as required.

Prognosis
The prognosis depends on the age of the patient, the duration of fitting and the aetiology of SE.
- Overall 30 day mortality is 15–20%
  - elderly patients have a mortality of 30% compared with 3% in children.
- Refractory SE has a worse prognosis than that responding to first line treatment.
- Idiopathic SE has a better prognosis that that due to a primary brain disease.
- SE caused by a combined severe hypoxaemic and hypotensive insult is almost invariably fatal.

Tips and pitfalls
- SE requires urgent treatment; it is a condition with high mortality and morbidity if left untreated.
- Non-convulsive SE is almost impossible to diagnose without neurophysiological monitoring.
- Sedative infusions should be reviewed regularly in order to prevent overtreatment and subsequent complications.
- Muscle relaxation should be avoided if possible.
- SE caused by a combined severe hypoxaemic and hypotensive insult is almost invariably fatal.

Death

There is no legal definition of death in the UK and practice is guided by published Codes of Practice (for example, *A Code of Practice for the Diagnosis of Death*, Academy of Medical Royal Colleges, 2008). The legal situation in other countries or states is varied and should be carefully ascertained before the outline described below is followed.

Death entails the irreversible loss of those essential characteristics which are necessary to the existence of a living human person. Death must, therefore, include the irreversible loss of the capacity for:
- consciousness
- spontaneous respiration.

Irreversible cessation of *brainstem* function equates with this definition such that brainstem death is human death.

Brainstem death vs. whole brain death

Some countries (USA, Australia, Canada, Holland) use the term whole brain death either as analogous to brainstem death or to seek to establish that there has been irreversible cessation of *all* brain function, including brainstem function, before death is declared. This may require the use of additional confirmatory tests to assess cerebral electric activity (e.g. EEG) and/or cerebral blood flow (e.g. angiography or TCD) and/or sensory or motor pathways (evoked potentials).

In reality many countries which use the term whole brain death still only carry out clinical testing of the brain stem and whole brain death is assumed. These additional confirmatory tests are time-consuming, require considerable local expertise and if used without appropriate clinical testing of the brain stem can lead to misdiagnosis. There is no evidence that using brain stem criteria alone without additional confirmatory tests has led to misdiagnosis.

Persistent vegetative states

A person in a persistent vegetative state is not brainstem dead because spontaneous ventilation is retained as are many brainstem functions.

Certification of brainstem death (in the UK)

- Two doctors are present one performing, one observing
  - who have been registered >5 years
  - who are competent in the performance and interpretation of brainstem testing
  - neither of whom has a conflict of interest (e.g. transplant surgeons are excluded)
  - one should be a consultant.
- A total of two complete sets of tests should be performed:
  - a short period of time between tests will be necessary, to allow return of blood gases to normal, and rechecking of blood glucose
  - there is no minimum time interval between tests.
- The legal time of death is after the first confirmatory set of tests.

Pre-conditions for brainstem death

Cause
- Irreversible brain damage of known aetiology consistent with resultant brainstem death.

Unconscious
- Exclusion of all other causes of unconsciousness including:
  - medications
  - other drugs
  - hypothermia (temperature must be >34°C)
  - circulatory, metabolic and endocrine causes. Blood glucose should be between 3.0 and 20 mmol l^{-1}.

Plasma levels of sedative drugs may need to be tested (e.g. midazolam levels should be <10 µg l^{-1}) and/or antagonists administered.

Ventilated
- No (or assumed no) spontaneous ventilation
- No medications (muscle relaxants) causing apnoea.

Diagnosing brainstem death

The pre-conditions listed above must all be satisfied **and** all brainstem reflexes (as described below) are absent

- Pupils fixed and unreactive to light
- Corneal reflex absent
- Vestibular-ocular reflex absent
  - 50 ml ice-cold water squirted over 1 min via syringe against each ear drum, with the head flexed 30° and absent eye response observed. The normal response is nystagmus, with the fast component away from the ear tested
- Motor response (limb or facial) absent after a painful stimulus in a cranial nerve distribution
- Gag and cough reflexes absent:
  - no response to bronchial suctioning or pharyngeal stimulation
- Apnoea test
  - after pre-oxygenation with 100% O2, adjust the minute ventilation to ensure $PaCO_2$ >6.0 kPa and pH < 7.40.
  - disconnect the patient from the ventilator and observe over five minutes. Supplemental oxygen is often required and the test should be stopped if hypoxia, hypotension or arrhythmias develop.
  - no spontaneous respiration should be observed. Confirm that the $PaCO_2$ has risen a minimum of 0.5 kPa
  - at the conclusion of the first apnoea test a period of ventilation will be required to normalise parameters.

Ancillary tests (not required in the UK)
- Doll's eyes movement (occulocephalic reflex):
  - with lateral movement of the head the eyes remain fixed in position
- Cerebral electrical activity:
  - Absent EEG activity is required in some countries; false positives are common in an intensive care setting

- Cerebral blood flow/metabolism
  - contrast angiography, isotope scans (^{99}Tc-HMPAO), TCD or PET scanning. All can show the cessation of cerebral blood flow
- Cerebral evoked responses (sensory and motor evoked potentials).

Difficult situations

Spinal reflexes
Spinal reflexes may persist in the period following brain death. Reflex movements of the limbs and torso may occur in response to peripheral stimulation. The family should be warned of this before testing takes place.

Children
Children should be a minimum of 37 weeks gestation plus 2 months. Less than this age ancillary testing (e.g. cerebral angiography) is often required.

Apnoea test
- Patients with chronic obstructive pulmonary disease who are chronically hypercapnic require consultation with an expert in respiratory disease.
- If the patient becomes hypoxic during the apnoea test the use of a CPAP circuit (+/– recruitment maneouvres) may allow testing to proceed.

Facial/ocular trauma preventing full cranial nerve examination
- In these uncommon situations senior consensus may allow diagnosis to proceed or testing may have to be abandoned.
- With bilateral injury or disease, ancillary testing should be considered.

Managing the physiological consequences of brainstem death

There is a high incidence of complications in brainstem dead patients.

Cardiovascular
- Following the hypertensive storm often seen during 'coning', hypotension and arrhythmias are common secondary to loss of sympathetic tone. This may result in subendocardial ischaemia.
- Organ supportive treatment includes fluids (CVP 4–10 mmHg), norepinephrine (aim for MAP 60–80 mmHg) and vasopressin (argipressin bolus 1 IU then 1–5 IU h^{-1}).

Respiratory
- Neurogenic pulmonary oedema is a common consequence of brainstem death necessitating high inspired concentrations of oxygen and PEEP.

Endocrine
- Anterior and posterior pituitary failure may require replacement with thyroid hormone (liothyronine bolus 4 μg and then 3 μg h^{-1}), hydrocortisone (50 mg 6-hourly) and vasopressin.
- Insulin secretion is reduced resulting in hyperglycaemia.

Temperature
- Poikilothermia results and the patient approaches room temperature (active warming is required).

Coagulation
- Disseminated intravascular coagulation is common.

Long-term consequences

Even with full cardiovascular and endocrine support asystole generally occurs over the following days to weeks. None of these prolonged brainstem dead cases have 'woken up'.

If the patient's next of kin wish their relative to become an organ donor, aggressive donor resuscitation and optimization are crucial to maximize both the number of organs suitable for retrieval and post-transplant function of these organs. Many transplant units have developed their own management protocols, which may include 3-hormone donor support (steroids, T3/T4, and vasopressin) and targets for MAP and oxygenation.

Tips and pitfalls

- The process of brainstem testing and diagnosis of death is an emotionally difficult time for both relatives and staff.
- Reliable diagnosis of brain death requires that the preconditions are met before testing takes place.
- Two sets of tests must be performed. Testing should be undertaken by the doctors together and must always be performed completely and successfully.
- Clearance of sedatives may be delayed in these patients; if there is any concern then levels should be measured and discussed with a clinical chemist before testing takes place.
- Organ support will often need to continue following diagnosis of brain death in order to maximize donor organ function.

Chapter 12

Postoperative management

Postoperative analgesia *384*
Postoperative fluid management *388*
Postoperative seizures *392*
Postoperative levels of care *394*

Postoperative analgesia

Pain after neurosurgical procedures is common and may be severe. Traditionally strong opioids have been avoided because of concerns over respiratory depression and interference with the assessment of conscious level in the postoperative period. More recently many units have found that strong opioids can be used safely in a wide range of patients.

Alleviating postoperative pain is a humanitarian issue. It may also be of benefit in reducing complications in both the short and long term.

Acute pain following craniotomy

Cohort studies suggest that 60–80% of patients experience moderate to severe pain following craniotomy.
- Numerous studies from different centres have demonstrated that post-craniotomy pain is poorly managed, and under-recognized.
- The pain is usually superficial and related to soft tissue and muscle damage, though some patients experience a less well-localized 'deep' headache.
- Most pain resolves within 48 h but around one-third of patients will have pain beyond this time.

Pain intensity is associated with the site of craniotomy, age, and gender.
- Frontal and parietal craniotomies have the lowest rates of moderate and severe pain.
- Occipital, posterior fossa, and pterional craniotomies have the highest rates.
- Increasing age is associated with less pain.
- Females report more pain than males.
- Pre-operative pain or analgesic use does not appear to affect the degree of postoperative pain after craniotomy.

Not all pain following craniotomy is directly due to the wound.
- Common alternate causes of pain are:
  - Low-pressure headache if there is an ongoing CSF leak
  - Cervicogenic pain associated with degenerative cervical spine disease
  - Intra-operative head and neck positioning.
- Functional aspects must always be considered.

Assessment of pain in patients following craniotomy may be challenging, particularly when acute or chronic cognitive impairment, reduced consciousness, or dysphasia are present.

Analgesic approaches

There is no consensus on the ideal approach to postoperative analgesia following craniotomy. However, the following points should be considered.
- Codeine phosphate, although traditional, is relatively ineffective in treating pain following craniotomy.
  - Variable metabolism results in unpredictable pharmacokinetics and inadequate pain relief in many patients.

- Morphine and oxycodone have been demonstrated to be safe in a wide range of craniotomy settings.
  - Various routes of administration have been used safely including intravenous, PCA, oral, intramuscular, and subcutaneous.
  - Nausea and vomiting and urinary retention are common side-effects.
- Tramadol is not recommended for post-craniotomy analgesia.
  - It is associated with poorer pain control and higher PONV rates
  - There are theoretical concerns about increased seizure activity.
- Use of intra-operative remifentanil is associated with increased analgesic requirements in the early postoperative period.
  - Morphine takes up to 20 min to achieve peak effect so needs to be administered around 30 min before the remifentanil infusion is stopped to prevent severe 'rebound' pain.
- Paracetamol alone is generally not sufficient to provide adequate analgesia, but is a very safe component of multimodal analgesic techniques.
- The use of non-steroidal anti-inflammatory drugs is controversial due to their detrimental effect on platelet function.
  - Many units use them postoperatively from day 1 or day 2 onwards.
  - Others do not use them at all in the postoperative period.
- Local anaesthetic infiltration may be a useful adjunct either as discrete nerve blocks or scalp infiltration.
  - Early analgesia is better when local anaesthesia is used, but overall analgesic consumption has not been convincingly demonstrated to be reduced.
  - 0.75% ropivicaine may provide up to 48 h analgesia.
  - Pre-incision local anaesthesia provides no or minimal postoperative benefit, though it may be of advantage in reducing haemodynamic responses to skin incision.
- Non-pharmcological approaches are also important.
  - Reassurance and discussion may be beneficial to some patients if they have particular concerns or beliefs about their pain.
  - Certain postures may exacerbate or relieve pain.

Chronic pain following craniotomy

A significant number of patients will suffer longer-lasting pain following craniotomy. This is often multifactorial including:
- Neuropathic pain mechanisms common to other types of post-surgical pain
- CSF leak
- Post-traumatic syndrome in survivors of TBI
- Cervicogenic pain
- Increased pericranial muscle tension
- Scar tissue affecting occipital nerves or dura
- Epilepsy
- Aseptic meningitis
- Infection.

Some of these problems may be directly amenable to surgical or pharmcological intervention, such as tricyclic antidepressants, anti-epileptics (gabapentin, sodium valporate or lamotrigine) or sumatriptan. Others may require a multidisciplinary approach, usually offered by a chronic pain service.

Acute pain following spine surgery

The amount of pain patients feel following spinal surgery is operation and patient-specific.
- Some procedures, such as microdiscectomy, can be performed as a day-case, without the need for strong opioids postoperatively.
  - Some patients with sciatic pain report an immediate reduction in symptoms postoperatively.
- Others, such as extensive laminectomy and spinal deformity correction, may result in severe and prolonged pain.
- The amount of pain reported correlates with the number of operated vertebrae and degree of surgical insult.
- Pre-operative analgesic use appears to influence the amount of postoperative pain that patients experience.
- Severe postoperative pain is associated with an increased risk of chronic pain.
- Occasionally, surgical release of long-standing cord or nerve compression can result in an intense, but relatively short-lived neuropathic pain, which may be relatively insensitive to opioids.

Analgesic approaches

- There is less concern about respiratory depression in spinal surgery patients compared with intracranial surgery, but patients with high cervical cord lesions, pre- or postoperatively, should be given opioids with caution.
- The route of opioid administration is probably unimportant provided the patient has timely access to an appropriate dose.
- Paracetamol is a useful adjunct, but unlikely to be sufficient alone.
- Non-steroidal anti-inflammatory drugs can be used safely following most spinal surgery provided there are no concerns about coagulopathy, ongoing bleeding or hypovolaemia.
  - ❶ Intra-medullary tumours are at risk from even small amounts of bleeding so NSAIDs should be **avoided** in the early postoperative period.
  - There is little evidence that there is a clinically significant impact on bone formation with the use of peri-operative NSAIDs.
- Gabapentin, as a single oral, pre-operative dose of 900–1200 mg reduces pain scores and morphine requirements following spinal surgery.
  - PONV may be reduced when gabapentin is used.
- Local anaesthetic techniques may be useful adjuncts.
  - Following laminectomy, local anaesthetic infiltrated deep in the wound has been shown to reduce postoperative pain.
  - Intrathecal and epidural techniques have been used to good effect in more extensive surgery. These techniques require careful monitoring, clear guidelines and multidisciplinary management.

Chronic pain following spinal surgery

A significant number of patients will experience worsening or recurrence of neurological or back pain symptoms following spinal surgery. A few of these will have disease that is amenable to re-operation. Most patients with persistent postoperative pain are best managed by a multidisciplinary pain clinic.

Tips and pitfalls
- Assume that patients are at risk of pain postoperatively and plan for it.
- Don't use codeine.
- Carefully titrate strong opioids such as morphine in the immediate postoperative period.
- Use strong opioids cautiously, if at all, in patients who may be predicted to have impaired consciousness postoperatively, e.g. elderly patients with subdural haematoma.
- V-P shunts are more painful than often appreciated.
- Early, strong, analgesia is often needed if remifentanil has been used.

Postoperative fluid management

Patients undergoing neurosurgery may have very different postoperative fluid requirements. Pre-operative fluid restriction, administration of mannitol and other diuretics, intra-operative bleeding, diabetes insipidus, and cerebral salt-wasting syndrome may all contribute to disturbed fluid balance.

How much fluid?

There is no single prescription which is appropriate for all patients.

The rate of fluid administration in neurosurgical patients should be guided by the same principles as for other postoperative patients.

- Restoration and maintenance of circulating blood volume
- Avoidance of hypovolaemia
- Avoidance of sodium overload
- Avoidance of water overload
- Traditionally neurosurgical patients have been fluid restricted on the assumption that reducing circulating blood volume would reduce brain volume. There is little evidence that, within clinically tolerable limits, such a reduction in brain volume occurs. Most patients are probably more at risk from the deleterious systemic effects of hypovolaemia.
- Most postoperative patients will be able to drink fairly soon after operation, and this is the most appropriate way to provide fluids. This does require that patients have access to drinks and are able to reach them.
- Patients who have had significant fluid loss intra-operatively (whether through bleeding or diuresis) will need close monitoring, including a urinary catheter. Fluids should be prescribed on the basis of restoring lost volume and matching ongoing losses. This can only be achieved safely through ongoing, regular review.

Which fluid?

Again, there is no 'one-size-fits-all' prescription. Clinical judgement is required to match the prescription to the need. Movement of fluid across the blood–brain barrier is determined by osmotic rather than oncotic pressure.

Crystalloids

Dextrose-containing solutions are traditionally avoided for two reasons:
- Hyperglycaemia is deleterious to the injured brain
- 5% dextrose is 'free' water, which may cause hyponatraemia.

There is little evidence in favour of one crystalloid solution over another in the postoperative period.
- Some units favour Hartmann's solution based on the better acid-base profile and 'balanced' electrolyte composition.
- Other units favour 0.9% saline (with added potassium if needed) due to its slightly hyperosmolar composition (effective osmolarity ~285 mOsm l^{-1}; Hartmann's is slightly hypo-osmolar with an effective osmolarity ~250–260 mOsm l^{-1}).

Colloids

There is little evidence to assist in deciding which colloid should be used if urgent volume replacement is required.

- Similar considerations apply to the carrying solution as for pure crystalloids.
- Some studies have suggested that large-volume colloid infusions impair the coagulation process.
- The use of albumin in patients with TBI has been associated with increased mortality.

Electrolytes

Hypokalaemia and hypomagnesaemia are common in the postoperative period, through a combination of pre-operative starvation, inadequate replacement and diuretic use. Replacement and maintenance electrolytes should be prescribed in a similar fashion to other surgical patients.

Blood

Acute blood loss is managed during neurosurgery in much the same way as other specialties. In the postoperative period, intracranial bleeding presents with neurological rather than cardiovascular complications. Bleeding after spinal surgery may be hidden as there is plenty of space for the blood to go without it appearing at the wound or the drain.

There is no clear consensus on the 'ideal' postoperative haemoglobin concentration.

- Traditionally haemoglobin concentrations >8 g dl^{-1} have been advocated as the best compromise between oxygen carrying capacity and blood viscosity.
- More recently, higher haemoglobin concentrations have been advocated, as evidence has emerged of the deleterious effects of anaemia on neurological outcome.

Diabetes insipidus

This is covered in more detail in Pituitary tumours, p. 200, and Systemic complications of brain injury, p. 370. Diabetes insipidus can usually be adequately managed by:
- allowing the patient free access to water
- a urinary volume matched intravenous infusion of 0.9% saline.

Only if these measures are insufficient should desmopressin be used.

Triple-H therapy

This is covered in more detail in Systemic complications of brain injury, p. 370. This should only be undertaken with:
- clear therapeutic goals
- close monitoring.

There is little evidence to support any particular fluid regime for this technique.

Tips and pitfalls
- The amount of fluid is probably more important than the individual fluid used.
- Although the aim should be for normovolaemia intra-operatively, this may not always be achieved. Restoration of fluid volumes may be required in the postoperative period.
- Bleeding may be hidden following spinal surgery.
- A urinary catheter not only provides accurate urine output monitoring, but may also relieve the discomfort of bladder distension after periods of high urine production.

Postoperative seizures

Postoperative seizures are relatively common after cranial neurosurgery. The exact incidence varies according to surgical pathology, the procedure undertaken and previous seizure history. Clinicians are faced with two questions:
- What, if any, seizure prophylaxis should be given?
- How should postoperative seizures be managed?

Seizures are associated with a worsened postoperative course. They may also be confused with other causes of rapid deterioration in conscious level such as shunt blockage, acute hydrocephalus, cerebral oedema, and intracranial bleeding.

Pathology
- Around 60% of patients with brain tumours will have a seizure at some point following presentation.
- Seizures may occur in up to 20% of patients following SAH, most commonly in the first 24 h.
- Seizures following traumatic brain injury are relatively common both in the acute (<7 days) and late phases. The seizure rate if untreated is similar in both phases (around 15%).
- Seizure following burr hole for acute subdural haematoma is less common (around 5%).
- A small proportion of patients present for surgical treatment of epilepsy and clearly have a high risk of postoperative seizures.
- Postoperative seizures may occur for non-neurosurgical reasons, such as hypoxia, infection, and hypoglycaemia.

Prophylaxis
- There is some evidence in favour of prophylactic anticonvulsants in the immediate period following SAH. Long-term prophylaxis is not recommended unless risk factors are present (previous seizure, intracerebral haematoma or infarct, MCA aneurysm).
- Phenytoin is effective in reducing the number of seizures in the early phase of TBI. It has no effect on long-term seizure rate or neurological outcome.
- Meta-analysis of the limited number of studies regarding prophylactic anti-epileptic drugs for patients with brain tumours concluded that 'the best evidence available at present is neither in favour nor against prophylaxis in brain tumours'.
- Most of the evidence concerns phenytoin, carbamazepine, and sodium valproate. There are few data for the newer drugs.

Treatment
Postoperative seizures should be treated along the same lines as any other seizure, but with a high index of suspicion for a treatable surgical cause.
- ABC ... including 100% O_2.
- Check the blood glucose.
- Liaise with neurosurgeons, in particular whether the patient needs an urgent CT.

POSTOPERATIVE SEIZURES

- Lorazepam (0.1 mg kg^{-1}) or diazepam (0.1 mg kg^{-1}) is the first line treatment.
- Phenytoin 15 mg kg^{-1} (loading dose) is used as second line treatment if there are no contraindications; administer as a slow iv infusion (<50 mg min^{-1}).
- Fosphenytoin (a prodrug of phenytoin) can be used; 1.5 mg fosphenytoin is equivalent to 1 mg phenytoin and faster infusion rates can be used: 225 mg min^{-1}.
- Maintain normoxia, normocapnia and normotension.

Tips and pitfalls

- Assume that a treatable cause is present. Always consider the possibility that the patient has bled, swollen, developed hydrocephalus or become hypoglycaemic.
- Some units avoid use of tramadol postoperatively due to its association with seizures in a small number of patients.
- Postoperative seizures in the recovery ward may be subtle due to the effects of residual anaesthetic drugs.
- Non-convulsive seizures are difficult to spot, particularly if patients are pharmacologically sedated. If suspected, for example because of a reduced conscious level, EEG monitoring may be necessary.

Postoperative levels of care

Different neurosurgical units have different policies regarding where and how postoperative patients are managed. These are largely determined by historical practice and resource availability rather than good evidence for improvements in outcome.

For some patients the decision on where they should be managed is relatively straightforward. Simple lumbar discectomies can be cared for on a normal ward; a patient with traumatic brain injury and the need for ICP monitoring will be going to critical care. For a significant group of patients, it is a matter of clinical judgement where they should go. If in doubt, senior advice should be sought.

Levels of care

A variety of names may be used for postoperative care areas, and many will provide differing levels of care within the same location. The UK Intensive Care Society has produced guidance on the interpretation of these levels. The criteria specifically relevant to neuroanaesthesia have been included below.

Level 0
- Normal ward care in an acute hospital.

Level 1
- Patient at risk of their condition deteriorating, or those recently relocated from higher levels of care, whose needs can be met on an acute ward with additional advice and support from the critical care team.
- Patients requiring a minimum of 4-hourly GCS assessment.
- Ideally a designated area within a neurosurgical ward with dedicated nursing staff and regular critical care outreach and physiotherapy cover.
- Should be able to manage tracheostomy suctioning and care.

Level 2
- Patients requiring more detailed observation or intervention including support for a single failing organ system or postoperative care and those 'stepping down' from higher levels of care.
- Patients where there is a risk of postoperative complications or a need for enhanced interventions and monitoring.
- Central nervous system depression sufficient to prejudice the airway and protective reflexes.
- Invasive neurological monitoring or treatment e.g. ICP, jugular bulb sampling, external ventricular drain.
- Continuous intravenous medication to control seizures and/or continuous cerebral monitoring.
- A 'high-dependency' unit capable of providing respiratory care, at a high level, for neurologically impaired patients.

Level 3
- Patients requiring either:
  - advanced respiratory support alone or
  - basic respiratory support together with support of at least two other organ systems.
- This level includes all complex patients requiring support for multi-organ failure.
- There is some evidence that patients admitted to a specialized neuro-intensive care unit have a better outcome than those cared for on a general ICU.

Who should go where?
There is no convincing evidence that where patients are managed postoperatively alters outcome. What appears to be most important is that the area has appropriate systems in place to care for the sicker patients. This will include:
- Staffing levels.
- Education and training of staff.
- Clinical experience of the patient population.
- Clear, well formulated, policies and procedures regarding:
  - monitoring
  - medication
  - access to senior review.

Most intracranial neurosurgery patients fall into the definitions for level 1 and 2 care.
- Some centres send all craniotomies routinely to HDU.
- Others use HDU only for selected cases.
- Others use an extended stay in the recovery ward as a triage tool.

Factors which suggest a requirement for level 2 care include:
- pre-existing comorbidity (e.g. poor cardiorespiratory reserve)
- a history of obstructive sleep apnoea (acromegalics)
- significant predicted or actual blood loss
- large tumour resection
- intra-operative brain swelling
- surgical expectation of postoperative brain swelling
- prolonged or marked intra-operative brain retraction
- prolonged surgery
- significant cardiovascular instability intra- or postoperatively
- impaired GCS pre- or postoperatively
- high risk of postoperative seizures.

Common factors suggesting a need for level 3 care include:
- more significantly impaired GCS pre- or postoperatively
- requirement for continued sedation or controlled ventilation
- multiple comorbidities or trauma.

Tips and pitfalls
- It is not possible to predict with certainty who will need a particular level of care.
- Always seek senior advice, particularly if higher level care is unavailable, before starting an elective case.

Appendix

Guidance for transfers *398*
Drug infusions for ICU use *400*

Guidance for transfers

Remember 'ACCEPT'.

Assess
- A thorough assessment of the patient is mandatory. During the transfer the patient should have the same level of care as when they left. This requires adequate knowledge of the patient's history and clinical condition.

Control
- A team leader for the transfer should be nominated.
- This leader should make sure the necessary tasks for a safe transfer are completed, in addition to ensuring continuation of clinical care.

Communicate
- Ensure that relevant individuals at both transferring and receiving hospitals know what is going on.
  - Surgery
  - Anaesthesia
  - Critical care
  - Ambulance service
  - Relatives.
- Keep meticulous written records.

Evaluate
- Is the transfer is appropriate for the patient?
- How urgent is the transfer?
- How is the transfer going to occur?
- Who is going to go with the patient?
- When is it going to happen?

Prepare and package
- Patient
  - Are the airway and all cannulae secured?
  - Have you got the notes, scans and other essential documents?
  - Have you completed the pre-transfer checklist?
- Personnel preparation
  - Do you have adequate training, a charged mobile phone, money and contact details?
- Equipment preparation
  - Do you have enough oxygen, airway equipment, drugs and suction?
  - Is your monitoring equipment going to work for the duration of the journey?

Transportation
- Road transport is first choice.
- Specific 'transfer trolleys' may be available, but these may only be compatible with a limited number of ambulances.

Suggested targets for transfer of the brain injured patient

Airway and breathing
Tracheal intubation and controlled ventilation should be used for patients with:
- GCS ≤8
- Significantly deteriorating GCS
- Loss of protective pharyngeal reflexes
- Hypoxaemia
- Hypercarbia
- Spontaneous hyperventilation
- Bilateral fractured mandible
- Copious bleeding into the mouth (e.g. from skull base fracture)
- Seizures.

Aim for:
- PaO_2 >13 kPa;
- $PaCO_2$ 4.5-5.0 kPa;
- Blood gases should be checked prior to departure.

Circulation
- Mean arterial pressure should be maintained ≥80 mmHg.
- Any causes of hypotension should be identified and treated prior to transfer.
- Major haemorrhage should be stopped and significant clotting derangements treated.
  - If blood is likely to be required it should be cross-matched and taken with the patient in the ambulance.
- Urine output should be monitored by urinary catheter.

Disability (neurology)
- Pupil size and reactivity should be checked prior to departure.
- If possible the patient should be positioned with 20° head-up tilt, whilst maintaining spinal immobilization if appropriate.
- A patient who has had a seizure may be loaded with phenytoin or other anticonvulsants prior to departure.

Other injuries
- Have other major injuries been treated or excluded? In particular check:
  - Cervical spine
  - Chest (pneumothorax)
  - Pelvis
  - Abdomen
  - Long bones.

Equipment and monitors
- Ensure that adequate primary and reserve power is available for essential devices.
- Check adequacy of oxygen supply.
- FiO_2, SpO_2 and $ETCO_2$ must be monitored throughout.
- Invasive arterial blood pressure monitoring should be used.

Drug infusions for ICU use

Doses, compatibility and routes of administrations given below should always be checked against a national formulary (e.g. BNF) and against local guidelines before being prescribed.

DRUG INFUSIONS FOR ICU USE

Drug	Infusion concentration	Compatible Infusion fluid G = 5% Glucose S = 0.9% NaCl H = Compound sodium lactate solution (Hartmann's) W = Water for injection	Route C-Central P-Peripheral	Usual dose range (adults) [Rate range for a 50 kg adult (ml h^{-1})]	Indications & Notes
Alfentanil	0.5 mg ml^{-1} (25 mg in 50 ml)	S, G, H	C / P	Bolus 10–50 µg kg^{-1} Maintenance 0.5–1 µg kg^{-1} min^{-1} [3–6 ml h^{-1}]	Analgesic and/or sedative agent.
Atracurium	10 mg ml^{-1} (500 mg in 50 ml)	Neat, G, S, H	C / P	0.3–0.6 mg kg^{-1} h^{-1} [1.5–3 ml h^{-1}]	Neuromuscular blocker. Monitor with a peripheral nerve stimulator. Incompatible with propofol.
Clonidine	30 µg ml^{-1} (1500 µg in 50 ml)	S, G	C / P	0–2 µg kg^{-1} h^{-1} [0–3.5 ml h^{-1}]	Antihypertensive agent. Also used in the management of agitation. α_2 adrenergic agonist. Monitor for hypotension and bradycardia. Risk of accumulation in renal failure.
Dobutamine	0.5–1 mg ml^{-1} (max 5 mg ml^{-1}) (250 mg in 250 ml)	G, S	C preferred (risk of phlebitis)	0.5–20 µg kg^{-1} min^{-1} (rarely up to 40 µg kg^{-1} min^{-1} has been required) [1.5–60 ml h^{-1} of 1 mg ml^{-1} solution]	Inotropic agent. Predominately β1 agonist.

Continued

Appendix

Drug	Infusion concentration	Compatible Infusion fluid **G** = 5% Glucose **S** = 0.9% NaCl **H** = Compound sodium lactate solution (Hartmann's) **W** = Water for injection	Route C-Central P-Peripheral	Usual dose range (adults) [Rate range for a 50 kg adult (ml h^{-1})]	Indications & Notes
Epinephrine	80 μg ml^{-1} (8 mg in 100 ml or 20 mg in 250 ml)	G	C ONLY	0.04-0.4 μg kg^{-1} min^{-1} [1.5-15 ml h^{-1}]	Inotropic agent β > α. Adrenergic action at low doses.
Fentanyl	25-50 μg ml^{-1} (1250-2500 μg in 50ml)	S	C / P	Bolus 1-5 μg kg^{-1} Maintenance 25-200 μg h^{-1} [1-8 ml h^{-1} of 25 μg ml^{-1} solution]	Analgesic and/or sedative agent.
Hypertonic saline	30, 50 & 75 mg ml^{-1} (3, 5 & 7.5% solutions)	Neat	C ONLY	2 ml kg^{-1} (7.5% solution) 250 ml bolus (3% solution)	For cerebral oedema. Aim for serum [Na$^+$] 145-155 mmol l^{-1}
Labetalol	5 mg ml^{-1} (300 mg in 60 ml)	Neat, G, S	C / P	20-160 mg h^{-1} [4-32 ml h^{-1}]	α & β adrenergic blocker. For peripheral administration dilute to 1 mg ml^{-1} with G (preferred) or S. Contra-indicated in asthmatics.

Mannitol	100 mg ml^{-1} (10% solution) 200 mg ml^{-1} (20% solution)	Neat	C preferred	0.25–1 g kg^{-1} [125–500 ml of 10% solution]	For cerebral oedema. Monitor serum and urine osmolality. Serum osmolality should be < 315 mOsm l^{-1}
Midazolam	1–2 mg ml^{-1} (50–100 mg in 50 ml)	G, S	C / P	0–20 mg h^{-1} [0–20 ml h^{-1} of 1 mg ml^{-1} solution]	Sedative agent. Also used in status epilepticus.
Morphine	1–2 mg ml^{-1} (50–100 mg in 50 ml)	S	C / P	0–20 mg h^{-1} [0–20 ml h^{-1} of 1 mg ml^{-1} solution]	Analgesic and/or sedative agent
Nimodipine	200 µg ml^{-1} (10 mg in 50 ml)	Neat, G, S, H	C ONLY	Start at 1 mg h^{-1} for first 2 h increasing to 2 mg h^{-1} provided BP permits (if BP unstable or <70 kg start at 0.5 mg h^{-1}). Administer centrally with a co-infusion via a 3-way tap or G, S or H running at a minimum of 40 ml h^{-1}.	Only calcium channel blocker shown to reduce risk of vasospasm after SAH. Incompatible with PVC. Infuse via syringe and dedicated polyethylene coated giving set.
Norepinephrine	80 µg ml^{-1} (8 mg in 100 ml) or 20 mg in 250 ml)	G, S	C ONLY	0.1–1 µg kg^{-1} min^{-1} [3.75–37.5 ml h^{-1}]	Vasoconstrictor. $\alpha > \beta$ adrenergic action.
Phenytoin (loading dose)	Not to exceed 10 mg ml^{-1}	S	C / P	Load 15 mg kg^{-1} over 1 h Max rate 50 mg min^{-1}. Maintenance 100 mg tds.	Anti-epileptic. Loading dose based on ideal body weight. Average sized patients often receive 1 g.

Continued

Appendix

| Drug | Infusion concentration | Compatible Infusion fluid
G = 5% Glucose
S = 0.9% NaCl
H = Compound sodium lactate solution (Hartmann's)
W = Water for injection | Route
C-Central
P-Peripheral | Usual dose range (adults)
[Rate range for a 50 kg adult (ml^{-1})] | Indications & Notes |
|---|---|---|---|---|---|
| Propofol | 10 mg ml^{-1} (1% solution)
20 mg ml^{-1} (2% solution) | Neat, G or S | C / P | 1-5 mg kg^{-1} h^{-1}
[5-25 ml h^{-1} of 1% solution] | Anaesthetic/Sedative agent. Higher doses, especially in children, have been linked with propofol infusion syndrome. |
| Remifentanil | 25-50 μg ml^{-1} (1-2 mg in 40 ml) | G, S, W | C / P | 0.0125-1 μg kg^{-1} min^{-1}
[1.5-120 ml/hr of 25 μg/ml solution] | Analgesic and/or sedative agent. |
| Thiopental | 25 mg ml^{-1} (1500 mg in 60 ml) *via a syringe driver* | W | C preferred (extravasation can cause pain and tissue necrosis) | **1-3 mg/kg bolus (max 500 mg) followed by infusion:**
For status epilepticus: 1.5 mg kg^{-1} h^{-1} [2-10 ml/hr]
Increase to 8mg/kg/hr if burst suppression not achieved on EEG. Continue for 12-24 h post-seizure control then consider weaning.
For traumatic brain injury: 1-8 mg kg^{-1} h^{-1} [2-16 ml h^{-1}]
(Up to 12 mg kg^{-1} h^{-1} has been used). | Anaesthetic agent. Also used in status epilepticus and for burst suppression. EEG monitoring required for continuous infusions. |

Index

A

α₂ agonists 46
  clonidine 47
  dexmedetomidine 47
abducent nerve 8
accessory nerve 9
ACE inhibitors 47
acoustic neuroma 196
  intra-operative issues 197
    CVS instability 198
    NBAs, avoidance of 198
  management 197
  postoperative care 198
acute brain injury 334
  brainstem death 379
  cerebral protection 358
  complications, systemic 371
  general management 352
    ICP/CPP management algorithm 357
    monitoring 355
    positioning 353
    sedation/analgesia 354
    TBI management protocols 355
  immediate care 340
    neurosurgeon, discussion with 345
    neurosurgical unit, transfer to 346
  pathophysiology 334
    Glasgow Coma Scale, outcome after 1 year 337
    Marshall classification 338
    outcome 337
  status epilepticus (SE) 374
  subarachnoid haemorrhage (SAH) 363
acute intermittent porphyria 80
air embolism 142
  monitoring 143
  postoperative care 143
  posterior fossa surgery 210
  prognosis 144
  treatment 143
anaemia, effects of acute 16
anatomy 2

autonomic nervous system 8
  blood supply 4–5
  brain 2
  central nervous system 2
  cranial nerves 8
  meninges 4
  nerve tracts 6–7
  spinal cord 3
aneurysms see intracerebral aneurysms, coiling of; intracranial aneurysms
anterior cervical discectomy 294
anti-emetics 62
  systemic effects 63
antibiotics 117, 353
antioxidants 360
Arnold-Chiari Malformation Type II 317
arteriovenous fistula (AVF) 327
arteriovenous malformations (AVMs) 271
  embolization of 327
atracurium 56
autonomic nervous system 8, 15
  parasympathetic nervous system 16
  sympathetic nervous system 15
  trigeminovascular nerves 16

B

β antagonists 44
baclofen pump
  implantation 314
  complications 315
  intra-operative management 315
balloon angioplasty 369
barbiturates 77, 354
benzodiazepines 37
blood loss and cell salvage 146
  acute normovolaemic haemodilution (ANH) 148
  allogenic transfusion 148
  blood loss, minimizing 148
  intra-operative cell salvage 147

blood-brain barrier (BBB), in neonates 120
botulism 80
brain injury see acute brain injury
brain, anatomy of 2–3
brainstem auditory evoked potentials (BAEP) 77, 78
brainstem death 378
  diagnosis of 379
  physiological consequences, management of 380
  pre-conditions for 380
  versus whole brain death 378

C

calcium antagonists 361
calcium channel antagonists 45
cardiotogram (CTG) monitoring 158
cardiovascular system see CVS (cardiovascular system)
carotid endarterectomy (CEA) 278
  anaesthesia, conduct of 279
  associated conditions 280
  blood pressure management 281, 284
  hyperfusion syndrome 282
  monitoring 280
  pre-operative assessment 281
  postoperative care 282
  recovery room management 284
  ward management 284
CBF (cerebral blood flow)
  autonomic nervous system 15
  cerebral circulation, control of 10–14
  inhalational anaesthetics 30
  monitoring 92
  paediatric neuroanaesthesia 120

405

INDEX

CBV (cerebral blood volume)
  cerebral circulation, control of 10–14
  ICP, manipulation of 24
CEA see carotid endarterectomy (CEA)
central nervous system 2, 120
central sulcus 3
central venous pressure see CVP (central venous pressure)
cerebellum 2
cerebral abscesses 250
  diagnosis 251
  intra-operative issues 252
  monitoring 252
  postoperative care 252
  pre-operative assessment 251
  prognosis 252
  surgical approach 251
cerebral blood flow see CBF (cerebral blood flow)
cerebral blood volume see CBV (cerebral blood volume)
cerebral circulation, control of 10
  biochemical 12
  flow dynamics 16
  flow-metabolism coupling 15
cerebral extra-cellular fluid (ECF) 88
cerebral function analysing monitor (CFAM) 74–76
cerebral hemispheres 2
cerebral metabolism 18
  measurement of 19
cerebral microdialysis (CM) 88
cerebral perfusion pressure see CPP (cerebral perfusion pressure)
cerebral protection 130, 358
  drug therapies 360
  glycaemic control 131
  temperature control 358
cerebral salt-wasting syndrome (CSWS) 372
cerebral stroke 6
cerebrospinal fluid see CSF (cerebrospinal fluid)
cerebrovascular resistance see CVR (cerebrovascular resistance)

cerebrovascular surgery 257
  arteriovenous malformations 274
  carotid endarterectomy 278
  EC-IC bypass procedures 276
  extradural haematoma 258
  intracranial aneurysms 272
  intracranial haematoma 268
  subdural haematoma 262
cerebrum 2
cervical laminectomy 292
  cervical spine stenosis 300
  intra-operative management 296
  positioning 297
  postoperative management 297
  pre-operative assessment 296
channelopathies 81
clonidine 47
codeine 53, 128, 387
colloid cysts 222
compound muscle action potential (CMAP) 79, 80
computed tomography imaging see CT (computed tomography) imaging
corticosteroids 361
CPP (cerebral perfusion pressure)
  acute brain injury 355
  cerebral circulation, control of 10–11
  definition of 10
  derivation of 68
  ICP/CPP management algorithm 357
  maintenance of 44
  multimodal monitoring 86
cranial nerves 8
  cranial neuralgias 238
  intra-operative issues 240
  pre-operative assessment 239
  prognosis 240
  treatment options 239
craniectomy, decompressive 254
  intra-operative issuues 255
  monitoring 255
  positioning 255
  postoperative care 255
  prognosis 255

craniofacial surgery, children 288
  intra-operative management 289
  monitoring 290
  positioning 289
  postoperative care 290
  pre-operative assessment 288
craniopharyngioma 224
cranioplasty 286
craniotomy 384
  awake 242
  intra-operative issues 243
  positioning 243
  postoperative management 245
  Caesarean section preceding 157
CSF (cerebrospinal fluid)
  absorption 26
  composition 27
  flow 26
  ICP, manipulation of 25
  pressure 27
  volume 26
CT (computed tomography) imaging 344, 345
  Cushing's syndrome 200, 221
CVP (central venous pressure) 10
CVR (cerebrovascular resistance) 10
CVS (cardiovascular system) 198
cyclizine 62, 63

D

death, acute brain injury see brainstem death
decompressive craniectomy see craniectomy, decompressive
deep brain stimulation 234
desflurane 30, 32, 134
desmopressin 64
dexamethasone 42, 62
dexmedetomidine 47
diabetes insipidus
  acute brain injury 372
  craniopharyngioma 225
  neuroendoscopic surgery 221
  postoperative fluid management 389
diastematomyelia 317
diclofenac 60
diencephalon 2
diffusion weighted imaging (DWI) MRI 95

INDEX

DNA (deoxyrobonucleic acid) 42
DVT (deep vein thrombosis) 372
  prophylaxis 117, 353

E

EC-IC bypass procedures 276
  complications 277
EDH see extradural haematoma (EDH)
EEG (electroencephalography) 72, 281, 356
  anaesthetic drugs, effects of 73
  cerebral function analysing monitor (CFAM) 74–75
  electrocorticography (ECoG) 74
  pathological patterns 72
electroencephalography see EEG (electroencephalography)
electrolyte disturbances 372
electromyography (EMG) 72, 79
enalaprilat 47
ephedrine 48, 50
esmolol 44
etomidate 34, 36, 73, 112, 360
evoked potentials (EP) 77
  brainstem auditory evoked potentials (BAEP) 78
  motor evoked potentials (MEP) 77
  somatosensory evoked potentials (SEP) 78
  visual evoked potentials (VEP) 78
excitotoxicity 335
extradural haematoma (EDH) 258
  CT scan 259
  intra-operative issues 259
  monitoring 260
  positioning 259
  postoperative care 260
  prognosis 261
  surgical approach 259

F

facial nerve 9
fentanyl 52, 112, 124, 272

focal tissue oxygen tension ($PbrO_2$) 98
frontal lobe 2
functional MRI (fMRI) 95
functional neurosurgery 234
  deep brain stimulation 235
  intra-operative issues 236
  intrathecal drug delivery 235
  monitoring 237
  positioning 236
  postoperative care 237
  prognosis 237
  spinal cord stimulation 236
  surgical approach 235

G

gabapentin 386
Glasgow Coma Score (GCS) 98, 269, 337
  children, use in 99–101
glossopharyngeal nerve 9
glucocorticoids 42
  systemic effects 43
glutamate antagonists 361
glycopyrrolate 56
Guillain-Barré syndrome (GBS) 80

H

haloperidol 62, 63
halothane 31
heparin 327
herpes encephalitis 73
hydralazine 46
hydrocephalus 69, 121, 214–5, 368
hypercapnia 342
hypernatraemia 372
hyperosmolar agents 38
  hypertonic saline 39
hyperperfusion syndrome 277, 282
hypertension, drugs used to treat 44
hypertonic saline 39
hypocapnia 31, 342
hypoglossal nerve 9
hypokalaemia 372
hyponatraemia 372
hypopituitarism 374
hypotension, drugs used to treat 48
hypoxia 342

I

ibuprofen 60
ICH see intracranial haematoma (ICH)
ICP (intracranial pressure) 22
  cerebral circulation, control of 10
  CSF 12
  ICP/CPP management algorithm 357
  intracranial elastance curve 23
  monitoring 68
  Monroe-Kellie doctrine 22
  paediatric neuroanaesthesia 121
  pressure-volume relationships 22
  temporal variation in 25
indomethacin 60
inhalational anaesthetics 30
  autoregulation 31
  carbon dioxide reactivity 31
intra-arterial papaverine 369
intracerebral aneurysms, coiling of 324
  complications 326
  interventional radiology 325
  monitoring 325
  radiation safety 325
intracranial aneurysms 272
  postoperative care 274
intracranial haematoma (ICH) 268
  associated conditions 269
  CT scan 269
  intra-operative issues 271
  monitoring 271
  positioning 270
  postoperative care 271
  pre-operative assessment 270
  presentation 269
  prognosis 271
  surgical management 270
intracranial pressure see ICP (intracranial pressure)
intracranial surgery, non-vascular 179
  acoustic neuroma 196
  awake craniotomy 242
  cerebral abscesses 250
  colloid cysts 222
  cranial neuralgias 238

INDEX

intracranial surgery, non-vascular (*cont.*)
 decompressive craniectomy 254
 functional neurosurgery 234
 midline surgery 224
 neuroendoscopic surgery 220
 pituitary tumours 200
 posterior fossa surgery 206
 seizure surgery 228
 shunts and ventricular drains 214
 stereotactic surgery 246
 tumours
  in adults 180
  in children 191
intravenous agents 34
 cerebral effects
  autoregulation 35
  carbon dioxide reactivity 35
  EEG activity 35
  ICP 35
  neuroprotection 35
  vasodilation/coupling 35
 tips and pitfalls 37
isoflurane 30, 32, 73, 134

J

jugular venous bulb oxygenation (S_jO_2) 87

K

ketamine 34, 36, 112, 134, 361

L

labetolol 44
lactate:pyruvate ratio (LPR) 88
laminectomy see cervical laminectomy
laser Doppler flowmetry 92
laudanosine 56
lignocaine 361
limbic system 3
lumbar surgery
 cauda equina compression 299
 indications 298
 neurosurgery *versus* orthopaedic spinal surgery 298
 peri-operative management 300
 positioning 301

postoperative management 301
pre-operative assessment 300
surgical procedures 299
Lund protocol 355

M

magnetic resonance imaging see MRI (magnetic resonance imaging)
mannitol 38, 117
MAP (mean arterial pressure) 10, 39, 45, 68
Marshall classification, acute brain injury 338
meninges, anatomy of 4
meningocele 316
meningomyelocele 316
metaraminol 48, 50
methylprednisolone 42
microdiscectomy 299
 positioning 178
midbrain 2
middle cerebral artery flow velocity (MCAFV) 280
monitoring techniques
 cerebral function analysing monitor (CFAM) 76
 electroencephalography (EEG) 74
 electromagnetic interference 81
 electromyography (EMG) 72
 evoked potentials (EP) 78
 Glasgow Coma Scale (GCS) 98
 nerve conduction studies (NCS) 80
 see also multimodal monitoring
Monroe-Kellie doctrine 23
morphine 52, 54, 385
motor evoked potentials (MEP) 77
motor unit potential (MUP) 79
Moya Moya syndrome 276
MRI (magnetic resonance imaging) 329
 angiography 95
 diffusion weighted imaging (DWI) 95
 environmental factors 329
 functional MRI (fMRI) 95
 patient factors 329

perfusion MRI 95
multimodal monitoring 86
 acute brain injury 356
 CBF 87
 cerebral microdialysis (CM) 88
 CPP 87
 focal tissue oxygen tension ($PbrO_2$) 88
 ICP 86
 jugular venous bulb oxygenation (S_jO_2) 87
 NIRS 89
 TCD 86
muscle relaxants 56
myasthenia gravis (MG) 81
myeloschisis 316

N

near infrared spectroscopy see NIRS (near infrared spectroscopy)
neostigmine 56
nerve conduction studies (NCS) 72
 indications 80
nerve tracts 6–7
neural tube defects 316
 anaesthetic considerations 317
 associated conditions 317
 cranial malformations 317
neuroanaesthesia, general principles of 110
 airway management 113
  asleep/awake intubation 114
  throat pack 114
 blood pressure control 115
  hypertension 116
 consent 110
 emergence 117
 induction of anaesthesia 111
 intra-operative fluids 116
 intra-operative management 115
 maintenance of anaesthesia 115
 perioperative drugs, other 117
 postoperative care 118
 premedication 110
 pre-operative issues 110
 temperature control 117
 see also paediatric neuroanaesthesia

neurodiagnostics,
    and interventional
    procedures 323
  embolization
    procedures 327
  intracerebral aneurysms,
    coiling of 324
  MRI/CT scans, anaesthesia
    for 326
neuroradiology,
    anaesthesia for 324
neuroendoscopic
    surgery 220
  complications 221
  monitoring 221
neuroendoscopic third
    ventriculostomy
    (NTV) 220
  pre-operative
    assessment 220
neurogenic pulmonary
    oedema 370
neuromuscular blockades
    (NMBs) 198
neuroradiology, anaesthesia
    for 324
neurosurgery, general
    principles of
  air embolism 142
  blood loss, and cell
    salvage 146
  brain swelling,
    management of 140
  glycaemic control 150
  investigations 107
  neurosurgical
    imaging 108
  patient counselling 109
  postoperative care 108
  pre-operative
    assessment 104
  temperature control 136
  thromboprophylaxis 152
  TIVA 134
  see also cerebral
    protection;
    neuroanaesthesia,
    general principles of;
    pregnancy
nifedipine 45
nimodipine 368
NIRS (near infrared
    spectroscopy) 89–90,
    281, 356
nitrates 45–6
  neurological effects 46
  systemic effects 46
nitrous oxide 30, 73,
    134, 325
non-steroidal anti-
    inflammatory drugs
    (NSAIDs) 60, 128, 386
norepinephrine 48

normal pressure perfusion
    breakthrough
    (NPPB) 275
normocapnia 352
normoglycaemia 353
normotension 352
normothermia 353
normoxia 352
NSAIDs see non-steroidal
    anti-inflammatory
    drugs (NSAIDs)

O

occipital lobe 3
oculomotor nerve 8
oedema 336
olfactory nerve 8
ondansetron 62, 63
opioids 52, 73, 112, 128
  alfentanil 52
  codeine 53
  fentanyl 52
  morphine 52, 54
  remifentanil 52, 53
optic nerve 8
orthopaedic spinal
    surgery 298
oxycodone 385

P

paediatric
    neuroanaesthesia 120
  anaesthesia 122
  blood conservation
    strategies 127
  central nervous system
    development 120
  consent 123
  fluid management
    126, 129
  induction, and tracheal
    intubation 123
  intra-operative blood
    loss 126, 129
  maintenance of
    anaesthesia 124
  monitoring 125
  neuropharmacology 122
  neurophysiology 120
  positioning 124–5
  postoperative
    care 127
  pre-medication 123
  pre-operative
    assessment 123
  temperature
    maintenance 127
  see also tumours, in
    children
paracetamol 128, 385, 386

parasympathetic nervous
    system 8, 16
parietal lobe 3
perfusion CT 95
perfusion MRI 95
persistent vegetative
    states 378
PET (positron emission
    tomography)
    techniques 20, 94
PFUCD see posterior
    fossa upper cervical
    decompression
    (PFUCD)
pharmacology 29, 44
  anti-emetics 62
  glucocorticoids 42
  hyperosmolar
    agents 38
  inhalational
    anaesthetics 30
  intravenous agents 34
  muscle relaxants 56
  NSAIDs 60
  opioids 52
  paracetamol 61
  vasoactive drugs 44
phenylephrine 48, 50, 157
pineal gland tumours 225
  anaesthetic
    considerations 226
  postoperative
    complications 227
  pre-operative
    considerations 226
  presentation 225–6
  prognosis 227
pituitary gland 2
pituitary tumours 200
  anaesthetic
    considerations 203
  complications 204
  pituitary apoplexy 201
  postoperative
    management 203
  pre-operative
    assessment 202
  prognosis 204
  treatment options 201
  visual disturbance 201
pneumonia 351, 370
PONV (postoperative
    nausea and vomiting) 62
  postoperative care 188
  posterior fossa
    surgery 211
  see also anti-emetics
porphyria 80
positioning, and surgical
    approaches 161
  biocoronal flap
    craniotomy 172–3
  burr hole 171

positioning, and surgical approaches (cont.)
 craniotomy, for trauma 171
 hair 171
 infiltration 171
 posterior fossa, midline craniectomy 174–5
 posterior fossa, retrosigmoid craniectomy 174
 principles 162, 171
 prone position 163–6
 sitting position 169–70
 small craniotomies, pterional and straight 173
 spinal procedures 174–8
  anterior cervical approach 175
  laminectomy 176
  lumbar microdiscectomy 177
 supine position 162–3
positive end-expiratory pressure (PEEP) 143
positron emission tomography see PET (positron emission tomography) techniques
postoperative management 383
 analgesia 384–7
 care levels 294
 fluid management 388
 seizures 392–3
postoperative nausea and vomiting see PONV (postoperative nausea and vomiting)
posterior fossa surgery 206
 associated conditions 207
 complications 212
 intra-operative issues 209–11
 monitoring 211
 pathology 206
 positioning 209
 postoperative care 211
 pre-operative assessment 207–8
 presentation 207
 prognosis 212
 surgical approach 209
 urgency 208
posterior fossa upper cervical decompression (PFUCD) 296
 indications 296
 intra-operative management 296
 positioning 297
 postoperative management 297
 pre-operative assessment 296
 symptomatic Chiari malformation 296
precentral gyrus 3
pregnancy 156
 Caesarean section, preceding craniotomy 157
 craniotomy, fetus in utero 158
 intracerebral haemorrhage, incidence of 156
 intracranial haemorrhage, incidence of 156
 meningioma, incidence of 156
 neurosurgical intervention, timing of 156
 physiological concerns 156
 postpartum conditions 158
 pre-eclampsia 157
 regional analgesia/anaesthesia, in presence of intracranial lesions 158
 spinal surgery 158
 subarachnoid haemorrhage, incidence of 156
primitive neuroectodermal tumours (PNET) 206
prone position
 at risk areas 164
 key issues 163
 variations of 166
  bolsters 168
  knee-chest 166
  Montreal mattress 167
  park bench/lateral recumbent position 168–9
  Wilson frame 166–7
propofol 34, 36, 73, 112, 134, 231, 325, 361
pulmonary embolism 371

R

radiology, interventional 326, 328
ranitidine 157, 158
regional cerebral blood flow (rCBF), monitoring 92
remifentanil 52, 53, 112, 124, 272, 383, 404
RNA (ribonucleic acid) 42

rocuronium 56, 57
Rosner protocols, acute brain injury 354–5

S

SAH see subarachnoid haemorrhage (SAH)
SDH see subdural haematoma (SDH)
SE see status epilepticus (SE)
seizure surgery 228
 intra-operative issues 231
 monitoring 232
 pathology 228
 patient population 229
 positioning 231
 postoperative care 232
 pre-operative assessment 229
 presentation 229
 prognosis 232
 surgical approach 230
sensory cortex 3
sevoflurane 30, 32, 124, 134, 325
shunts and ventricular drains 214
 intra-operative issues 217
 monitoring 217
 pathology 214–5
 postoperative care 218
 pre-operative assessment 217
 presentation 215
 purpose of 214
 surgical considerations 215–6
single photon emission computed tomography see SPECT (single photon emission computed tomography)
sitting position 169–70
somatosensory evoked potentials (SEP) 77, 78
SPECT (single photon emission computed tomography) 94
spina bifida occulta 316
spinal cord masses, and AVM 302
 arteriovenous malformations 303
 intra-operative management 304–5
 monitoring 305
 positioning 304
 postoperative management 305
 pre-operative assessment 304

surgical management 304
thoracic intramedullary lesion 303
spinal cord, anatomy of
 blood supply to 5
 cerebrospinal fluid (CSF) 3
 dura mater 4
 representative anatomy, cervical level 7
spinal cord stimulation 236
spinal dermal fistula 316
spinal dermal sinus 316
spinal haematoma and abscess 316
 postoperative management 317
 pre-operative assessment 317
spinal injury 291, 308
 anterior cervical discectomy 294
 associated conditions 308
 baclofen pump implantation 314–5
 cervical laminectomy 292
 intra-operative managment 311
 lumbar surgery 298–301
 monitoring 313
 neural tube defects 316–8
 pathology 308
 patient population 309
 positioning 311
 postoperative management 313
 posterior fossa upper cervical decompression (PFUCD) 296
 preoperative assessment 309
 presentation 308–9
 prognosis 313
 spinal cord masses, and AVM 302
 spinal haematoma and abscess 320–1
 surgical approaches 310–1
spinal surgery 386–7
SSEP (somatosensory evoked potentials) 281
status epilepticus (SE) 374
 aetiology 374
 diagnosis 375
 pathophysiology 374
 prognosis 377
 systemic effects of 375
 treatment 376–7
stereotactic surgery 246–9
 framed 246
 frameless 247, 248

intra-operative issues 247–8
 monitoring 248
 positioning 247
 postoperative care 248
 procedures using 246
 stereotactic biopsy 247
 steroids 117
stress ulcer prophylaxis, acute brain injury 354
stump pressure 281
subarachnoid haemorrhage (SAH) 362–9
 classification of 364–5
 CT image 363
 epidemiology 362
 hydrocephalus 368
 intracerebral aneurysms, coiling of 324
 intracranial aneurysms 272
 investigations 365
 medical complications 366–7
 neurological complications 367–8
 pathophysiology 363
 presentation 363–4
 prognosis 362
 rebleeding, prevention of 366
subdural haematoma (SDH) 262
 associated conditions 262
 CT scan 264
 intra-operative issues 265
 monitoring 265
 pathology 262
 patient population 263
 positioning 264
 postoperative care 265
 pre-operative assessment 263
 presentation 262
 prognosis 266
 surgical approach 264
succinylcholine 157
sugammadex 56, 57
supine position 162–3
suxamethonium 57
Sylvian fissure 3
sympathetic hyperactivity 371
sympathetic nervous system 8, 15
sympathomimetics 48
 neurological effects 49
 systemic effects 49
syndrome of inappropriate antidiuretic hormone secretion (SIADH) 372
systemic arterial hypotension 342

T

TBI (traumatic brain injury)
 ICP monitoring 68
 incidence of 334
 see also acute brain injury
TCD (transcranial Doppler ultrasonography) 82, 86, 280, 282
 acute brain injury 356
 advantages of 82
 cerebral arteries, TCD trace 83
 embolism 85
 principles of 82
 regulatory capacity, tests of 84
 technique 82
 values, measured and derived 83
temporal lobe 3
terlipressin 64
thalamus 2
thermal diffusion flowmetry 92
thiopental 34–5, 112, 134, 157
thromboprophylaxis 152
 guidelines for 153
 non-pharmacological options 153
TIVA (total intravenous anaesthesia) 30, 34, 115, 134
tramadol 385
transcranial Doppler ultrasonography see TCD (transcranial Doppler ultrasonography)
transfer guidelines
 acute brain injury 348
 airway and breathing 350, 399
 circulation 350, 399
 disability (neurology) 342, 399
 equipment and monitors 349, 399
 indications 348
 injuries, other 399
 principles (ACCEPT) 348, 399
traumatic brain injury see TBI (traumatic brain injury)
trigeminal nerve 8
trigeminovascular nerves 16
triple-H therapy 389
trochlear nerve 8
tromethamine (THAM) 362

tumours, in adults 180–90
  associated conditions 183
  epidemiology 180
  intra-operative issues 186
  monitoring 187–8
  pathology 180
    patient population 184
  positioning 186
  postoperative care 188–9
  pre-operative
    assessment 184
  presentation 183
  prognosis 189–90
  surgical approach 185–6
tumours, in children
  191–9
  associated conditions 191
  incidence of 191
  intra-operative
    management 193–4
  monitoring 194–5
  pathology 191
  positioning 193
  postoperative care 195
  pre-operative
    assessment 191–2
  presentation 191
  prognosis 195
  surgical approach 192

V

vagus nerve 9
vasopressin 50, 64
  analogues 49
  argine vasopressin (AVP)
    antidiuretic hormone
    (ADH) 64
vecuronium 56

ventricular drains see shunts
  and ventricular drains
vestibula schwannomas see
  acoustic neuroma
vestibulocochlear (auditory)
  nerve 9
visual cortex 3
visual evoked potentials
  (VEP) 77, 78
volatile agents 361
VTE (venous
  thromboembolism) 152
  risk factors 154

X

Xenon 93–4

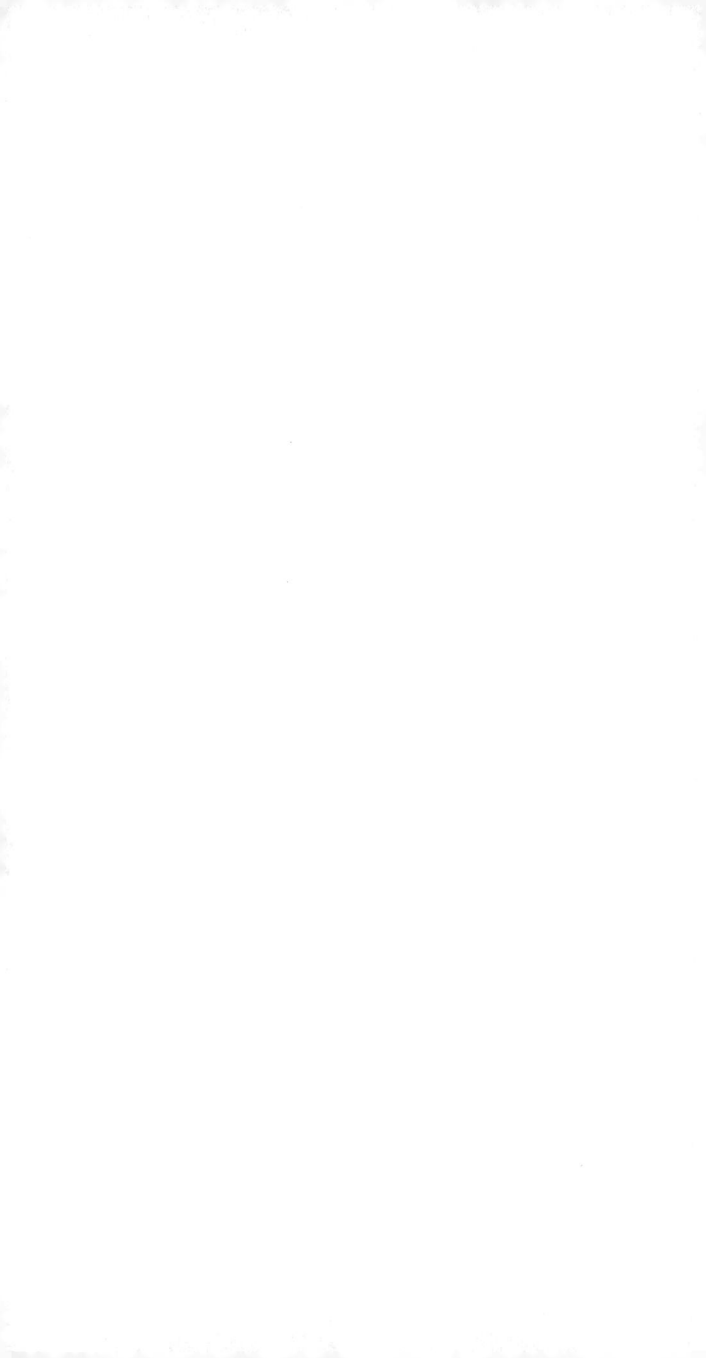

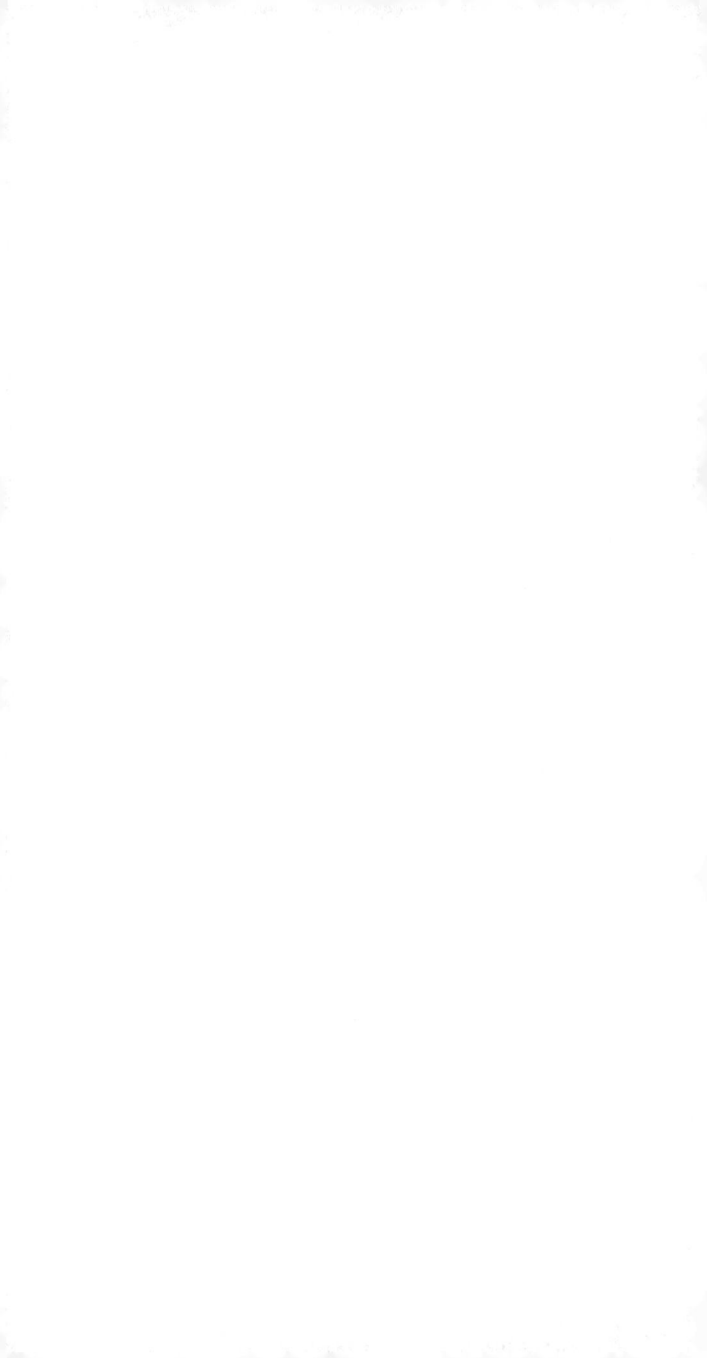